2024

ADVANCES IN
SMALL ANIMAL CARE

EDITOR-IN-CHIEF
Philip H. Kass

SECTION EDITORS
Larry D. Cowgill
Chiara Mariti
Angela J. Marolf
Silke Salavati Schmitz
Jonathan Stockman

ELSEVIER

Publishing Director, Medical Reference: Dolores Meloni
Editor: Stacy Eastman
Developmental Editor: Sukirti Singh

Reprints: For copies of 100 or more of articles in this publication, please contact the Commercial Reprints Department, Elsevier Inc., 360 Park Avenue South, New York, NY 10010-1710. Tel: 212-633-3874; Fax: 212-633-3820; E-mail: reprints@elsevier.com.

Editorial Office:
Elsevier, Inc.
1600 John F. Kennedy Blvd,
Suite 1800
Philadelphia, PA 19103-2899

International Standard Serial Number: 2666-4518
International Standard Book Number: 978-0-443-24672-2

ADVANCES IN SMALL ANIMAL CARE

EDITOR-IN-CHIEF

PHILIP H. KASS, BS, DVM, MPVM, MS, PhD,
Diplomate, American College of Veterinary Preventive Medicine (Specialty in Epidemiology)
Vice Provost for Academic Affairs
Professor of Analytic Epidemiology
Department of Population Health and Reproduction,
School of Veterinary Medicine
Department of Public Health Sciences,
School of Medicine University of California,
Davis Davis, California, USA
phkass@ucdavis.edu

SECTION EDITORS

LARRY D. COWGILL, DVM, PhD, Dipl. ACVIM
Professor, Department of Medicine & Epidemiology
2108 Tupper Hall School of Veterinary Medicine
University of California-Davis
Davis, CA 95616
Office/Voice Mail: 530-752-8367
FAX: 530-752-0414

Director, UC Veterinary Medical Center-San Diego
10435 Sorrento Valley Road,
Suite 101 San Diego, CA 92121
Office/Voice Mail: 858-875-7505
FAX: 858-875-7578
Email: ldcowgill@ucdavis.edu

CHIARA MARITI, DVM, PhD, MSC, EBVS
Professor, Department of Veterinary Sciences,
University of Pisa, Italy
Chiara.mariti@unipi.it

ANGELA J. MAROLF, DVM, DACVR
Professor, Environmental and Radiological
Health Sciences College of Veterinary Medicine and
Biomedical Sciences Colorado State
University Fort Collins, Colorado, USA
angela.marolf@colostate.edu

SILKE SALAVATI SCHMITZ, DR.MED.VET., PhD,
DIPL.ECVIM-CA, FHEA, MRCVS
Senior lecturer in Small Animal Internal Medicine
University of Edinburgh Royal (Dick)
School of Veterinary Studies and
The Roslin Institute Hospital for Small Animals
Easter Bush, Midlothian, UK
Silke.Salavati@ed.ac.uk

JONATHAN STOCKMAN, DVM, DACVN
Associate Professor, Department of Veterinary
Clinical Sciences, College of Veterinary Medicine,
Long Island University, Old Brookville, New York,
USA; Affiliate Faculty, Department of Clinical
Sciences, College of Veterinary Medicine and
Biomedical Sciences at Colorado State University,
Fort Collins, Colorado, USA
jonathan.stockman@liu.edu

CONTRIBUTORS

EDITOR
PHILIP H. KASS, BS, DVM, MPVM, MS, PhD
Diplomate, American College of Veterinary Preventive
Medicine (Specialty in Epidemiology), Vice Provost for
Academic Affairs, Professor of Analytic Epidemiology,
Department of Population Health and Reproduction,
School of Veterinary Medicine, Department of Public
Health Sciences, School of Medicine, University of
California, Davis, California, USA

AUTHORS
RYAN B. APPLEBY, DVM, DACVR
Assistant Professor, Department of Clinical Studies,
Ontario Veterinary College, University of Guelph,
Guelph, Ontario, Canada

PARMINDER S. BASRAN, PhD, FCCPM
Associate Research Professor, Section of Medical
Oncology, Department of Clinical Sciences, Cornell
University College of Veterinary Medicine, Ithaca,
New York, USA

SIMONE MOREIRA BERGAMINI, DVM, MSc, Dipl
CLEVE-CVLBAMC
Veterinary Behaviorist, Behavioral Clinic, Etoclinvet,
Scientific Coordinator and Professor of the Postgraduate
Program, Veterinary Clinical Ethology at the Qualittas
Institute of Graduate Studies, Rio de Janeiro, Brazil

KATHRIN BUSCH, DVM, Dr Med Vet, DECVIM
Consortium Working Group Lead and Member,
Centre for Clinical Veterinary Medicine, Ludwig-
Maximilian University Munich, Munich, Germany

PAOLA CAZZINI, DVM, MS, DiplACVP (Clin Path),
MRCVS
Senior Lecturer, Easter Bush Pathology, The Royal
(Dick) School of Veterinary Studies, The Roslin Institute,
University of Edinburgh, Roslin, United Kingdom

JENNIFER CHAITMAN, VMD, DACVIM (Small
Animal Internal Medicine)
Consortium Member, President, Veterinary Internal
Medicine and Allergy Specialists, New York,
New York, USA

LAKHMIR S. CHAWLA, MD
Professor of Medicine, Department of Anesthesiology
and Critical Care Medicine, George Washington
University Medical Center, Washington, DC, USA;
Department of Research and Development, ExThera
Medical Corporation, Martinez, California, USA;
Veterans Affairs Medical Center, San Diego,
California, USA

EMILY L. COFFEY, DVM, DACVIM (Small Animal
Internal Medicine), PhD
Consortium Member, Assistant Professor, Department
of Veterinary Clinical Sciences, University of
Minnesota College of Veterinary Medicine, Saint Paul,
Minnesota, USA

MARCIO C. COSTA, DVM, DVSc, PhD
Consortium Member, Associate Professor,
Department of Veterinary Biomedical Sciences,
University of Montreal, Saint-Hyacinthe, Québec,
Canada

LARRY D. COWGILL, DVM, PhD, Dipl ACVIM
(SAIM), ACVNU (President)
Professor, Department of Medicine and
Epidemiology, University of California, Davis School
of Veterinary Medicine, Davis, California, USA

JULIEN R.S. DANDRIEUX, BSc, Dr med vet, PhD,
SFHEA, GCUT, Diplomate of American College of
Veterinary Internal Medicine (Small Animal Internal
Medicine), MRCVS
Senior Lecturer in Small Animal Medicine, University
of Edinburgh, Roslin, Scotland, United Kingdom;
Consortium Member, Senior Lecturer, Hospital for
Small Animals, The Royal (Dick) School of Veterinary
Studies, The Roslin Institute, College of Medicine and
Veterinary Medicine, University of Edinburgh,
Midlothian, United Kingdom

ARNON GAL, DVM, MSc, PhD, DACVIM, DACVP
Consortium Member, Assistant Professor, Department
of Veterinary Clinical Medicine, University of Illinois
at Urbana-Champaign, Champaign, Illinois, USA

FREDERIC GASCHEN, DrMedVet, Drhabil, DACVIM (Small Animal Internal Medicine), DipECVIM-CA
Consortium Working Group Lead and Member, Professor, Department of Veterinary Clinical Sciences, School of Veterinary Medicine, Louisiana State University, Baton Rouge, Louisiana, USA

ANGELO GAZZANO, DVM, PhD, Dipl ECAWBM
Full Professor, Department of Veterinary Sciences, University of Pisa, Pisa, Italy

TRACY HILL, DVM, PhD, DACVIM (Small Animal Internal Medicine)
Consortium Member, Director of Science, Veterinary Science Consultancy, Ethos Veterinary Health, USA

CATHY E. LANGSTON, DVM, DACVIM (SAIM)
Professor, Department of Veterinary Clinical Sciences, College of Veterinary Medicine, The Ohio State University, Columbus, Ohio, USA

JANNE GRAARUP-HANSEN LYNGBY, DVM, PhD, DACVIM (SAIM)
Assistant Professor in Veterinary Clinical Pathology and Internal Medicine, Department of Veterinary Clinical Science, University of Copenhagen, Frederiksberg C, Denmark

ALEXANDRA MALBON, BVSc, BSc(hons), Dr med vet, PhD, DiplECVP, MRCVS
Senior Lecturer, Easter Bush Pathology, The Royal (Dick) School of Veterinary Studies, The Roslin Institute, University of Edinburgh, Roslin, United Kingdom

STANLEY L. MARKS, BVSc, PhD, Diplomate ACVIM (Small Animal Internal Medicine, Oncology, Nutrition)
Professor of Small Animal Medicine, Department of Medicine and Epidemiology, University of California, Davis, School of Veterinary Medicine, Davis, California, USA

SINA MARSILIO, Dr med vet, PhD, DACVIM (Small Animal Internal Medicine), DipECVIM-CA
Consortium Working Group Lead and Member, Assistant Professor, Department of Veterinary Medicine and Epidemiology, UC Davis School of Veterinary Medicine, Davis, California, USA

KEITH R. McCREA, PhD
Chief Science Officer, Department of Research and Development, ExThera Medical Corporation, Martinez, California, USA

MANUEL MENGOLI, DVM, MSc, PhD
Principal Chief Executive Officer, Néthos, Plan d'Orgon, France

LINDA MORRISON, BVMS, FRCPath, Dipl ECVP, MRCVS
Senior Lecturer, Easter Bush Pathology, The Royal (Dick) School of Veterinary Studies, The Roslin Institute, University of Edinburgh, Roslin, United Kingdom

LISE NIKOLIC NIELSEN, DVM, PhD, CertSAM
Professor (mso) in Veterinary Clinical Pathology, Department of Veterinary Clinical Science, University of Copenhagen, Frederiksberg C, Denmark

ASAHI OGI, DVM, PhD
Diplomate of European College of Animal Welfare and Behavioural Medicine, EBVS® European Veterinary Specialist in Behavioural Medicine, Post-doc researcher, Department of Neurobiology and Molecular Medicine, IRCCS Stella Maris Foundation, Pisa, Italy

TAMMY JANE OWENS, DVM, MS, DACVIM (Nutrition)
Assistant Professor, Department of Small Animal Clinical Sciences, Western College of Veterinary Medicine, University of Saskatchewan, Saskatoon, Saskatchewan, Canada

LUDOVICA PIERANTONI, DVM, MSc, Spec.EABA, Dipl ECAWBM
Principal Chief Executive Officer, Can-BS, Napoli, Italy

RACHEL PILLA, DVM, PhD
Consortium Member, Professor and Associate Director, Department of Small Animal Clinical Sciences, Gastrointestinal Laboratory, Adjunct Professor, Texas A&M University, College Station, Texas, USA; Professor, Department of Veterinary Medicine and Animal Sciences, Universita, Degli Studi di Milano, Lodi, Italy

FABIO PROCOLI, DVM, MedVet, DACVIM, DipECVIM-CA, MRCVS
Consortium Member, Anicura Ospedale Veterinario i Portoni Rossi, Zola Predosa, Bologna, Italy

JESSICA QUIMBY, DVM, PhD, DACVIM (SAIM)
Professor, Department of Veterinary Clinical Sciences, College of Veterinary Medicine, The Ohio State University, Columbus, Ohio, USA

MIRANDA J. SADAR, DVM
Diplomate of the American College of Zoological Medicine, Associate Professor, Department of Clinical Sciences, Veterinary Teaching Hospital, Colorado State University, Fort Collins, Colorado, USA

SILKE SALAVATI SCHMITZ, Dr MedVet, PhD, DipECVIM-CA, FHEA, FRCVS
Senior lecturer in Small Animal Internal Medicine, University of Edinburgh Royal (Dick), School of Veterinary Studies and The Roslin Institute Hospital for Small Animals, Easter Bush, Midlothian, UK

JIA WEN SIOW, BSc(VB), DVM, GradCert(SAUA), MVetStud, MVetClinStud, FANZCVS(Veterinary Radiology)
Veterinary Radiologist, Department of Diagnostic Imaging, Small Animal Specialist Hospital Adelaide, Kent Town, South Australia, Australia

JONATHAN STOCKMAN, DVM, DACVIM (Nutrition)
Associate Professor, Department of Veterinary Clinical Sciences, College of Veterinary Medicine, Long Island University, Old Brookville, New York, USA; Affiliate Faculty, Department of Clinical Sciences, College of Veterinary Medicine and Biomedical Sciences at Colorado State University, Fort Collins, Colorado, USA

JAN S. SUCHODOLSKI, DrMedVet, PhD, DACVM, AGAF
Consortium Working Group Lead and Member, Professor and Associate Director, Department of Small Animal Clinical Sciences, Gastrointestinal Laboratory, Texas A&M University, College Station, Texas, USA

M. KATHERINE TOLBERT, DVM, PhD, DACVIM (Small Animal Internal Medicine, Small Animal Nutrition)
Consortium Member, Assistant Professor, Department of Small Animal Clinical Sciences, Gastrointestinal Laboratory, Texas A&M University, College Station, Texas, USA

LINDA TORESSON, DVM, PhD
Consortium Member, Evidensia Specialist Animal Hospital, Helsingborg, Sweden

STEFANIA UCCHEDDU, DVM, PhD, MSc
Diplomate European College Animal Welfare and Behavioural Medicine, Behavioral Department, Behavioural Unit, San Marco Veterinary Clinic and Lav, Veggiano, Padua, Italy

TARINI V. ULLAL, DVM, MS, Diplomate ACVIM (Small Animal Internal Medicine)
Staff Veterinarian, Department of Medicine and Epidemiology, University of California, Davis, School of Veterinary Medicine, Davis, California, USA

STEFAN UNTERER, DVM, Dr med vet, Dr habil., DECVIM-CA
Consortium Member, Clinic for Small Animal Internal Medicine, Vetsuisse Faculty, University of Zurich, Zurich, Switzerland

SHELLY L. VADEN, DVM, PhD, DACVIM (SAIM)
Professor, Department of Clinical Sciences, College of Veterinary Medicine, North Carolina State University, Raleigh, North Carolina, USA

ÉRIKA VALVERDE-ALTAMIRANO, DVM
Consortium Member, Medical Director of Nutrinac Veterinary Digestive Health, Nutrinac, San Rafael, Escazu San José, Costa Rica

GUILHERME G. VEROCAI, DVM, MSc, PhD, DACVM (Parasitology)
Consortium Member, Clinical Assistant Professor, Department of Veterinary Pathobiology, Parasitology Diagnostic Laboratory, Texas A&M University, College Station, Texas, USA

LAUREN VON STADE, DVM
Diplomate of the American College of Veterinary Radiology, Radiologist, Veterinary Teaching Hospital, Colorado State University, Fort Collins, Colorado, USA

MELANIE WERNER, Dr Med Vet, Dipl ECVIM-CA (Internal Medicine)
Consortium Member, Small Animal Clinic Marigin Feusisberg, Feusisberg, Switzerland

JENESSA A. WINSTON, DVM, PhD, DACVIM (Small Animal Internal Medicine)
Consortium Chair and Member, Assistant Professor, Department of Veterinary Clinical Sciences, Comparative Hepatobiliary and Intestinal Research

Program (CHIRP), Veterinary Clinical Sciences, The Ohio State University College of Veterinary Medicine, Columbus, Ohio, USA

GLYNN WOODS, BVMS, MSc, SFHEA, Diplomate of the European College of Veterinary Internal Medicine, MRCVS
Senior Lecturer in Small Animal Medicine, University of Edinburgh, Roslin, Scotland, United Kingdom;

Hospital for Small Animals, The Royal (Dick) School of Veterinary Studies, Midlothian, United Kingdom

ANNA-LENA ZIESE, Dr med vet
Consortium Member, Veterinary Affairs and Product Development Manager, Terra Canis GmbH, Garching bei München, Germany

CONTENTS

SECTION I - BEHAVIOR

In dogs, an attentive mother can have a positive impact on the physical and mental growth of her puppies. Indeed, early life experiences could have a significant and lasting impact on an individual's behavioral development. Considering the relevance of this topic in breeding dogs, with this review we want to facilitate a better understanding of the neurophysiological mechanisms underlying maternal behavior in order to improve the selection of dams and manage their abnormal behaviors.

Recent advancements in our understanding of grief have led to the recognition that this complex emotion extends beyond human experience and encompasses animal behavior. Additionally, grief is conceptualized as a human response to the loss of companion animals, who hold a significant place in our lives and often become integral members of our families. These 2 factors have propelled grief to the forefront of both human psychology and veterinary medicine, requiring professionals to not only address the grief of clients but also manage their own personal grief responses.

▶ Video content accompanies this article at https://www.advancesinsmallanimalcare. com/

This review seeks to examine the intrinsic (animal) and extrinsic (environmental) factors influencing the indoor lifestyle of domestic cats. It also explores strategies for managing these factors and considers the potential consequences of inter-cat cohabitation.

SECTION II - DIAGNOSTIC IMAGING

Computed Tomographic Imaging of the Gastrointestinal Tract in Small Animals, 31

Jia Wen Siow

Gastrointestinal disease is a common cause for presentation to veterinary hospitals. Computed tomography (CT) is increasingly being used to investigate this. Few studies evaluate the normal gastrointestinal tract, but these highlight the importance of patient preparation and contrast medium administration technique to optimize evaluation. Despite clinical studies using widely variable contrast CT protocols, there are common features of several gastrointestinal diseases. In the future, the use of standardized patient preparation and contrast medium administration protocols may provide more robust data to aid in prioritizing differential diagnoses.

Advanced Imaging of Small Mammals, 51

Lauren von Stade and Miranda J. Sadar

Computed tomography (CT) and MRI are diagnostic imaging modalities employed in small mammal practice. A major advantage of these cross-sectional modalities is the ability to evaluate anatomy in multiple planes without superimposition of adjacent structures. CT provides excellent spatial resolution and detail of osseous and dental anatomy and is relatively fast to perform compared to MRI, which employs superior contrast resolution of soft tissues. The diagnostic capability of these technologies is widespread, and their use in clinical practice will continue to advance as their application for a wide range of diseases is further investigated.

Artificial Intelligence in Diagnostic Imaging, 67

Ryan B. Appleby and Parminder S. Basran

Artificial intelligence (AI) is rapidly developing as an important aspect of diagnostic imaging workflows in both human and veterinary medicine. AI can reshape aspects of care, but it is challenged by ongoing infrastructure limitations, appropriate development of use cases, and critical review of AI tools for veterinary imaging. AI can aid many aspects of the diagnostic imaging workflow including image acquisition, workflow optimization, computer-aided diagnosis, radiomic analysis, and other predictive modeling. This article describes the current state of AI in veterinary diagnostic imaging and establishes limitations and opportunities for developing this important and novel technology.

SECTION III - GASTROENTEROLOGY

Clinical Guidelines for Fecal Microbiota Transplantation in Companion Animals, 79

Jenessa A. Winston, Jan S. Suchodolski, Frederic Gaschen, Kathrin Busch, Sina Marsilio, Marcio C. Costa, Jennifer Chaitman, Emily L. Coffey, Julien R.S. Dandrieux, Arnon Gal, Tracy Hill, Rachel Pilla, Fabio Procoli, Silke Salavati Schmitz, M. Katherine Tolbert, Linda Toresson, Stefan Unterer, Érika Valverde-Altamirano, Guilherme G. Verocai, Melanie Werner, and Anna-Lena Ziese

▶ Video content accompanies this article at https://www.advancesinsmallanimalcare. com/.

The Companion Animal Fecal Microbiota Transplantation (FMT) Consortium is an international group of veterinary experts that are currently performing FMT in dogs and cats. Based on available evidence and expert opinions, the Companion Animal FMT Consortium developed the first clinical guidelines for FMT in companion animals aimed at increasing the accessibility of this microbial-directed therapeutic in veterinary medicine. These clinical guidelines include recommendations and protocols for fecal donor screening, FMT product processing and preparation, and current FMT clinical indications and administration. These clinical guidelines are intended to be utilized by veterinarians in all practice types.

MicroRNA as Biomarkers in Small Animal Gastrointestinal Inflammation and Cancer, 109

Janne Graarup-Hansen Lyngby and Lise Nikolic Nielsen

Gastrointestinal (GI) disease is common in companion animals. Extensive diagnostics are required for the differentiation between GI cancer and chronic inflammatory enteropathy. This diagnostic work-up is cost-prohibitive and potentially invasive. However, reaching a final diagnosis to initiate appropriate therapeutic intervention and improve patient outcome is imperative. Thus, there is a great need for diagnostic biomarkers. One could be microRNAs, as they are promising diagnostic biomarkers. MicroRNAs are small RNAs involved with post-transcriptional gene regulation in health and disease. In both dogs and cats, microRNA expression in tissue, serum, and feces has been investigated as diagnostic biomarkers in GI disease.

Vitamin D Metabolism in Canine Protein-Losing Enteropathy, *121*

Glynn Woods and Julien R.S. Dandrieux

▶ Video content accompanies this article at https://www.advancesinsmallanimalcare.com.

Hypovitaminosis D has long been associated with canine protein-losing enteropathy (PLE). Although hypovitaminosis D is widely accepted to arise secondary to PLE, its role as an initiator of PLE disease through immune dysregulation remains unanswered precipitating ongoing research. Within the context of canine GI disease, vitamin D concentration was first measured to investigate ionized hypocalcemia. Within this article, authors review literature pertaining to vitamin D metabolism with a particular focus on canine PLE and aim to highlight current practices, discuss limitations of publications to date, and assess whether vitamin D supplementation in canine PLE is warranted.

Comparative Cytology and Histology in Canine and Feline Gastrointestinal Neoplasia: Advantages and Challenges, *133*

Paola Cazzini, Alexandra Malbon, and Linda Morrison

This article evaluates advantages and disadvantages of cytology and histology of gastrointestinal (GI) neoplasia, from sampling to diagnosis. Available cytologic and histologic sampling techniques for the GI tract are summarized and discussed. The most common GI neoplasias are then described from both a cytologic and histologic point of view, highlighting the strengths and weaknesses of each technique and suggesting additional tests when appropriate. Understanding of the diagnostic process will help guide the clinician in the investigative process.

SECTION IV - NUTRITION

Conversations and Considerations Relevant to Nutrition for Senior Pets, *151*
Jonathan Stockman and Tammy Jane Owens

The population of geriatric pets is increasing and requires consideration. Aging is associated with chronic inflammation, sarcopenia, and declining immunity and sensory acuity in humans and pets alike. Nutritional strategies to address age-related concerns include maintaining optimal body composition, supporting gut microbial health, and supplementation of omega-3 fatty acids and medium-chain triglycerides to mitigate canine cognitive decline. There are no established nutritional requirements specific to senior pets; therefore, nutrient profiles of senior pet foods vary widely and must be evaluated for appropriateness for individual pets. Dietary phosphorus should be considered, given its contribution to chronic kidney disease.

Rational Approach and Dietary Considerations for Managing Dogs with Swallowing Impairment (Dysphagia), *165*
Stanley L. Marks and Tarini V. Ullal

Dietary modification plays a pivotal role in the management of dogs with swallowing impairment (dysphagia), and the anatomic categorization of the dog's swallowing impairment into oropharyngeal or esophageal causes followed by establishment of the underlying cause (structural vs. impaired motility) is important to formulate a personalized medical and dietary treatment plan. Swallowing fluoroscopy and contrast static esophagrams are particularly helpful in dogs with megaesophagus for optimizing dietary consistency and texture. In general, increasing bolus viscosity has anecdotally been observed to improve clinical signs and reduce laryngeal penetration and aspiration in dogs with pharyngeal weakness and cricopharyngeus muscle dysfunction.

SECTION V - UROLOGY

New Therapeutic Approaches to Management of Anemia and Iron Metabolism in Chronic Kidney Disease, *179*

Shelly L. Vaden, Jessica Quimby, and Cathy E. Langston

Anemia affects 30% to 65% of cats and dogs with chronic kidney disease (CKD). The resultant hypoxia promotes renal fibrosis, which further impairs diffusion of oxygen, and thus exacerbates the progression of CKD. Even small decreases in PCV are associated with progression (eg, median PCV 31% vs 35%). Hypoxia-inducible factor-prolyl hydroxylase inhibitors (HIF-PHIs) are a new category of drug. HIF causes erythropoietin to form when oxygen is low, but HIF is rapidly degraded by prolyl hydroxylase when oxygen is present. By stabilizing HIF, HIF-PHIs promote the production of erythropoietin by cells in the peritubular interstitium of the kidneys.

The Future of Veterinary Nephrology and Urology: Historical and Editorial Perspective, *189*

Larry D. Cowgill

Contrary to announcement of a late-breaking scientific discovery, this article chronicles the value and evolution of clinical specialization in veterinary nephrology and urology culminating in the establishment of the American College of Veterinary Nephrology and Urology as the American Veterinary Medical Association's newest provisionally recognized veterinary specialty. It offers an editorial perspective (rather than scientific results) on the value of clinical specialization in veterinary medicine and its future impact for urinary disease. I hope you will enjoy my perspectives.

Extracorporeal Removal of Viral and Bacterial Pathogens, *199*

Lakhmir S. Chawla and Keith R. McCrea

Managing sepsis and disseminated infections remains a challenge with current medical interventions. While antimicrobial drugs have significantly helped reduce morbidity and mortality caused by infectious disease, many patients will still experience poor outcomes. Additionally, emergence of drug resistance is a growing threat, and therapeutics for emerging infectious diseases rely on a slow discovery and approval process. This review presents an alternative approach at treating sepsis and disseminated infections. Instead of 'adding' drugs to fight infections, infectious organisms, damage-associated molecular patterns, and pathogen-associated molecular patterns can be 'subtracted' from the bloodstream through hemoperfusion.

Advances in Small Animal Care 5 (2024) xvii–xix

ADVANCES IN SMALL ANIMAL CARE

Preface

A Glimpse into the Future of Veterinary Medical Practice and Standards of Care

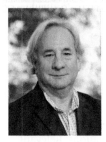

Philip H. Kass, BS, DVM, MPVM, MS, PhD

Editor

We have now reached the five-year mark of this journal, and it no longer is the novelty that it once was in 2020. But it occupies a special place among the ever-growing number of veterinary medical journals, because it lies at the confluence of original research, the discovery of new knowledge, and evidence-based medicine. It may be some time before we know how much the knowledge base recounted in the articles from this issue will eventually make their way into mainstream practice. Surely, though, much of what used to be considered futuristic is today part of accepted standard of care, and there is no reason to believe this will not continue to be the case. Last year, I wrote that this journal pushes the frontier of veterinary medicine forward, and this issue's contributions affirm that it is no less true today.

As I have said before, my aspiration for this journal is to bring the future closer to reality and expose veterinarians not only to what soon lies ahead but also to what is present in the here and now, and but for lack of awareness could encroach as a new part of our standards of practice. But for this information to be accessible to a wide readership that is not strictly in a specialty, this can only be accomplished through the sophisticated erudition of a distinguished roster of international authors. The time between receipt of the initial drafts of these manuscripts and the publication date is less than one year, guaranteeing that this new knowledge is truly cutting-edge veterinary medicine. Whether they are opinion pieces or review articles, all are extensively documented to ensure that they adhere to the highest scientific standards.

The first part of this issue, comprising three articles, addresses novel topics in animal behavior that are nevertheless likely to be experienced by owners and veterinarians alike. The article "Maternal Behavior in Domestic Dogs" addresses the issue of perinatal maternal behavior in dogs, underscoring the importance of having a better understanding of its determinants to allow for a propitious bearing on the physical and mental growth of a dam's puppies. It also directs the reader to potential future pharmacologic interventions pending additional research that will hopefully be forthcoming. The article "Mourning in Veterinary Medicine" is an

https://doi.org/10.1016/j.yasa.2024.07.002
2666-450X/24/   © 2024 Published by Elsevier Inc.

important contribution to the omnipresent emotional trauma that exists following the loss of a pet. What makes this article so novel is that it examines mourning not only from the perspective of the owners and veterinarian but also from the potential perspective of other animals, namely, that dogs may also exhibit grief-related behavioral and emotional reactions (readers may recall this embodied in the classic children's novel *Where the Red Fern Grows*). The article "Cats Living Together: How to Cope with a Multicat Household" addresses the familiar and vexing problem of the dysfunctionality that can occur when multiple cats share the same domicile and proposes strategies to mitigate inimical behavior.

The second part of this issue addresses new frontiers in veterinary imaging. The article "Computed Tomographic Imaging of the Gastrointestinal Tract of Small Animals" provides a comprehensive overview of the growing use of computed tomographic (CT) imaging to visualize gastrointestinal (GI) tract pathology, as well as the use of contrast media to improve visualization. The article "Advanced Imaging of Small Animals" extends the topic of CT scanning to zoologic medicine, addressing its use in small mammals as a lower-cost and more-rapid alternative to MRI, and discussing multiple modalities that are currently in use. "Artificial Intelligence in Diagnostic Imaging" looks into the future of using artificial intelligence in diagnostic imaging, including "image optimization, computer-aided diagnosis, radiomics, and workflow optimization." It represents an important introduction to this topic particularly for veterinarians with particular expertise or interests in radiology and diagnostic imaging.

The next four articles are focused on the GI tract, starting with the article "Clinical Guidelines for Fecal Microbiota Transplantation in Companion Animals," which provides guidance in the use of fecal microbiota transplantation (FMT) as a means of treating, at the present time, canine parvovirus enteritis, canine acute diarrhea, and chronic enteropathy in both dogs and cats. It builds upon the work by the international Companion Animal FMT Consortium in advocating FMT as a safe, well-tolerated, and minimally invasive method of treating GI disease of presumably infectious origin. "MicroRNA as Biomarkers in Small Animal Gastrointestinal Inflammation and Cancer" is more of a basic science article concerning the potential for small microRNA molecules to distinguish between chronic inflammatory bowel disease and neoplasia at or near incision sites. The article "Vitamin D Metabolism in Canine Protein-losing Enteropathy" is an exhaustive and authoritative literature review on the relationship between hypovitaminosis D and protein-losing enteropathy. The article underscores the many unanswered questions that remain about the therapeutic value of Vitamin D supplementation and provides evidence-based guidance about treatment under different pathologic scenarios. "Comparative Cytology and Histology in Canine and Feline Gastrointestinal Neoplasia: Advantages and Challenges" covers the cytologic and histologic characteristics of neoplastic lesions and includes differential diagnoses and other recommended diagnostic tests. Topics covered include GI neoplasia, including intestinal lymphomas, mast cell tumors, GI extramedullary plasma cell tumors/plasmacytomas, histiocytic sarcomas; epithelial neoplasia, including hyperplastic polyps, adenomas, and (adeno)carcinomas; neuroendocrine tumors (carcinoids), including nonneoplastic lesions; mesenchymal tumors, including GI stromal tumors, leiomyomas, and leiomyosarcomas; and nonneoplastic tumorlike lesions, including gossypibomas, feline infectious peritonitis, and feline GI eosinophilic sclerosing fibroplasia.

Nutritional topics comprise the following two articles. "Conversations and Considerations Relevant to Nutrition for Senior Pets" contains essential guidance on how veterinarians should approach the nutritional requirements of these pets as they grow older. The section on the advisability of supplementation with omega-3 fatty acids is particularly interesting given the ambiguity surrounding such supplementation in humans. "Rational Approach and Dietary Considerations for Managing Dogs with Swallowing Impairment (Dysphagia)" provides an up-to-date analysis of the major forms of swallowing impairments that veterinarians are most likely to be confronted with. These include oropharyngeal disorders, including pharyngeal weakness, cricopharyngeus muscle dysfunction when the upper esophageal sphincter fails to relax (achalasia) or there is asynchrony between pharyngeal contraction and upper esophageal sphincter relaxation. Common esophageal disorders include esophagitis typically secondary to gastroesophageal reflux disease under anesthesia, or sliding hiatal herniation, esophageal strictures, and megaesophagus.

Renal disease is a prominent component of veterinary medical practice, and veterinary nephrology is a specialization that is coming into its own right through professional recognition. The article "New Therapeutic Approaches to Management of Anemia and Iron Metabolism in Chronic Kidney Disease" provides a luminous explanation of the complex physiology underlying the anemia of chronic disease that is so often concomitant with the disease. Guidance is also provided for treating such anemia using darbepoetin, molidustat, and iron citrate. The article "The Future of Veterinary Nephrology" describes the genesis of the American Veterinary Medical Association's newest provisionally recognized veterinary specialty, the American College of Veterinary Nephrology and Urology (ACVNU). This rather momentous development portends a bright future for pets and pet owners alike; as the author writes, "The diagnostic expertise and specialized therapies currently limited to a handful of focal centers will become increasingly available throughout the world by highly skilled urinary specialists, eliminating disease risk and providing diversified therapeutic benefits … One can only speculate on the future advancements to be realized for veterinary nephrology and urology as a regiment of urinary specialists expands from this small cadre of its early and current pioneers."

The final article in this issue, "Extracorporeal Removal of Viral and Bacterial Pathogens", revisits a topic familiar to this journal: treatment of infectious disease. This time, though, an entirely new concept is proposed: instead of pharmacologic (ie, antimicrobial) interventions to immediately manage sepsis, a product has recently been developed to physically remove pathogens (bacteria, viruses, fungi, and parasites) and disease-causing molecules and cell fragments from the bloodstream using adsorbent beads. This is an emerging treatment to watch in the coming years.

As this journal continues to flourish, we remain committed to providing the most up-to-date and accessible resources for practitioners that bridge the gap between peer-reviewed scientific journals, publishing the discovery of new knowledge, and the textbooks that can be years in the making. I welcome your feedback about the contents of this journal and invite you to nominate new developing topics for forthcoming issues on emerging and new prospects that have the potential to revolutionize veterinary medicine.

Philip H. Kass, BS, DVM, MPVM, MS, PhD
Office of Academic Affairs
University of California, Davis
One Shields Avenue
Davis, CA 95616, USA

E-mail address: phkass@ucdavis.edu

SECTION I - BEHAVIOR

Advances in Small Animal Care 5 (2024) 1–7

ADVANCES IN SMALL ANIMAL CARE

Maternal Behavior in Domestic Dogs

Asahi Ogi, DVM, PhD, Dipl, ECAWBM[a],*, Angelo Gazzano, DVM, PhD, Dipl, ECAWBM[b]

[a]Department of Neurobiology and Molecular Medicine, IRCCS Stella Maris Foundation, Viale del Tirreno, 331, 56128 Pisa PI, Italy;
[b]Department of Veterinary Sciences, University of Pisa, Viale delle Piagge, 2, 56124 Pisa PI, Italy

KEYWORDS
- Attachment • Dog • Maternal behavior • Neurophysiology • Oxytocin

KEY POINTS
- Maternal behavior plays a crucial role in survival and well-being of the offspring. A caring and attentive mother could positively influence the physical and mental development of her puppies.
- There is a lack of consistent findings on the role of canine oxytocin as a neuromodulator of maternal behavior or, in general, of social behavior.
- Providing a quiet environment to dams–including the use of Dog Appeasing Pheromone–is probably the most effective available tool for preventing perinatal stress. Further studies on amniotic fluid, oxytocin, or even brexanolone may reveal novel approaches in improving maternal care in dogs.

INTRODUCTION

The reproductive cycle of female canids is distinct from that of other mammals because it involves extended periods of proestrus and estrus, followed by obligatory diestrus and prolonged anestrus [1]. Moreover, domestic dogs (*Canis familiaris*) differ from other species among genus *Canis* because they exhibit non-seasonal reproduction [2]. The domestic dog has also peculiar parental care. For example, dams do not regularly regurgitate food to puppies [3], while all members of a wolf pack contribute to pup-rearing by regurgitating food [4]. This behavioral difference, like many others, is probably grounded in the predatory motivation [5]. The food abundance granted by humans has changed the predatory motivation of proto-dogs and, consequently, both their social nature and their parental behavior [4]. Indeed, free-ranging dogs not only provide maternal care for a short period (compared to wolves), but also start to compete for food with their own offspring within a span of 4 to 6 weeks [6], an age at which wolf pups are still completely dependent on their mother [7]. Apart from these distinctions, all

Canidae are underdeveloped at birth and exhibit altricial characteristics during their early life stages.

In precocial species, the offspring are relatively mature and require minimal care from their parents [8]. In altricial species, on the contrary, the puppies are not born sufficiently developed to regulate their own temperature and need a nest where they can be left by the mother during her absence [9]. Parental care in dogs is mainly provided by the female, which ensures the well-being and development of the offspring [8]. Newborn puppies, in fact, depend entirely on their mother, as they need maternal stimulation for elimination; their movements are restricted to crawling; and their eyes and ears are closed. The canine species is also placentophagous. In fact, the female dog ingests the fetal membranes after their expulsion. This behavior helps to reduce the risk of attracting potential predators to the nest and it allows the mother to recover some energy without having to leave the puppies [10]. Moreover, the presence of amniotic fluid on the body of newborns triggers the first mother-infant contact, represented by the licking behavior toward the pups

*Corresponding author, *E-mail address:* a.ogi@hotmail.com

https://doi.org/10.1016/j.yasa.2024.06.001

2666-450X/24/

[11] – a fundamental step for stimulating breathing and ejections of the newborns [12].

Lactating dams are particularly attracted by pups bathed with amniotic fluid [13], and this attraction seems to be a crucial exogenous stimulus not only for the onset but also for maintenance of maternal care and, consequently, for mother-infant recognition and bond [14]. Instead, the endogenous stimulus pivotal for both the onset and maintenance of maternal behavior is regulated by the oxytocinergic system [8]. If the peripheral role of the hormone oxytocin (OXT) in stimulating myometrium contractility and regulating the release of prostaglandins during parturition is well-established [15], its central role–as neuromodulator–in regulating social and maternal behavior still needs a deeper exploration [16]. In dogs the sole study that correlates salivary OXT (sOXT) with maternal care indicates a weak correlation between hormone levels and behavior [17]. Indeed, the validity of hormonal regulation model of maternal behavior is widely discussed, and the views on this topic are conflicting. It was found, in fact, that some external stimuli can have an impact on maternal behavior without being influenced by the hormonal state of the animal. The sole exposure to pups, for example, was found to stimulate maternal behavior in ovariectomized female mice [18], rats [19], and ewes [20].

Already with Sigmund Freud, the idea that early experience–especially mother-infant bond could have a potent influence on adult behavior has inspired several psychologists [21]. In particular, starting from this concept, John Bowlby developed the attachment theory, a psychologic interpretation of the affective connections among individuals beyond the mother-infant relationship, a primary drive to intimate bonds "from the cradle to the grave" [22]. The attachment, "the lasting psychologic connectedness between human beings" [23], can be established also by adult dogs toward their human caregiver [24], and the owner can embody a "secure base" for their dogs, providing a sense of safety and security [25]. Regarding the intraspecific attachment bond, there is evidence that pups may experience proximity seeking and separation distress toward their own mothers [26]. Similarly, when adult dogs live with their biologic mothers, their bond appears to be stronger compared to their bond with an older female dogs they live with who are not their mothers [27].

Maternal behavior plays a crucial role in the survival and well-being of their offspring, and a caring and attentive mother could positively influence the physical and mental development of her puppies. With this review, we want to facilitate a better understanding of the mechanisms underlying dog maternal behavior.

Neurophysiology of Maternal Behavior

According to the Approach-Withdrawal model of Rosenblatt and Mayer, there are two contrasting motivational systems responsible for the onset, maintenance, and decline of maternal behavior [28]. And, as mentioned earlier, exposure to pups can change the motivation from initial avoidance (withdrawal) to acceptance (approach) in non-mother mammals. The assumptions that form the foundation of this model are represented by the existence of two antagonistic neural systems: the excitatory system, responsible for the "approach" motivation; and the inhibitory system, responsible for the "withdrawal" motivation [28]. However, the intricate neural pathways of these two opposite systems do not self-regulate on their own, but require the intervention of the medial prefrontal cortex (mPFC) [29].

Through the action of specific neurotransmitters–mainly dopamine, serotonin, and OXT–the mPFC also regulates maternal behavior [30]. In particular, the combination of two conceptual systems – the bio-behavioral feedback loop and the allostatic theory – emphasizes the importance of the oxytocinergic system in regulating maternal behavior [31]. The bio-behavioral feedback loop hypothesis proposes that OXT can stimulate positive social interactions, which in turn trigger the release of further OXT and so forth [32]. On the other hand, allostasis is the ability to maintain the stability of physiologic systems through change, the process of preserving equilibrium through transformation [33]. According to the allostatic theory, the oxytocinergic system would regulate physiologic setpoints facilitating also behavioral adaptation, and behavioral adaptation would enable the development of adaptive strategies by anticipating environmental changes [34]. It follows that, in an allostatic loop, a more functional oxytocinergic system would lead to better parenting and, therefore, to a better reproductive success. Moreover, better parenting would promote the adaptability of the offspring due to a more functional oxytocinergic system.

On one hand, the 2-fold role of OXT (hormone/neuromodulator) makes difficult to validate this nonapeptide as a biomarker of social, including maternal, behavior. Indeed, finding a peripheral mirror of the central activity of OXT is still a subject of scientific debate. Despite sOXT seeming to mirror central levels of OXT better than plasma [35], sampling the cerebrospinal fluid should be the goal–even though this is an invasive practice–because both sOXT and plasmatic OXT could have some limitations as effective biomarkers of central oxytocinergic system physiology [36]. In addition, urinary OXT was found not to be correlated with saliva and plasma [37].

On the other hand, the 2-fold role of OXT as a biomarker (retrospective/prospective) further complicates the picture. In fact, peripheral OXT increases after a single "acute" positive experience, but it does not seems to correlate with "chronic" prosocial aptitude influenced neither by lifestyle nor by domestication [38]. Salivary OXT, in particular, can be considered a valid retrospective marker of a positive human-dog interaction [16,39], but basal sOXT seems to fail as strong predictive biomarker of maternal behavior in dogs [17] and humans, in which the late pregnancy sOXT has not proved predictive of postpartum depression (PPD) [40]. To complicate the picture even further, serum OXT levels were found to be negatively related to maternal cannibalism in dogs [41]. However, according to this study, maternal cannibalism was also related to a number of stress behaviors attributable to a state of anxiety, and therefore, it is difficult to validate serum OXT as predictive of maternal cannibalism or retrospective of anxiety [41].

Similarly, the analysis of gene–behavior associations is still inconclusive. A study performed by Kis and colleagues indicates that polymorphisms in the OXT receptor gene affect friendliness in dogs in an opposite manner, depending on the breed [42]. Indeed, it was found that German Shepherds carrying the A allele in the rs8679684 SNP achieved higher scores on the friendliness scale compared to those with the T allele. Conversely, in Border Collies, individuals carrying the A allele were found to be less friendly. In a study on lactating Labrador Retriever dogs the presence of the A allele in the rs8679684 SNP seems to play a positive role in influencing maternal behavior of the dam [31].

In conclusion, if the connections among OXT secretion patterns, uterine contractility levels, and fetal expulsion progress in dogs need additional exploration [43], the lack of the consistent data in canine species on OXT as neuromodulator of maternal behavior–or, in general, of social behavior–does not allow for reaching any accurate conclusions.

Influence of Maternal Care on Puppy Development

The rearing environment of the litter might influence the behavior and disposition of dogs during their youth and adulthood. In a study conducted by Wilsson and Sundgren, the presence of a blanket in the whelping box had a significant positive effect on sleeping behavior of the puppies [44]. Moreover, it was found that in low temperatures the puppies were more active, attracting more attention from the mother. On the other hand, high temperatures possibly cause the mother discomfort from the proximity with the litter, reducing maternal care [44]. In addition to the temperature, other environmental stimuli, like incorporating a specific handling routine at a young age, could be beneficial particularly in circumstances where puppies are susceptible to inadequate tactile stimulation [45,46]; this includes situations like single-puppy litters, litters with mothers exhibiting poor maternal behavior, orphaned puppies, or those reared in kennel facilities [45]. Regarding social stimuli, it is well known that hypostimulation resulting from isolation could have a severe impact on adult dogs [47]. And, as could be expected, even if for just 1 week, the social isolation of puppies–also with minimal contact with humans–has a negative impact on their adaptability [46]. Furthermore, long-term isolation could lead the puppy to develop avoidance behavior due to fear [48].

Moreover, it was found that some litter traits could affect both mother and puppy behavior. Unexpectedly, the impact of the litter size on puppy behavior seems to be minimal [44], whereas its impact on maternal behavior is reported to be relevant [49,50]. Regarding the weight of the puppies, which normally decreases when the size of the litter increases, it was found that larger female puppies were more explorative than the smaller ones, while apparently there is no size effect on male puppies behavior [44]. Sex ratio of the litter is reported in some studies as a determining factor of maternal care [17] and puppy behavior [49].

Another critical aspect that can influence the behavior of puppies for an extended period of life is represented by mother-puppy interactions. Foyer and colleagues examined maternal care in a sample of military German Shepherds within the initial three weeks following birth, and their findings revealed a positive correlation between the amount of maternal care and offspring temperament (social/physical engagement and aggression) when they reach adulthood [51]. Similarly, Guardini and colleagues found in laboratory Beagles that a higher level of maternal care during the first three weeks post-partum has long-term positive consequences on puppies behavior [52]. Performing the arena and isolation test at 58 to 60 days of age, Guardini found that the care provided by dams can facilitate offspring to cope with stressful situations, making them more resilient individuals [52]. On the contrary, in a separate study by Guardini and colleagues conducted in a domestic environment, a higher degree of maternal care was linked to an increased exhibition of distress related to separation and less ability to cope with stress [53]. The rearing environment or the different breeds involved could have determined the contrasting results of these two studies conducted with a very similar rationale. Indeed, an increase in sensory stimulations from the environment of the puppies could mitigate the impact of maternal care [45], and it is widely shared within the scientific community that genetics could have a severe impact on maternal behavior [12,31].

In line with the findings of the later study of Guardini and colleagues [53], Bray and colleagues found that puppies that received a greater level of care from their mothers were less likely to excel in their guide dogs training program [54]. All these contrasting results on the impact of the quantity of maternal care in dogs can find an explanation previously stated by the present authors: it is not the quantity, but the quality of maternal care that matters. Indeed, the over-expression of some maternal behaviors could be associated with more anxious mothering [17]. The new experience of having pups in primiparous dams could stimulate a heightened attention toward the litter, resulting in higher total amount of maternal care. For example, it was observed that the frequency of licking the anogenital area was significantly higher in primiparous mothers compared to multiparous ones [55].

Even the nursing position (lateral, ventral, or vertical) appears to affect the puppy behavior. It has been hypothesized that lateral nursing, the easiest access to the milk, is not challenging enough for the puppies, and this could consequently lead to a detrimental impact on future performance [54]. As reported in the rat, handling and mild-stress stimuli in newborn positively modify their adult behavior, making them less prone to stress [56,57]. Maternal behavior can significantly modify the hypothalamic-pituitary-adrenal axis or stress responsiveness pathways of the litter and these modifications are maintained throughout adulthood, but like every other type of stimulus, the intensity needs to be balanced. When the mother is too protective, or conversely too uncaring, the resilience and adaptability of the puppies could not be maximized.

In conclusion, regarding puppy development the authors entirely agree with the statement of Pierantoni and colleagues [58]: the environment should offer an adequate level of stimulation, but the precise definition of "adequate" remains unclear.

Abnormal Maternal Behavior

Behavioral medicine is a relatively new field within veterinary medicine and is gaining greater significance alongside the growth of human attitudes toward

animals [59], but possible aberrant maternal behavior–maternal aggression, rejection of the offspring, and maternal infanticide or cannibalism–are not yet extensively studied in domestic dogs.

Maternal aggression, a crucial component of maternal behavior for protecting the offspring from potential threats, seems to be mainly regulated by the brain OXT and vasopressin systems [60]. This normal protective behavior could be aggravated by a perinatal stressful environment and directed toward familiar or unfamiliar people [61]. Maternal aggression could be displayed also during false pregnancy [62]. Stress reduction, minimizing handling of the puppies, and providing a secure and quite area should be the strategy to prevent undesirable aggressive behavior or other abnormal behaviors in dams [62]. Despite the use of pheromones being positively evaluated in certain specific behavioral problems, it appears that their efficacy could extend to stress reduction in multiple cases [63]. In addition, Santos and colleagues found that Dog Appeasing Pheromone (DAP) increases and prolongs the focus of lactating dogs on their puppies [64]. Therefore, the use of DAP could be suggested both for stress reduction in the dam and for maternal care increase, especially because any medications could pass into the milk [65].

Even though there are no specific pathologic conditions, if one or two puppies are frequently relocated from the nest or concealed, dams could exhibit rejection of the offspring [8]. Some primiparous dams, particularly with high nervousness or anxiety, could be more prone to rejection due to perinatal stress (PRS) [8]. Also, dams with litters born prematurely or delivered via cesarean section, and dams living in stressful environments could reject the offspring [66]. Although handling pups could be behaviorally healthy for them [62], removing the pups from the nest area and holding them for a brief duration can influence the behavior of the dam toward her litter [67]. For example, bathed neonates could be rejected by the dam due to amniotic fluid removal [11]. As mentioned earlier, the role of amniotic fluid in triggering maternal behavior is crucial and should be more deeply investigated in domestic dogs. The attraction toward this fluid could help to decrease the rejection of the offspring, or possibly increase the quantity of maternal care.

Maternal cannibalism could not only be expressed to remove any dead or sick puppy, decrease litter size, and balance sex ratio, but also when the environment is not suitable for the litter's growth [65,68]. As reported for rejection of the offspring, the experience and maturity of the dams could influence and reduce the incidence of this behavior [69]. In some cases, accidental cannibalism can occur. Specifically in prognathic breeds, where the mouth structure makes it challenging to sever the umbilical cord [70]. Also when a dam is exposed to constant threat, she could reach the point of eating her own pups [65].

PPD in dogs is not reported as possible abnormal maternal behavior, but understanding more deeply the pathogenetic mechanism underlying this condition could help to treat PRS in domestic species. In humans, several studies have shown that fluctuations in reproductive hormones during the postpartum phase (particularly allopregnanolone, the main metabolite of progesterone) play an important role in the pathophysiological processes of PPD [71]. The difficulty of GABA-A receptors in adapting to the abrupt decrease in allopregnanolone after childbirth has been considered one of the main factors in the onset of PPD [72]. For this mechanism, brexanolone, a neuroactive steroid and allosteric modulator of GABA-A receptors, has proven useful in the treatment of this condition and it is currently a US Food and Drug Administration approved treatment for PPD [73]. In addition, the metabolic profile of PRS has been recently studied in rats, and the involvement of the oxytocinergic system in the postpartum blues has revealed OXT treatment efficient to reverse the PRS at both behavioral and molecular levels [74].

Finally, the impact of genetic selection in preventing recurrences of inherited abnormal maternal behaviors, and assuring a quiet environment for the dams–including the use of DAP–are probably the most effective available tools for preventing PRS, but further study on amniotic fluid, OXT, or even brexanolone may reveal novel approaches in improving maternal care in dogs.

SUMMARY

Experiences in early life, including maternal nurturing, bonding, and social interactions, have profound and enduring effects on an individual's behavioral and physiologic growth [75]. But excessive care toward pups, even if apparently positive or enjoyable, can become detrimental because it does not contribute to increase the resilience of the litter. Essentially, it is beneficial for the puppy to experience a variety of social and environmental stimuli, but with the appropriate intensity. However, finding a clear definition of "appropriate" remains to be accomplished, and preventing behavioral disorders rooted in ontogenetic development are still goals to be achieved [58].

Despite the low incidence, dogs are not immune to abnormal maternal behaviors due to PRS, especially when they are primiparous, easily excitable, or anxious. Better comprehending neurophysiologic mechanisms underlying maternal behavior could help select dams, and eventually, treat possible aberrant behaviors. Currently there are no approved medical treatments for PRS in dogs, but brexanolone [73] and OXT [74] have proven effective in other species and could be possibly considered for further studies.

FUNDING

Dr Asahi Ogi is partially funded by the Italian Ministry of Health RC2024.

DISCLOSURE

The authors have nothing to disclose.

REFERENCES

[1] Nagashima JB, Songsasen N. Canid Reproductive Biology: Norm and Unique Aspects in Strategies and Mechanisms. Animals 2021;11:653.

[2] Concannon PW. Reproductive cycles of the domestic bitch. Anim Reprod Sci 2011;124:200–10.

[3] Lord K, Feinstein M, Smith B, et al. Variation in reproductive traits of members of the genus Canis with special attention to the domestic dog (Canis familiaris). Behav Process 2013;92:131–42.

[4] Marshall-Pescini S, Cafazzo S, Virányi Z, et al. Integrating social ecology in explanations of wolf–dog behavioral differences. Curr Opin Behav Sci 2017;16:80–6.

[5] Riggio G, Mariti C, Boncompagni C, et al. Feeding Enrichment in a Captive Pack of European Wolves (Canis Lupus Lupus): Assessing the Effects on Welfare and on a Zoo's Recreational, Educational and Conservational Role. Animals 2019;9:331.

[6] Paul M, Majumder SS, Bhadra A. Selfish mothers? An empirical test of parent-offspring conflict over extended parental care. Behav Process 2014;103:17–22.

[7] Mech LD, Boitani L. Wolves: behavior, ecology, and conservation. Chicago, IL: University of Chicago Press; 2019.

[8] Lezama-García K, Mariti C, Mota-Rojas D, et al. Maternal behaviour in domestic dogs. Int J Vet Sci Med 2019;7: 20–30.

[9] Numan M, Insel TR. The Neurobiology of parental behavior. New York: Springer-Verlag; 2003.

[10] Beaver B. Canine behavior: insights and answers. St. Frisco, CO: Elsevier Health Sciences; 2009.

[11] Abitbol ML, Inglis SR. Role of Amniotic Fluid in Newborn Acceptance and Bonding in Canines. J Matern Neonatal Med 1997;6:49–52.

[12] Santos NR, Beck A, Fontbonne A. A review of maternal behaviour in dogs and potential areas for further research. J Small Anim Pract 2020;61:85–92.

[13] Dunbar I, Ranson E, Buehler M. Pup retrieval and maternal attraction to canine amniotic fluids. Behav Process 1981;6:249–60.

[14] Lévy F, Keller M, Poindron P. Olfactory regulation of maternal behavior in mammals. Horm Behav 2004;46: 284–302.

[15] Gram A, Boos A, Kowalewski MP. Uterine and placental expression of canine oxytocin receptor during pregnancy and normal and induced parturition. Reprod Domest Anim 2014;49:41–9.

[16] Ogi A, Mariti C, Baragli P, et al. Effects of Stroking on Salivary Oxytocin and Cortisol in Guide Dogs: Preliminary Results. Animals 2020;10:708.

[17] Ogi A, Mariti C, Pirrone F, et al. The Influence of Oxytocin on Maternal Care in Lactating Dogs. Animals 2021;11:1130.

[18] Gandelman R. The ontogeny of maternal responsiveness in female Rockland-Swiss albino mice. Horm Behav 1973;4:257–68.

[19] Rosenblatt JS. Nonhormonal Basis of Maternal Behavior in the Rat. Science 1967;156:1512–4.

[20] Poindron P, Le Neindre P. Endocrine and sensory regulation of maternal behavior in the ewe, . Advances in the Study of BehaviorVol. 11. Cambridge, MA: Academic Press; 1980. p. 75–119.

[21] Chisholm JS. The evolutionary ecology of attachment organization. Hu Nat 1996;7:1–37.

[22] Bowlby J. The Making and Breaking of Affectional Bonds. Br J Psychiatry 1977;130:201–10.

[23] Bowlby J. Attachment and loss, (Vol. 1), Basic Books, New York, NY, 1969.

[24] Payne E, DeAraugo J, Bennett P, et al. Exploring the existence and potential underpinnings of dog–human and horse–human attachment bonds. Behav Process 2016; 125:114–21.

[25] Mariti C, Ricci E, Zilocchi M, et al. Owners as a secure base for their dogs. Behaviour 2013;150:1275–94.

[26] Previde EP, Ghirardelli G, Marshall-Pescini S, et al. Intraspecific attachment in domestic puppies (Canis familiaris). J Vet Behav 2009;4:89–90.

[27] Mariti C, Carlone B, Ricci E, et al. Intraspecific attachment in adult domestic dogs (Canis familiaris): Preliminary results. Appl Anim Behav Sci 2014;152:64–72.

[28] Rosenblatt JS, Mayer AD. An analysis of approach/withdrawal processes in the initiation of maternal behavior in the laboratory rat. Routledge: Behavioral Development; 2013. p. 199–252.

[29] Li M. The medial prefrontal regulation of maternal behavior across postpartum: A triadic model. Psychol Rev 2023;130:873.

[30] Sabihi S, Dong SM, Durosko NE, et al. Oxytocin in the medial prefrontal cortex regulates maternal care, maternal aggression and anxiety during the postpartum period. Front Behav Neurosci 2014;8:1–11.

[31] Ogi A, Naef V, Santorelli FMFM, et al. Oxytocin Receptor Gene Polymorphism in Lactating Dogs. Animals 2021; 11:1–10.

[32] Brooks J, Kano F, Yeow H, et al. Testing the effect of oxytocin on social grooming in bonobos. Am J Primatol 2022;84:1–7.

[33] Sterling P. Allostasis: A model of predictive regulation. Physiol Behav 2012;106:5–15.

[34] Quintana DS, Guastella AJ. An Allostatic Theory of Oxytocin. Trends Cogn Sci 2020;24:515–28.

[35] Martin J, Kagerbauer SM, Gempt J, et al. Oxytocin levels in saliva correlate better than plasma levels with concentrations in the cerebrospinal fluid of patients in neurocritical care. J Neuroendocrinol 2018;30:e12596.

[36] Martins D, Gabay AS, Mehta M, et al. Salivary and plasmatic oxytocin are not reliable trait markers of the physiology of the oxytocin system in humans. Elife 2020;9: 1–19.

[37] Feldman R, Gordon I, Zagoory-Sharon O. Maternal and paternal plasma, salivary, and urinary oxytocin and parent-infant synchrony: considering stress and affiliation components of human bonding. Dev Sci 2011;14: 752–61.

[38] Ogi A, Gazzano A. Biomarkers of Stress in Companion Animals. Animals 2023;13:660.

[39] MacLean EL, Gesquiere LR, Gee NR, et al. Effects of affiliative human-animal interaction on dog salivary and plasma oxytocin and vasopressin. Front Psychol 2017; 8:1–9.

[40] Cevik A, Alan S. Are pregnancy and postpartum oxytocin level a predictive biomarker for postpartum depression? J Obstet Gynaecol Res 2021;47:4280–8.

[41] Kockaya M, Ercan N, Demirbas YS, et al. Serum oxytocin and lipid levels of dogs with maternal cannibalism. J Vet Behav 2018;27:23–6.

[42] Kis A, Bence M, Lakatos G, et al. Oxytocin Receptor Gene Polymorphisms Are Associated with Human Directed Social Behavior in Dogs (Canis familiaris). PLoS One 2014; 9:e83993.

[43] Klarenbeek M, Okkens AC, Kooistra HS, et al. Plasma oxytocin concentrations during late pregnancy and parturition in the dog. Theriogenology 2007;68:1169–76.

[44] Wilsson E, Sundgren P-E. Effects of weight, litter size and parity of mother on the behaviour of the puppy and the adult dog. Appl Anim Behav Sci 1998;56:245–54.

[45] Gazzano A, Mariti C, Notari L, et al. Effects of early gentling and early environment on emotional development of puppies. Appl Anim Behav Sci 2008;110: 294–304.

[46] Fox MW, Stelzner D. Behavioural effects of differential early experience in the dog. Anim Behav 1966;14: 273–81.

[47] Cozzi A, Mariti C, Ogi A, et al. Behavioral modification in sheltered dogs. Dog Behav 2016;2:1–12.

[48] Fisher AE. The effects of differential early treatment on the social and exploratorybehavior of puppies. University Park, PA: The Pennsylvania State University; 1955.

[49] Foyer P, Wilsson E, Wright D, et al. Early experiences modulate stress coping in a population of German shepherd dogs. Appl Anim Behav Sci 2013;146:79–87.

[50] Bray EE, Sammel MD, Cheney DL, et al. Characterizing Early Maternal Style in a Population of Guide Dogs. Front Psychol 2017;8:1–13.

[51] Foyer P, Wilsson E, Jensen P. Levels of maternal care in dogs affect adult offspring temperament. Sci Rep 2016; 6:1–8.

[52] Guardini G, Mariti C, Bowen J, et al. Influence of morning maternal care on the behavioural responses of 8-week-old Beagle puppies to new environmental and social stimuli. Appl Anim Behav Sci 2016;181:137–44.

[53] Guardini G, Bowen J, Mariti C, et al. Influence of Maternal Care on Behavioural Development of Domestic Dogs (Canis Familiaris) Living in a Home Environment. Animals 2017;7:93.

[54] Bray EE, Sammel MD, Cheney DL, et al. Effects of maternal investment, temperament, and cognition on guide dog success. Proc Natl Acad Sci USA 2017;114: 9128–33.

[55] Guardini G, Bowen J, Raviglione S, et al. Maternal behaviour in domestic dogs: a comparison between primiparous and multiparous dogs. Dog behavior 2015;1(1): 22–33.

[56] Meerlo H, Nagy B, Koolhaas JM. The influence of postnatal handling on adult neuroendocrine and behavioural stress reactivity. J Neuroendocrinol 1999;11:925–33.

[57] Vallee M, Mayo W, Dellu F, et al. Prenatal stress induces high anxiety and postnatal handling induces low anxiety in adult offspring: correlation with stress-induced corticosterone secretion. J Neurosci 1997;17:2626–36.

[58] Pierantoni L, Amadei E, Pirrone F. Factors to Consider when Selecting Puppies and Preventing Later Behavioral Problems. Adv Small Anim Care 2022;3:1–11.

[59] Gazzano A, Giussani S, Gutiérrez J, et al. Attitude toward nonhuman animals and their welfare: Do behaviorists differ from other veterinarians? J Vet Behav 2018;24: 56–61.

[60] Bosch OJ, Neumann ID. Both oxytocin and vasopressin are mediators of maternal care and aggression in rodents: From central release to sites of action. Horm Behav 2012; 61:293–303.

[61] Horwitz DF, editor. Blackwell's five-minute veterinary consult clinical companion: canine and feline behavior. Hoboken, NJ: John Wiley & Sons; 2018.

[62] Landsberg G, Hunthausen W, Ackerman L. Behavior problems of the dog and cat. St. Frisco, CO: Elsevier Health Sciences; 2011.

[63] Pageat P, Gaultier E. Current research in canine and feline pheromones. Vet Clin Small Anim Pract 2003;33: 187–211.

[64] Santos NR, Beck A, Blondel T, et al. Influence of dog-appeasing pheromone on canine maternal behaviour during the peripartum and neonatal periods. Vet Rec 2020;186:449.

[65] Overall K. Manual of clinical behavioral medicine for dogs and cats-E-book. St. Frisco, CO: Elsevier Health Sciences; 2013.

[66] Horwitz D, Mills D. BSAVA manual of canine and feline behavioural medicine. Lincoln, UK: BSAVA; 2009.

[67] Battaglia CL. Periods of Early Development and the Effects of Stimulation and Social Experiences in the Canine. J Vet Behav 2009;4:203–10.

[68] Agrell J, Wolff JO, Ylönen H. Counter-Strategies to Infanticide in Mammals: Costs and Consequences. Oikos 1998;83:507.

[69] Kustritz MVR. Reproductive behavior of small animals. Theriogenology 2005;64:734–46.

[70] Evans JM. Parental injuries to the offspring in various anomal species. Proc Roy Soc Med 1968;61:1292.

[71] Schiller CE, Meltzer-Brody S, Rubinow DR. The role of reproductive hormones in postpartum depression. CNS Spectr 2015;20:48–59.

[72] Paoletti AM, Romagnino S, Contu R, et al. Observational study on the stability of the psychological status during normal pregnancy and increased blood levels of neuroactive steroids with GABA-A receptor agonist activity. Psychoneuroendocrinology 2006;31:485–92.

[73] Balan I, Patterson R, Boero G, et al. Brexanolone therapeutics in post-partum depression involves inhibition of systemic inflammatory pathways. EBioMedicine 2023;89:104473.

[74] Morley-fletcher S, Gaetano A, Gao V, et al. Postpartum Oxytocin Treatment via the Mother Reprograms Long-Term Behavioral Disorders Induced by Early Life Stress on the Plasma and Brain Metabolome in the Rat. Int J Mol Sci 2024;25(5):3014.

[75] Dietz L, Arnold A-MK, Goerlich-Jansson VC, et al. The importance of early life experiences for the development of behavioural disorders in domestic dogs. Behaviour 2018;155:83–114.

Advances in Small Animal Care 5 (2024) 9–20

ADVANCES IN SMALL ANIMAL CARE

Mourning in Veterinary Medicine

Stefania Uccheddu, DVM, PhD, MSc*

Behavioral Department, San Marco Veterinary Clinic and Lab, Viale dell'Industria 3, Veggiano, Padova 35030, Italy

---

KEYWORDS
- Mourning • Grief • Domestic animal • Professional grief • Caregiver

KEY POINTS
- *Recognize the prevalence of grief in nonhuman animals*: Grief is a complex emotion that may extend beyond human experience and encompass the behavior of companion animals.
- *Address the unique characteristics of pet grief*: Veterinarians and caregivers should be aware of the distinct features of pet grief to effectively support and validate the bereavement experiences of their companions.
- *Emphasize the significance of pet grief*: Grief associated with the loss of a companion animal is a valid and often profound experience that should be acknowledged and addressed.

INTRODUCTION AND BACKGROUND

Grief has traditionally been regarded as a natural human experience. On the one hand, basic characteristics of our response to loss reflect our evolution as biological and social creatures and are founded in the break of attachment relationships that are necessary for our survival. On the other hand, we respond to grief on both symbolic and physiologic levels, imputing meaning to the symptoms of separation we experience as well as the changes in personal and collective identity that precede the death of a member of the family or a member of the larger community [1].

Grief has recently been linked not just to human experience but also to animal experience. Furthermore, grief is regarded also as a human experience as a result of separation that follows the separation from pets, which are considered family members. Because of these 2 factors, mourning has become an aspect that is not only significant for human psychology but has also become a major topic for veterinary medicine, particularly for 3 major points that will be covered in further detail. A veterinarian should be aware of (1) grief in nonhuman animals; (2) grief in the caregiver after the animal has passed; and (3) professional grief.

GRIEF IN ANIMALS

Current research shows that at least some animals experience a wide range of feelings, such as fear, joy, happiness, anger, disgust, and grief [2]. Researchers interested in animal emotions investigate questions like, "Do animals experience emotions?" What emotions do they have, if any? Is there a clear dividing line between species that experience emotions and those that do not? Many current studies follow Charles Darwin's (1872) lead, which he outlined in his book *The Expression of Emotions in Man and Animals*. Darwin maintained that there is continuity between our emotional life and those of other animals, and that many animal differences are in degree rather than kind.

Numerous studies have documented instances of nonhuman animals displaying behaviors that suggest they possess an understanding of death, and engaging in mourning rituals [3,4]. Elephants, for instance, have been observed covering the bodies of their deceased companions with branches and dirt, a behavior that could be interpreted as a form of burial [5]. Additionally, elephants have been reported lifting and manipulating the bones of their relatives, suggesting a connection to their deceased kin even after their

---

*Corresponding author, *E-mail address:* comportamento@sanmarcovet.it

https://doi.org/10.1016/j.yasa.2024.06.002

2666-450X/24/

physical bodies have decomposed [5]. Magpies, ravens, and crows have also been observed engaging in similar behaviors, including bringing grass and laying it beside a dead conspecific, standing vigil, and returning to the site repeatedly [6].

Beyond these specific behaviors, numerous anecdotal reports suggest that a wide range of nonhuman animals exhibit signs of grief following the death of a close companion. Chicks, cows, pigs, and many other species have been observed exhibiting behaviors such as decreased activity, reduced appetite, and vocalizations reminiscent of mourning [7]. King's book "How Animals Grieve" provides a comprehensive collection of these anecdotes, further highlighting the prevalence of grief-related behaviors in the animal kingdom. While nonhuman animals' experiences of grief are largely confined to localized effects, as described in King's book, human grief, enabled by language, transcends spatial and temporal boundaries. Language fosters cognitive niches that nurture a normative explosion, governing our mourning practices and allowing grief's impact to permeate diverse communities and generations.

Cetaceans, including whales and dolphins, have also been observed displaying behaviors that suggest a deep understanding of death and associated grief [8]. In one instance, a killer whale was observed carrying the body of its dead calf for over 6 hours [9].

These observations collectively provide compelling evidence that nonhuman animals possess an awareness of death and the capacity to experience grief. These findings challenge traditional anthropocentric views of emotions and intelligence in the animal kingdom, highlighting the rich emotional lives of many species. In the future, skeptics of animal emotions will be expected to provide compelling evidence to support their positions, shifting the burden of proof to those who contend that animals experience a wide range of emotions. It will no longer be acceptable to acknowledge that chimpanzees or ravens exhibit behaviors indicative of love, or elephants display signs of grief, while simultaneously asserting that animals cannot truly experience emotions. Explanations regarding animal emotions often possess a comparable foundation to numerous other theories we readily accept, such as evolutionary concepts.

GRIEF IN PET ANIMALS
However, when we discuss grief in domestic animals, or animals that share our environment and might be identified as family members, we realize that knowledge and study on grief are scarce. Paradoxically, our understanding of grief-like behavioral patterns is more limited for familiar companion animals than for non-domestic species. Despite dogs and cats sharing lives with humans, relatively few publications have focused on their mourning [10]. What have we learned thus far?

Behavioral responses to a deceased conspecific have only been seen on rare occasions in wild canids, and there is no scientific evidence of grieving in companion dogs. A multidisciplinary research team conducted a quantitative analysis of the responses regarding mourning in dogs and their owners using the validated online Mourning Dog Questionnaire [11]. The purpose of the study was to investigate whether, how, and what a dog might go through after losing a companion dog. The main predictors of negative behavioral changes included not just the owner's grief and fury, but also the fact that dogs used to share food and had a friendly or paternal relationship. Dog owners' responses indicate that following the companion dog's death, the surviving dog underwent changes in behavior (such as "playing," "sleeping," and "eating") as well as feelings (such as fearfulness), which were related to how well the 2 animals got along. On the other hand, the remaining dog's behavior was unaffected by the time the 2 canines had spent together. Perceptions held by owners regarding their dog's responses and feelings were unrelated to the pain or recollection of the incident, which tended to fade with time. These results suggest that when a close conspecific dies, a dog may exhibit grief-related behavioral and emotional patterns; however, some of the latter may be connected to the emotional state of the owner. As there is currently a lack of evidence, a number of constraints must be taken into account, such as the possibility of anthropocentric interpretation and the challenge of creating representative and replicable scientific research. But this study is unique in that it takes into account and compares owners' reports on both themselves and their dog companions. This makes it possible for the assessment of the possibility of biased responses. However, not only may anthropomorphism play a role in attributing a specific function to the dogs' behavior, but attention to a deceased individual might also occur as a result of the owners' increasing attention (stimulus enhancement) [12]. Not surprisingly, an emotional contagion might also be considered, since stress seems contagious between dogs and owners [13]. These results might suggest that the dogs are responding to the "loss" of an affiliate, more than their "death" per se.

Because of their highly sociable nature, dogs, according to Bekoff, may exhibit mourning as a result of a close relationship [6]. Given that domestic dogs have either no access to the corpse or very limited access, only the response to being separated from the bonded individual may be assessed if viewing the corpse is a component of the death rite. From a biological standpoint, dogs that display grief-like behavioral patterns may be reacting to being split off from an attachment figure [14–16].

Behavioral responses to deceased or dying-dead conspecifics have hardly ever been documented in wild canids [17,18]. Boyd and colleagues [18] briefly provided evidence showing that 2 week old pup carcasses were buried by wild wolves (*Canis lupus*). Appleby detailed the passing of a 3 month old dingo puppy and the reactions of its mother and other littermates, including the puppy's transportation in the days that followed [17]. Regarding pets, owners have long reported anecdotally individuals mourning the death of a companion dog; nonetheless, there is a lack of published scientific research confirming grief-like behavioral responses in domestic dogs [19]. Even defining grief and the "ability to mourn" in dogs is challenging, and the same challenges occur in humans, particularly young children. It is important to note that a dog's mind can be compared, on certain levels, to that of a human child between the ages of 2 and 3 years [20]. We might also begin discussing a grief-like reaction only if the exposure to the body produced a noteworthy difference when compared to "simply" separation stress. Children between the ages of 2 and 5 years may not understand what death is, but they will definitely experience the pattern of behaviors known as grieving and mourning if they lose a caregiver. Dogs do develop emotional ties with other people and animals in their home, so it is reasonable to expect that losing a companion may result in behavioral changes that closely resemble the behaviors we typically associate with bereavement and grieving.

Other studies have documented behavioral changes in grieving dogs, such as decreased appetite, lethargy, and changes in sleep patterns [21]. Dogs may also exhibit destructive behaviors, withdraw from social interactions, and engage in searching behaviors, suggesting they are experiencing emotional distress in response to their loss. The underlying mechanisms of grief in dogs remain an area of active research. Neuroscientific studies have shown that dogs possess the same brain structures involved in processing emotions in humans. Changes in activity within these brain regions may contribute to the behavioral manifestations of grief in dogs.

WHAT ABOUT CATS?

There was agreement among cat owners that companion animal behavior changed in response to the loss of a feline companion [19]. These behavioral changes could indicate that the loss had an effect on the remaining cat.

The 2 most common types of behavioral changes described in cats were affectionate (78% of cats) and territorial (63% of cats). Cats were reported to demand more attention from their owners, exhibit affiliative behavior, and spend time seeking out the deceased's favorite area. Following the death of a companion, cats were shown to increase the frequency (43%) and volume (32%) of vocalizations. The median length of reported behavioral alterations was shorter than 6 months.

RECOGNIZING DEATH

Chemical cues emanating from deceased conspecifics may trigger fascination with death, potentially serving as a source of information regarding potential hazards in the surrounding environment [4]. From an evolutionary standpoint, the presence of a deceased conspecific could serve as a valuable indicator of potential threats, prompting subsequent behavioral modifications aimed at mitigating risks [22].

Moreover, animals like primates, when faced with loss, may seek solace and support from their peers, leading to enhanced collective coping mechanisms [23]. Analogously, a surviving dog might perceive a threat associated with the death of its companion and seek solace from its owner. However, if the owner is grappling with grief or anger, they may be less equipped to provide the necessary support, potentially exacerbating the dog's anxiety and fear.

Comparable behavioral interactions with carcasses of conspecifics have been documented in other species, particularly those considered to possess exceptionally high cognitive abilities, such as elephants. Elephants display approach and exploratory (sniffing and inspecting) behaviors toward the remains of their fallen comrades [24]. Cetaceans and primates have also been observed engaging in complex rituals surrounding death, further bolstering the notion of this phenomenon transcending species boundaries [25].

With respect to domestic animals, intriguingly, the surviving dogs exhibited no discernible behavioral differences based on whether they had encountered the deceased dog's body [11]. This observation aligns with previous reports on companion dogs, wherein 58%

of surviving dogs reportedly viewed the deceased companion's remains [19]. However, based on the authors' experience, it is recommended to provide dogs with the opportunity to see or visit the body of their companion dog, even in cases of euthanasia (Fig. 1). The dog may need to explore the body and process the fact that their companion dog is deceased.

Moreover, animals like primates, when faced with loss, may seek solace and support from their peers (Figs. 2 and 3), leading to enhanced collective coping mechanisms. Analogously, a surviving dog might perceive a threat associated with the death of its companion and seek solace from its owner. However, if the owner is grappling with grief or anger, they may be less equipped to provide the necessary support, potentially exacerbating the dog's anxiety and fear.

At present, we do not have a definitive answer to the question that is often asked by families about whether to show the body of a deceased pet to the other companion animal. However, it is certain that, from an ecological perspective, the recognition of death comes through the recognition of the body, so it would be appropriate to indicate that the nonhuman members of the family should be shown the body itself.

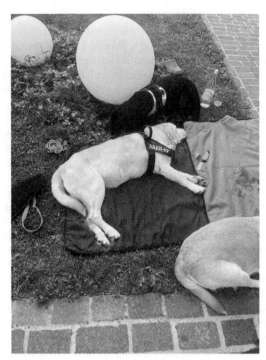

FIG. 2 The mother and 2 sons (Amleto and Ametis) few days before the euthanasia.

HEALING

In the context of grief healing, a recurring question pertains to the assistance we can offer dogs remaining after the passing of one companion. While the literature remains inconclusive on this matter, it is crucial to

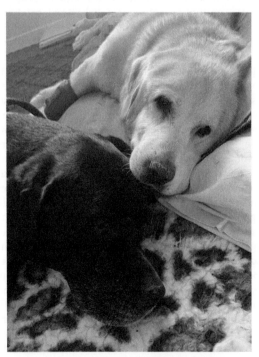

FIG. 1 Amleto and Nayk. Amleto (the black Labrador) was present during his mother's euthanasia.

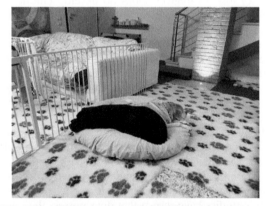

FIG. 3 Despite having the option to sleep in separate places, Amleto chose to share his sleeping quarters with the sister Ametis. This behavior was unexpected, as Amleto was not previously accustomed to sharing his sleeping space with any other member of the family.

recognize that mourning in dogs is not a pathologic condition. The surviving canine may experience a period of adjustment as they adapt to the loss of their familiar companion and the disruption of their established group dynamics [26,27]. Domestic dogs, like other social animals, exhibit strong tendencies toward cooperation and behavioral synchronization. This coordinated interaction is crucial for maintaining group cohesion and reaping the benefits of social living. However, when a member of the group passes away, this synchronization can be disrupted, potentially leading to behavioral changes in the surviving animal.

In light of this, it is suggested that changes to the surviving dog's routine should be introduced gradually, allowing for the gradual reestablishment of a new synchronized pattern of behaviors. This approach can help minimize the potential stress associated with sudden changes and facilitate a smoother adjustment process for the grieving dog.

It is essential to rule out any underlying medical conditions before attributing a dog's behavioral changes to grief. While there are no definitive diagnostic tests for canine grief, a thorough medical examination can identify potential organic causes of behavioral alterations, such as pain, anxiety, or neurologic disorders. By eliminating these medical factors, we can more accurately assess whether the dog's behavior aligns with the characteristics of grief-like patterns.

EUTHANASIA

Euthanasia, derived from the Greek words for "good" (eu) and "death" (thanatos), signifies a humane procedure that painlessly induces death in animals [28]. Even if euthanasia it is a common practice in veterinary medicine, particularly for geriatric pets or those suffering from terminal or chronic illnesses, the decision to euthanize remains ethically complex and emotionally challenging for both pet owners and veterinarians [29].

A crucial aspect of this ethical dilemma lies in determining the appropriate endpoint for euthanasia [30]. Veterinarians must weigh the animal's physical and physiologic health against the potential for prolonged suffering when making life-extending treatment decisions. Additionally, ethical frameworks for veterinary practice are not consistently integrated into veterinary education, potentially hindering effective navigation of these complex situations [31].

Furthermore, the veterinarian's professional obligation extends to advocating for both the animal's well-being and the owner's interests [32]. Owner-initiated euthanasia requests often involve factors beyond solely medical considerations, such as behavioral issues or financial constraints, adding another layer of complexity for veterinarians. The emotional and moral burden of euthanasia decisions weighs heavily on veterinarians [33]. To ensure an objective evaluation, a comprehensive approach is necessary. This includes ethical considerations, physical examinations, laboratory analyses, behavioral assessments, and a holistic evaluation of the animal's quality of life (QOL) [30,34]. Open communication between veterinarians and pet owners regarding treatment options, potential outcomes, and the animal's overall well-being is essential for informed decision-making [34].

A significant factor influencing euthanasia decisions is caregiver burden, defined as the physical, emotional, and social challenges experienced by individuals caring for a sick pet [35]. Studies have shown that owner satisfaction with veterinary care can act as a buffer against caregiver burden, potentially influencing euthanasia decisions [36]. Veterinarians who prioritize client communication and provide comprehensive support can potentially lessen caregiver burden and its impact on euthanasia choices. Caregiver burden manifests differently depending on the pet's condition: Spitznagel and colleagues explored caregiver burden in owners of dogs with chronic or terminal illnesses [35]. They identified signs like weakness, sadness, anxiety, and personality changes as potential indicators of burden. Furthermore, they found a correlation between caregiver burden and increased depression and stress, suggesting a significant impact on mental health [37]. Changes in daily routines due to the pet's illness and the difficulty of implementing new management strategies were also linked to heightened burden. Recognizing caregiver burden and its contributing factors allows veterinarians to provide empathetic responses that foster better communication and potentially alleviate the downstream effects on decision-making [38].

MOURNING IN THE CAREGIVER

The bond between humans and their pets is profound and enduring, often surpassing the connections we share with even our closest human companions. Our animal companions provide us with unconditional love, companionship, and comfort, becoming integral members of our families. When we lose a beloved pet, the grief experienced can be profound and multifaceted, leaving an emotional void that is often underestimated and misunderstood.

This analysis of pet bereavement thus poses 2 distinct problems to pet owners: factors related to the death of a pet that are not often associated with human death, and a culture that does not appear to recognize and support grief for pets in the same way that it does for humans. This can result in a pet bereavement experience that is influenced by both of these issues [39]: disenfranchised grief. The lack of an appropriate pet grieving routine indicated a lack of cultural significance toward pet mortality. This caused participants to deal with their tremendous loss in the face of society judgment, and even to suppress or conceal their actual grief in order to conform to societal norms. Cordaro [40] argued that this disenfranchised grief has 3 major causes: considering the bereavement over a companion animal unacceptable, believing that the individual can quickly cope with grief and easily replace the lost companion animal, and not considering the mourning experience as authentic.

Extant literature suggests that human–dog bonds can foster a level of comfort, security, and affection that rival or even surpass those experienced in close human relationships [41]. Several factors influence individuals' experiences following the loss of their canine companions, including the nature and strength of their attachment bond, the quality of social support received during bereavement, and the circumstances surrounding the pet's demise [42]. Notably, dogs have significantly shorter lifespans compared to humans. Consequently, human guardians may encounter multiple bereavements and recurrent grief experiences, which can potentially strain their adaptive capacities. In particular, the nature and intensity of the attachment link between the human and the pet, the level of social support offered to the bereaved, and the circumstances surrounding the pet's death are some of the factors that significantly impact the experience of canine loss that adult humans have. The inclusion of items like "How traumatic do you think it will be for you when your dog dies?" within the validated Monash Dog Owner Relationship Scale that has been translated and validated across multiple countries and languages (see, eg, ref. [43]) is unsurprising. These items, alongside others related to dog–owner interaction, reside within the same subscale. This subscale captures the emotional dimension of the relationship, reflecting not only time spent together but also opportunities for shared experiences and reciprocal interactions. Such elements are recognized as crucial for the formation of an affectional bond between humans and dogs, a bond present throughout life and extending even to the anticipation of loss [44]. Furthermore, the owner's gender and age [45] and the cause of loss [46] have been identified as potential influencing factors of grief intensity and predictors of profound grief. Life events, which can be classified as either positive or negative stressors, can also influence how a person deals with loss [47]. As a result, dog owners may experience multiple losses leading to repeated grief, which might overwhelm the person's normal coping ability [48].

Despite the relatively high frequency and intensity of grieving among pet owners, this process has been socially underrecognized and understudied in research [49]. Only a few studies have specifically focused on grief related to the loss of pet dogs and are limited either by the small sample sizes [50], the conceptualization of an individual's grief solely within an attachment framework [51,52], or the lack of a standardized, well-validated measure designed specifically to assess pet loss-related bereavement [53–56].

Individuals' responses to the death of a companion animal varied greatly, and the explanation for this variance is still unknown. People's responses to grief [45] range from sorrow to the most extreme suicide reaction [57]. People's responses to the death of a companion animal have received little attention, with most studies focusing on identifying characteristics such as gender, age, education, and marital status that may assist predict who is likely to feel intense or pathologic grief (eg, [46,56,58–60]).

When a person's pet animal dies, they may experience intense grief. In fact, the primary characteristics that reflect mourning in humans (guilt, grief, anger, and intrusive thoughts) are present following the death of a pet. Dog owners saw animals and people as being on the same continuum rather than as different individuals, and they had a pessimistic outlook on life after their pet died [61].

The decision to euthanize a pet is often viewed as a necessary and compassionate act, a way to alleviate the suffering of a beloved companion. However, this decision is not without its complexities and emotional challenges. Unlike decisions to end human suffering, which often evoke intense societal debate and controversy, the decision to euthanize a pet is generally supported and considered culturally acceptable. This acceptance stems from the unique bond that humans form with their pets, a bond that can be as strong or even stronger than the relationships they have with other humans [62]. The deep attachment we have to our pets can make the decision to euthanize even more difficult, as it involves the loss of a cherished companion and the acknowledgment of our own mortality [40].

The management of prolonged illness in companion animals can be intricate and time-consuming. Recent research highlights the prevalence of caregiver burden—the distress experienced while providing care for an individual with an illness—among human guardians and those caring for animals with chronic or terminal illness. This burden is associated with a range of negative psychosocial consequences, including elevated stress levels, symptoms of depression and anxiety, and diminished QOL. Understanding clients' experiences in caring for elderly or sick animals is of paramount importance. Caregiver burden not only contributes to client stress but also plays a significant role in influencing euthanasia decisions [42]. When clients feel overwhelmed, it is crucial to validate their experiences, both in the context of the companion animal's prolonged illness and in the decision-making process surrounding euthanasia. The psychological impact of euthanasia on pet owners has been extensively studied, with many studies reporting feelings of guilt, sadness, and anger [63]. These emotions are often exacerbated by the closeness of the human–pet bond, as owners may feel as though they have failed their pets by allowing them to suffer or by making the decision to end their lives [64]. The guilt associated with euthanasia can be particularly intense for owners who believe they may have contributed to their pet's illness or who feel like they could have done more to prolong their pet's life [65].

Mourning may begin in the veterinary clinic but does not end there. Caregivers may experience grief for 6 weeks after the death of a pet. But subclinical levels of grief and sadness can last for 6 months and more for 30% of people following the loss of a pet, with 4.3% experiencing complicated grief. Almost all owners believed their veterinarians should provide emotional support before and after their pet death. Even if the caretaking burden should be considered in the veterinary setting, the veterinarian is not the professional figure with the appropriate expertise. Psychological counseling is useful in providing insights into the decision-making and coping processes for chronic illness, end-of-life care, and mourning [66].

It is important to remember that grief is not only related to what happens when a dog passed away. Recent studies suggest that companion animal owners may exhibit depressive symptoms following a diagnosis with negative prognosis. However, caregiver burden may extend beyond mere diagnoses and encompass the challenges associated with caring for a sick pet, including the companion animal's treatment plan. Additionally, emotional distress may arise from anticipated bereavement, a phenomenon termed "anticipatory grief."

ANTICIPATORY GRIEF

Anticipatory grief, also known as prospective or pre-bereavement grief, is the emotional distress experienced by pet owners when they anticipate the impending loss of their pet due to a terminal illness or other life-threatening condition. This type of grief can be particularly challenging as it extends beyond the actual loss and involves the gradual adjustment to the inevitable separation.

The awareness of pet owners regarding for likely outliving their companion animals due to their shorter lifespans can induce anticipatory grief, which often manifests from the early stages of the relationship [67]. This shorter lifespan and anticipatory grief can also lead to the accumulation of multiple bereavement experiences associated with subsequent pets. This repeated bereavement, accompanied by a sense of disenfranchised grief, can pose substantial mental health challenges for individuals seeking to navigate loss. Moreover, pet loss differs from human loss in the unique experience of euthanasia, where owners assume a direct role in determining the timing and manner of their pet's death, and decisions may be influenced by factors not typically associated with human deaths, such as treatment costs [39].

The strength of the human–animal bond directly influences the expected outcomes of bereavement, including feelings of guilt, sadness, and the adoption of rituals and ceremonies to facilitate grief processing. Availability and quality of social support networks also play a crucial role in determining the intensity of grief experienced. Notably, pet grief exhibits unique characteristics, such as the accumulation of multiple bereavement experiences across an individual's lifetime, anticipatory grief arising from the shorter lifespans of companion animals, the decision-making process surrounding euthanasia, and the potential for disenfranchised grief due to societal perceptions that pet loss is less significant than human loss. In light of the inherent connection between euthanasia and veterinary practice, veterinarians play a pivotal role in minimizing negative experiences and mitigating grief severity for pet owners facing decisions regarding euthanasia.

Pet owners sometimes express to veterinarians their apprehension about experiencing profound grief upon the passing of their beloved animal companions. The ability of support services to anticipate and identify this type of anticipatory grief, along with its potential intensity, enables them to tailor their responses more effectively and provide individuals with the necessary support to positively manage their bereavement journey.

MOURNING IN THE VETERINARIAN

Veterinarians, as the caregivers of these cherished companions, are not immune to the emotional impact of pet loss. The intimate nature of their profession often brings them face-to-face with the raw emotions of pet owners, making them firsthand witnesses to the depths of human grief. While veterinarians are trained to provide expert medical care, they also play a crucial role in supporting pet owners through the grieving process. Understanding the nuances of pet loss and its impact on both pet owners and veterinarians is essential for fostering empathy, providing compassionate care, and promoting healing. The emotional impact of a patient's death on veterinarians is an intriguing topic that deserves a consideration because of the potential consequences. The death of a pet can be a very difficult experience for both the owner and the veterinarian who provides care. Veterinarians need to be aware of the potential professional psychological issues that can arise from this experience. Unlike many other problems that have been extensively researched in human medicine and later repeated in veterinary medicine, this has gotten minimal attention in the scientific human literature, presumably because of the small number of countries that permit physician-assisted suicide [68].

Veterinary practitioners' routines involve consultations with clients about euthanasia and the end of an animal's life. According to our research, the majority of veterinarians are emotionally affected when they have to inform the client of the animal's death, with many of them mentioning severe distress. It is established that veterinarians have a strong emotional relationship with their patients and are distressed when the animal-patient dies. It also means that the veterinarians suffer when observing the suffering of the animals and human families [33]. According to Figley [69], professionals who frequently care with animals or people who are dying may be influenced by other people's sadness and suffering, resulting in health difficulties such as burnout and secondary traumatic stress. Sleep and eating disorders are common emotional responses to stress, and they can result in feelings of guilt for everything that goes wrong [70]. Members of the veterinary team suffer from depression and other psychological problems at a high incidence [71], and professionals who are female and younger and work in small or mixed practices are more likely to experience work stress and consider suicide [72]. Among the areas of specialization, generalists were found to be more sensitive to patient loss than specialists. As a result of a greater number of animals with serious and/or fatal diseases or violent and unexpected animal deaths that do not reach specialists, generalists may be more emotionally affected [33].

The duration of time since graduation is another factor that affects the emotional status of veterinarians. The death of a patient has less of an impact on veterinarians who have been in practice for a long time (>20 years) than on those who have just graduated (<5 years). The professional's expertise appears to be a crucial role in the veterinarian's actions. Having graduated more recently leads in a better appropriate response and firmer control of the situation compared to individuals with less experience. This outcome, however, may reflect protective behavior in a professional as a result of extended exposure to stress-inducing stimuli.

Euthanasia and patient death are emotionally taxing experiences for veterinarians. These events can lead to a variety of psychological problems, including compassion fatigue, burnout, and depression. Mandatory instruction in veterinary degree programs should especially train future veterinarians to deal with death and communicate death or other unpleasant news to their patients' owners. Furthermore, veterinarians should be trained to spot signs of compassion fatigue and other psychological problems that may be created by having to cope with pain and death on a regular basis. This may also enhance their chances of obtaining medical and psychological guidance at an early stage of the condition and identifying colleagues who may be more vulnerable, such as female or young veterinarians.

Euthanasia and patient death can lead to a variety of psychological problems for veterinarians, including

- *Compassion fatigue*: Compassion fatigue is a form of burnout that can develop in people who work with people or animals who are suffering. It is characterized by feelings of emotional exhaustion, cynicism, and detachment.
- *Burnout*: Burnout is a state of physical, emotional, and mental exhaustion caused by prolonged stress. It can lead to a variety of symptoms, including fatigue, irritability, difficulty concentrating, and changes in sleep patterns.
- *Depression*: Depression is a mental illness that can cause a variety of symptoms, including sadness, loss of interest in activities, changes in appetite, and difficulty sleeping.

There are a number of actions that can be done to help prevent psychological problems in veterinarians, including

- *Mandatory instruction in veterinary degree programs*: Mandatory instruction in veterinary degree programs should especially train future veterinarians to deal with death and communicate death or other unpleasant news to their patients' owners. This training should cover topics such as the emotional impact of euthanasia and patient death, the signs of compassion fatigue and other psychological problems, and coping mechanisms for dealing with stress.
- *Support for practicing veterinarians*: Practicing veterinarians should have access to support services, such as counseling and therapy. These services can help veterinarians cope with the emotional challenges of their work.
- Because companion animals cannot express their needs and desires verbally, making decisions about their care, particularly euthanasia, can be emotionally and ethically problematic for both owners and veterinarians. Understanding the client's opinions and experiences may help a veterinarian modify their communication strategy to obtain the best potential outcomes for the client and their pet while also protecting their own mental health [38].

The emotional toll on veterinarians following a patient's death warrants further investigation due to its potential impact on professional well-being and the human–animal bond within veterinary medicine.

SUMMARY

The grieving process is a complex and multifaceted phenomenon. Recognizing the potential impact on caregivers, veterinarians, and other pets can help people better support those who are grieving the loss of a beloved animal.

The extensive neural similarities in emotional processing between humans and other animals, the profound psychological and physical impact of attachment relationships, and the intricate social structures and interpersonal connections that many species establish, provide compelling evidence that grief may be a fundamental aspect of social group experience. Caregivers, veterinarians, and companion animals might be affected by loss:

1. Caregivers experience a range of emotions during a pet's loss, including anticipation of loss, grief after death or euthanasia, and the burden of caregiving that can decrease QOL.

2. Veterinarians are also at risk for emotional distress and compassion fatigue due to the complex ethical considerations surrounding euthanasia and the frequent witnessing of animal suffering.
3. Other pets in the household may exhibit behavioral changes associated with loss, such as decreased activity, vocalization, and appetite.

Independent of any economic considerations, the well-being of living beings, encompassing both their physical and mental states, stands as a compelling ethical concern that warrants profound consideration and effective remedial measures.

CLINICS CARE POINTS

- *Grief may be a fundamental aspect of nonhuman animal experiences, and for welfare reason, veterinarians and caregivers should take care of that.*
- *Veterinarians should be cognizant of the unique characteristics of this form of grief to effectively accommodate, support, and validate the authenticity of human guardians' bereavement experiences.*
- *Understanding the multifaceted nature of pet loss and its consequences for veterinary professionals is crucial. Such knowledge can inform the development of empathetic communication strategies, compassionate care practices, and ultimately, the promotion of healing for all parties involved.*

ACKNOWLEDGMENTS

The authors express their sincere gratitude to all the caregivers who have shared stories and emotions with our research group. Their contributions have allowed us to gain a deeper understanding of this difficult topic and, in turn, develop methods to better support people grieving the loss of their pets, as well as pets experiencing the loss of their companions. A special thanks to Sabrina Turlon for providing the images but above all for sharing her and her family's (Amleto and Ametis) intimate experience of grieving the loss of their unforgettable Nayk.

DISCLOSURE

The authors have nothing to disclose.

REFERENCES

[1] Neimeyer RA, Prigerson HG, Davies B. Mourning and Meaning 2002;46(2):235–251+191+193.

[2] Bekoff M. Animal Emotions: Exploring Passionate NaturesCurrent interdisciplinary research provides compelling evidence that many animals experience such emotions as joy, fear, love, despair, and grief—we are not alone. Bioscience 2000;50(10):861–70.

[3] Monsó S, Osuna-Mascaró AJ. Death is common, so is understanding it: the concept of death in other species. Synthese 2021;199(1–2):2251–75.

[4] Anderson JR. Responses to death and dying: primates and other mammals. Primates 2020;61(1):1–7.

[5] Rutherford L, Murray LE. Personality and behavioral changes in Asian elephants (Elephas maximus) following the death of herd members. Integr Zool 2021;16(2):170–88.

[6] Marc Bekoff. The emotional lives of animals : a leading scientist explores animal joy, sorrow, and empathy–and why they matter. CA, USA: New World Library; 2007.

[7] King BJ. Animal Grief. Animal Sentience 2016.

[8] Pedrazzi G, Giacomini G, Pace DS. First Report of Epimeletic and Acoustic Behavior in Mediterranean Common Bottlenose Dolphins (Tursiops truncatus) Carrying Dead Calves. Biology 2022;11(2):337.

[9] Bearzi G, Kerem D, Furey NB, et al. Title: Whale and dolphin behavioural responses to dead conspecifics Whale and dolphin behavioural responses to dead conspecifics. Zoology (Jena) 2018. https://doi.org/10.1016/j.zool.2018.05.003.

[10] Park RM, Royal KD, Gruen ME. A Literature Review: Pet Bereavement and Coping Mechanisms. J Appl Anim Welfare Sci 2023;26(3):285–99.

[11] Uccheddu S, Ronconi L, Albertini M, et al. Domestic dogs (Canis familiaris) grieve over the loss of a conspecific. Sci Rep 2022;12(1):1–9.

[12] Huber L, Range F, Virányi Z. Dog imitation and its possible origins. In: Domestic dog cognition and behavior: the scientific study of Canis familiaris. Verlag Berlin Heidelberg: Springer; 2014. p. 79–100.

[13] Sundman AS, Van Poucke E, Svensson Holm AC, et al. Long-term stress levels are synchronized in dogs and their owners. Sci Rep 2019;9(1):1–7.

[14] Bowlby J. Attachment. Attachment and loss: Vol. 1. Loss. Published online 1969.

[15] József T, Miklósi Á, Csányi V, et al. Attachment Behavior in Dogs (Canis familiaris): A New Application of Ainsworth's (1969) Strange Situation Test. J Comp Psychol 1998;112(3):219–29.

[16] Cronin KA, van Leeuwen EJC, Mulenga IC, et al. Behavioral response of a chimpanzee mother toward her dead infant. Am J Primatol 2011;73(5):415–21.

[17] Appleby R, Smith B, Jones D. Observations of a free-ranging adult female dingo (Canis dingo) and littermates' responses to the death of a pup. Behav Process 2013;96:42–6.

[18] Boyd D, Pletscher D, W B. Evidence of wolves, Canis lupus, burying dead wolf pups. Canadian FieldNaturalist 1993;107:230–1.

[19] Walker J, Waran N, Phillips C. Owners' Perceptions of Their Animal's Behavioural Response to the Loss of an Animal Companion. Animals 2016;6(11):68.

[20] Stanley Coren. The intelligence of dogs : a guide to the thoughts, emotions, and inner lives or our canine companions. New York: Free Press; 2006.

[21] Walker JK, Waran NK, Phillips CJC. Owners' perceptions of their animal's behavioural response to the loss of an animal companion. Animals 2016;6(11). https://doi.org/10.3390/ani6110068.

[22] Iglesias TL, McElreath R, Patricelli GL. Western scrub-jay funerals: Cacophonous aggregations in response to dead conspecifics. Anim Behav 2012;84(5):1103–11.

[23] Ein-Dor T, Hirschberger G. Rethinking Attachment Theory: From a Theory of Relationships to a Theory of Individual and Group Survival. Curr Dir Psychol Sci 2016;25(4):223–7.

[24] Sharma N, Pokharel SS, Kohshima S, et al. Behavioural responses of free-ranging Asian elephants (Elephas maximus) towards dying and dead conspecifics. Primates 2020;61(1):129–38.

[25] Alderton D. Animal grief : how animals mourn. India: Hubble & Hattie; 2011.

[26] Ferrari PF, Palanza P, Parmigiani S, et al. Serotonin and aggressive behavior in rodents and nonhuman primates: predispositions and plasticity. Eur J Pharmacol 2005;526(1–3):259–73.

[27] Wright HF, Mills DS, Pollux PMJ. Behavioural and physiological correlates of impulsivity in the domestic dog (Canis familiaris). Physiol Behav 2012;105(3):676–82.

[28] Mota-Rojas D, Domínguez-Oliva A, Martínez-Burnes J, et al. Euthanasia and Pain in Canine Patients with Terminal and Chronic-Degenerative Diseases: Ethical and Legal Aspects. Animals 2023;13(7):1265.

[29] Deelen E, Meijboom FLB, Tobias TJ, et al. Handling End-of-Life Situations in Small Animal Practice: What Strategies do Veterinarians Contemplate During their Decision-Making Process? J Appl Anim Welfare Sci 2023. https://doi.org/10.1080/10888705.2023.2268516 Published online October 13.

[30] Pierce J, Shanan A. Quality of Life Assessments. Hospice and Palliative Care for Companion Animals 2023;26–43. https://doi.org/10.1002/9781119808817.CH4.

[31] Cooney K, Kipperman B. Ethical and Practical Considerations Associated with Companion Animal Euthanasia. Animals 2023;13(3):430.

[32] Brown CR, Edwards S, Kenney E, et al. Family Quality of Life: pet owners and veterinarians working together to reach the best outcomes. J Am Vet Med Assoc 2023;261(8):1238–43.

[33] Moreira Bergamini S, Uccheddu S, Riggio G, et al. The Emotional Impact of Patient Loss on Brazilian Veterinarians. Veterinary Sciences 2023;11(1):3.

[34] Spitznagel MB, Carlson MD, Caregiver Burden and Veterinary Client Well-Being. Vet Clin Small Anim Pract 2019;49(3):431–44.

[35] Spitznagel MB, Marchitelli B, Gardner M, et al. Euthanasia from the Veterinary Client's Perspective: Psychosocial Contributors to Euthanasia Decision Making. Vet Clin Small Anim Pract 2020;50(3): 591–605.

[36] Matte AR, Khosa DK, Coe JB, et al. Impacts of the process and decision-making around companion animal euthanasia on veterinary wellbeing. Vet Rec 2019;185(15): 480.

[37] Spitznagel MB, Carlson MD. Caregiver Burden in the Companion Animal Owner. Hospice and Palliative Care for Companion Animals. 2023:349-359. doi: 10.1002/9781119808817.CH26.

[38] Uccheddu S. Improving vet-client communication through understanding the client perspective. Vet Rec 2021;188(9):349–51.

[39] Cleary M, West S, Thapa DK, et al. Grieving the loss of a pet: A qualitative systematic review. Death Stud 2022; 46(9):2167–78.

[40] Cordaro M. Pet Loss and Disenfranchised Grief: Implications for Mental Health Counseling Practice. J Ment Health Counsel 2012;34(4):283–94.

[41] Lykins AD, McGreevy PD, Bennett B, et al. Attachment styles, continuing bonds, and grief following companion animal death. Death Stud 2023. https://doi.org/10.1080/07481187.2023.2265868.

[42] Testoni I, De Vincenzo C, Campigli M, et al. Validation of the HHHHHMM Scale in the Italian Context: Assessing Pets' Quality of Life and Qualitatively Exploring Owners' Grief. Animals 2023;13(6):1049.

[43] Riggio G, Piotti P, Diverio S, et al. The Dog–Owner Relationship: Refinement and Validation of the Italian C/DORS for Dog Owners and Correlation with the LAPS. Animals 2021;11(8):2166.

[44] Dwyer F, Bennett PC, Coleman GJ. Development of the Monash Dog Owner Relationship Scale (MDORS). Anthrozoös 2006;19(3):243–56.

[45] Blazina C, Boyraz G, Shen-Miller D. The psychology of the human–animal bond. New York: Springer; 2011.

[46] McCutcheon KA, Fleming SJ. Grief Resulting from Euthanasia and Natural Death of Companion Animals. Omega: J Death Dying 2002;44(2):169–88.

[47] Kimura Y, Kawabata H, Medical M. Frequency of neurotic symptoms shortly after the death of a pet. Journal of Veterinary 2013;76(4):499–502.

[48] Thomas J, Sours T. Multiple lacerations of the heart: when grief accumulates. VA, USA: Faculty Publications and Presentations; 2007. p. 15.

[49] Packman W, Carmack B. Therapeutic implications of continuing bonds expressions following the death of a pet. Omega (Westport) 2011;64(4):335–56. Available at: https://journals.sagepub.com/doi/abs/10.2190/OM.64.4.d?casa_token=w5vKnLFYY4sAAAAA:w9JN-jzBZbPUb1dyUIqhc7oP4UOrgqvkzkV2Heamp10nxx2Ak9O2swTPcrXa3TR1LedLSQyS1zCW. [Accessed 6 April 2019].

[50] Wrobel TA, Dye AL. Grieving Pet Death: Normative, Gender, and Attachment Issues. Omega: J Death Dying 2003;47(4):385–93.

[51] King LC, Werner PD. Attachment, Social Support, and Responses following the Death of a Companion Animal. Omega: J Death Dying 2012;64(2):119–41.

[52] Sable P. Pets, attachment, and well-being across the life cycle. Soc Work 1995;40(3):334.

[53] Gosse GH, Barnes MJ. Human Grief Resulting from the Death of a Pet. Anthrozoös 1994;7(2):103–12.

[54] Brown BH, Richards HC, Wilson CA. Pet Bonding and Pet Bereavement Among Adolescents. J Counsel Dev 1996;74(5):505–9.

[55] Jarolmen J. A Comparison of the Grief Reaction of Children and Adults: Focusing on Pet Loss and Bereavement. Omega: J Death Dying 1998;37(2):133–50.

[56] Gerwolls MK, Labott SM. Adjustment to the Death of a Companion Animal. Anthrozoös 1994;7(3): 172–87.

[57] Archer J, Winchester G. Bereavement following death of a pet. Br J Psychol 1994;85(2):259–71.

[58] Davis H, Irwin P, Richardson M, et al. When a pet dies: Religious issues, euthanasia and strategies for coping with bereavement. Anthrozoös 2003;16(1):57–74.

[59] Field N, Orsini L, Gavish R, et al. Role of Attachment in Response to Pet Loss. Death Stud 2009;33(4):334–55.

[60] Stokes S, Templer D, Planchon L, et al. Death of a Companion Cat or Dog and Human Bereavement: Psychosocial Variables. Soc Anim 2002;10(1):93–105.

[61] Uccheddu S, De Cataldo L, Albertini M, et al. Pet Humanisation and Related Grief: Development and Validation of a Structured Questionnaire Instrument to Evaluate Grief in People Who Have Lost a Companion Dog. Animals 2019;9(11):933.

[62] Testoni I, De Cataldo L, Ronconi L, et al. Pet Loss and Representations of Death, Attachment, Depression, and Euthanasia. Anthrozoös 2017;30(1):135–48.

[63] Tzivian L, Frigera M, Kushnir T. Associations between Stress and Quality of Life: Differences between Owners Keeping a Living Dog or Losing a Dog by Euthanasia. PLoS One 2015;10(3):e0121081.

[64] Kogan LR, Bussolari C, Currin-Mcculloch J, et al. Disenfranchised Guilt—Pet Owners' Burden. Animals 2022; 12(13):1690.

[65] Kogan L, Kogan LR, Bussolari C, et al. Dog owners: Disenfranchised guilt and related depression and anxiety. Human-Animal Interactions 2023. https://doi.org/10.1079/HAI.2023.0016.

[66] Campigli M, Strizzolo G, Furlanello T, et al. Pet owners' feedback on psychological support service in an Italian veterinary hospital. Acta Vet Hung 2022. https://doi.org/10.1556/004.2022.00011.

[67] Hamilton N. A psycho educational intervention program for veterinary practitioners:learning to cope with being a veterinarian. Queensland: University of Southern Queensland; 2016.

[68] Andriessen K, Krysinska K, Castelli Dransart DA, et al. Grief After Euthanasia and Physician-Assisted Suicide. Crisis 2019;41(4):255–72.

[69] Figley C. Treating compassion fatigue. J Clin Psychol 2002;58(11):1433–41.

[70] Seligman M. Flourish: A Visionary New Understanding of Happiness and Well-Being.; 2011.

[71] Quain A. The Gift: Ethically Indicated Euthanasia in Companion Animal Practice. Veterinary Sciences 2021; 8(8):141.

[72] Hartnack S, Springer S, Pittavino M, et al. Attitudes of Austrian veterinarians towards euthanasia in small animal practice: Impacts of age and gender on views on euthanasia. BMC Vet Res 2016;12(1):1–14.

Advances in Small Animal Care 5 (2024) 21–30

ADVANCES IN SMALL ANIMAL CARE

Cats Living Together

How to Cope with a Multi-cat Household

Simone Moreira Bergamini, DVM, MSc, Dipl CLEVE-CVLBAMC[a,b,*],
Ludovica Pierantoni, DVM, MSc, Spec.EABA, Dipl ECAWBM[c], Manuel Mengoli, DVM, MSc, PhD[d]

[a]Behavioral Clinic, Etoclinvet, Rua da Quitanda 19/911, Rio de Janeiro 20011-030, Brazil; [b]Veterinary Clinical Ethology at the Qualittas Institute of Graduate Studies, Rio de Janeiro 20011-030, Brazil; [c]CAN-BS, Via Tasso 9/A, Napoli, Italy; [d]Néthos, 84 Route de Cavaillon, Plan d'Orgon 13750, France

KEYWORDS
• Cat behavior • Indoor cats • Multi-cat households • Behavioral problems in multi-cat households

KEY POINTS

- The understanding of certain individual factors of both the adopted and resident cat can assist in making a better choice and decision during adoption.
- In multi-cat households, a comprehensive approach to environmental enrichment is essential to mitigate stress and improve the quality of life for all animals involved.
- Client education before adoption and before introducing a new cat is important to decrease the risk of having problems related to cohabitation in multi-cat households.
- Problems in multi-cat households can include compulsive problems, elimination problems, and urinary marking, as well as intraspecific and redirected aggression.

Video content accompanies this article at https://www.advancesinsmallanimalcare.com/

INTRODUCTION

Cats are still regarded as low-maintenance domestic pets compared to dogs due to their lower expenses, lack of need for daily walks, reduced food consumption, greater independence, and self sufficiency. Additionally, cats are perceived as capable of enduring longer periods alone, sometimes for days if required, and they also thrive in smaller living spaces.

In Brazil, a study stimated the presence of 33.6 million domesticated cats in 2023, representing a 6% increase compared to the year 2022 [1].

Cats, by nature, show a blend of solitary and social behavioral traits inherited from their ancestors, which can lead to varied interactions when housed together.

Furthermore, as urbanization increases and outdoor spaces become less accessible, more cats are kept strictly indoors. Compared to dogs, cats have a distinct evolutionary background with minimal selection for domesticated traits and their behavior and needs remain similar to their wild ancestors [2].

An indoor life also brings benefits to the cat, providing greater protection against diseases such as feline leukemia, feline immunodeficiency virus (FIV), and peritonitis, as well as reducing territorial disputes with neighboring cats, risks of accidents, mistreatment, and even theft. However, living indoors can also bring negative emotions, such as watching a neighbor's cat through the window without being able to chase it

*Corresponding author. Behavioral Clinic, Etoclinvet, Rua da Quitanda 19/911, Rio de Janeiro 20011-030, Brazil. E-mail address: smb_6@hotmail.com

https://doi.org/10.1016/j.yasa.2024.06.014
2666-450X/24/

away, a predictable and monotonous environment, reduced exploration, increased boredom, and frustration [3]. As a result, this radical change in cats' lifestyle from living outdoors may impact their behavior and welfare, particularly in terms of their natural behaviors and needs, which include hunting, territoriality, and social interactions [4]. Very little is currently known about how well cats adapt to an indoor lifestyle and when their behavioral needs are unmet, cats can develop poor welfare and problematic behaviors [5]. Cats that are kept exclusively indoors or are only allowed limited access outdoors are more protected from accidents and diseases, but they are also more prone to exhibit behaviors related to stress and disease with typical behavioral issues including unsuitable elimination, marking with urine, high levels of vocalization, damaging furniture through scratching, and aggression toward owners, unfamiliar individuals, or other animals more prevalent in indoor-only cats than in those with both indoor and outdoor access [6].

In families with multiple cats, a study showed that 50% of the respondents reported fights (scratching and biting) when a new cat was introduced, and approximately half of the people introduced the cats by simply bringing them together immediately [7]. In another study involving 2492 owners of multiple cats, 73.3% reported signs of conflict from the outset upon introducing the cats. The more cats there are in the household, the more frequent the signs of conflict are shown. Staring was the most commonly observed conflict sign, occurring at least daily in 44.9% of households, followed, in descending order of frequency, by chasing, fleeing, tail twitching, hissing, and yowling [8].

While the ancestors of the domestic cat were solitary hunters, today domestic cats have shown remarkable adaptability in forming various social structures. These can range from solitary living to forming loose colonies when resources are abundant [9].

In multi-cat households, behavioral issues such as inter-cat aggression, stress, territorial disputes, and anxiety are prevalent. These behaviors often stem from the forced cohabitation of unrelated individuals forced to live together. Common stressors include competition for resources, insufficient personal space, and the lack of escape routes. For instance, Clark [10] emphasizes that many behavioral problems are misinterpreted by owners who believe that their cats get along without recognizing underlying stress signs. This significantly affects the welfare of cohabitating animals, as they are compelled to live alongside unrelated individuals in a populous household, posing a potential source of feline stress [10]. Furthermore, a study concluded that

knowledge about cat needs was greater among veterinarians, followed by veterinary nurses, and finally, cat owners [11] who often mistakenly believe that cats living together in the same house, sharing food and sleeping spaces, inherently get along. The owners only recognize issues when behavioral problems, such as overt aggression between problematic cats, become apparent [10]. One study also demonstrated that in a multi-cat environment, the relationship among the animals (agonistic or not) influenced the relationship with the owner, as cats experiencing fighting issues also showed higher negative interaction with the owner (growling and hissing) [12].

This review aims to observe how intrinsic factors of the individual (feline), environmental management, and an unstructured introduction can affect the cat social interaction.

FACTORS TO CONSIDER BEFORE INTRODUCING A NEW CAT
Socialization

Early socialization, particularly before 9 weeks of age, results in an increase in the kitten's willingness to approach people and remain bonded to a person, which persists into adulthood [13]. Familiarity, relationship, and social exposure during the sensitive period (approximately between 2 and 7 weeks of age) have also been associated with differences in specific social behaviors (Video 1). Sibling cats from the same litters spent more time in physical contact with each other, were more likely to feed together, and groom each other. Higher rates of affiliative behaviors were linked to siblings from the same litter being socialized with each other during their sensitive periods [14].

In addition to kitten socialization, kittens from friendly fathered cats were not only friendlier toward unfamiliar people but also less distressed when approached and handled by them [15]. Cats living alone or with one cat were more fearful than cats living with multiple cats. On the other hand, this association may indicate that owners of fearful or aggressive cats may not be willing to acquire more cats as it could increase the likelihood of aggressive behavior among the cats [16]. Furthermore, because fearful behavior is partially hereditary, breeders can theoretically reduce average fear by favoring non-fearful parents in breeding [16]. Therefore, kittens from unsocialized cats may be more fearful.

Personality

Personality is considered the interactive product of genetic, cognitive, and environmental factors; identifying and evaluating personality traits in cats are potentially important because they are relatively stable and enduring, making each individual unique. Six dimensions of personality have been assessed in cats: playfulness, nervousness, amiability, dominance, demandingness, and gullibility. In the dimension of playfulness, a correlation with the cat's age was identified, suggesting that younger cats are perceived to be more energetic, playful, quick, mischievous, and curious than older ones [17]. Personality traits and environmental variables can affect feline fear, aggression toward humans, and excessive grooming [18] However, overall, the individual effects of environmental variables were smaller than the effects of personality, behavior, or breed. Fear is an important personality trait that can affect other dimensions of personality [16]. Knowledge of the cat's personality can be used as a strategy; for example, extroverted cats can be stimulated and encouraged in physical activity through playing with objects at home, aiming to reduce motivation for hunting. Cat owners may also be more inclined to adopt strategies that they believe best suit their perceptions of their cat's personality [19].

Sex and age

In wild cats, cooperative behavior in raising offspring is observed, for either related and not related cats. This can be observed when cats give birth to kittens with days or weeks of intervals. Care may include cleaning the perineum of the birthing cat, which will also clean the kittens and consume the amniotic membrane [20]. Free-ranging male and female domestic cats are typically solitary, but females may also form small groups of closely related individuals associated with human habitats and cooperate in rearing offspring. In rare cases, infanticide by males has been reported in rural areas among domestic cats, but the same has not been reported in urban areas. It is believed that in high-density colonies, defense of the offspring by females may provide an explanation [21]. Additionally, in free-ranging adult males, the spacing pattern of the home range corresponds to 2 or 3 home ranges of adult females [21].

The age at which a kitten is adopted and weaned can affect its relationship with conspecifics due to the importance of sensitive periods in the behavioral development of the kitten. In cats, weaning typically occurs around 8 weeks after birth, which also coincides with the period of socialization with littermates. It has been reported that littermate interaction is necessary for the development of appropriate social play patterns, the absence of which may result in higher levels of aggression in adulthood, even when raised by the mother. Early weaning in cats has been associated with stress and stereotypical behaviors. Additionally, sensory and social stimuli from the mother and littermates shape physiologic and behavioral phenotypes during sensitive postnatal periods, contributing significantly to stable individual differences in adulthood [22].

With an increased lifespan, owners can expect age-related changes. Aging is not a pathologic condition, but it will lead to deterioration in the function and morphology of body systems. By 10 years of age, cats may begin to experience sensory (eg, vision and direction), cognitive, and motor decline, as well as cerebral atrophy, contributing to behavioral changes. In animals with cognitive dysfunction, alterations related to vocalization, disorientation, changes in interactions, changes in the sleep–wake cycle, house soiling, alterations in activity level, and anxiety can be observed [23].

Health

Inflammation and stress can cause nonspecific clinical and behavioral signs, such as fatigue, drowsiness, vomiting, diarrhea, anorexia or decreased food and/or water intake, fever, reduced general activity and body hygiene, social withdrawal, or loss of interest in social activities, and altered cognition. It is important to understand that the stress response can be triggered by external environmental events, such as sudden changes, unfamiliar or loud noises, new and unfamiliar places and objects, and the approach of strangers, or even psychological factors [24].

Pain can lead to defensive aggressive behaviors to avoid contact, induce fear and anxiety, and trigger stress responses. Additionally, a decrease in physical activity may further reduce serotonin activity in the central nervous system, which has been linked to aggressive behaviors. Other clinical problems related to aggression, such as hyperthyroidism and vomeronasalitis, may also be observed. In the case of hyperthyroidism, alterations in neurotransmitters dopamine, norepinephrine, and serotonin are related, while in vomeronasalitis, inflammatory changes in the vomeronasal organ (VNO) can lead to social and behavioral alterations related to communication [25]. Therefore, the evaluation of potential clinical problems and stress in cats (adopted and resident) is important before adoption.

ENVIRONMENTAL ENRICHMENTS IN MULTI-CAT HOUSEHOLDS

In an era where pet ownership trends show a significant increase in multi-cat households, the importance of understanding the unique dynamics within these environments has never been more critical. Cat welfare organizations advise providing environmental enrichments such as food and water bowls, litter boxes, and scratching posts for basic cat's care. Additional enrichments like hiding places, elevated lookouts, and toys that mimic hunting behaviors had also been considered in enhancing the welfare of the indoor cat [3]. However, given that environments are intricate and vary both physically and socially, these structural and object-based provisions may contribute minimally to overall positive welfare. The way cats perceive their daily interactions with humans or other cats may significantly influence their behavior and could be as crucial as the physical amenities provided. Here, we explore strategic interventions through environmental enrichment aimed to enhance the welfare and cohabitation of multiple cats.

Environmental enrichment is defined as a concept aimed at modifying the environments of captive animals to benefit their well-being. It is also described as a process to enhance animal environments and care by aligning with the animals' behavioral biology and natural needs. This dynamic approach involves adjustments to structures and husbandry practices with the objective of providing animals more behavioral options, eliciting species-specific behaviors and skills, and thereby improving their welfare [26]. Cats can be considered captive animals when their owners confine them to spaces much smaller than their natural territory, often keeping cats indoors or with limited access to outdoor spaces. The objectives of environmental enrichment are to expand the variety, quantity, and diversity of normal behavioral patterns; decrease the frequency of abnormal behaviors; enhance positive engagement with the environment; and improve the ability of animals to handle challenges in a more typical manner [26].

Control and predictability

A key factor in a cat's environment that could impact their welfare is how much control and predictability they perceive they have. The sense of, or actual absence of, control over their environment is likely the most significant stressor for animals in captivity [26].

Control and predictability play crucial roles in an animal's capacity to adjust to different environments, as they allow for behavioral responses that enhance adaptation abilities.

As with all other aspects of confinement, control and predictability of caretaker behaviors are also of great importance to the animal's perceptions of humans [27].

Cat–caregiver relationship

The personality of cat owners can significantly affect the behavior and well-being of their cats. For instance,

neurotic owners are more likely to have cats with behavioral problems and stress-related sickness behaviors. In contrast, owners who score high in agreeableness, conscientiousness, and openness tend to have cats that exhibit less aggressive and anxious behaviors [28]. Cats are sensitive to their owners' emotional states, which can affect their own stress levels and general well-being. The perception of cats by their owners—whether as a family member, a child, or merely a pet—influences how cats are treated and can lead to variations in their living environment and access to outdoor space [29]. Furthermore, the interactions of cats with owners impact their ability to handle stress and unfamiliar situations. Cats that have positive interactions with their owners tend to develop a secure attachment, which significantly benefits their overall welfare [30]. To avoid tension in homes with multiple cats, it is essential that each cat receives individual attention without interference from others [31].

Trained human behaviors can increase cats' comfort and reduce aggression during interactions: when humans follow best practices in handling cats, it leads to more positive and affiliative behaviors from the cats. Key guidelines include giving cat's choice and control, paying attention to their body language, and gentle handling, especially around sensitive areas like the head and the back [32]. Furthermore, owners play a crucial role in providing environmental enrichment, which is vital for the physical and mental health of cats. The involvement of the owner in interactive play and providing a stimulating environment is key to preventing behavioral issues.

Resource distribution

In homes with multiple cats, ensuring that there are sufficient resources is critical. These resources should be plentiful and distributed throughout the home to avoid forcing cats into unnecessary competition. Ensuring ample and strategically placed resources such as food bowls, water stations, and multiple litter boxes can prevent resource guarding and reduce conflict. The ideal number is typically one per cat plus an extra one to ensure there is always an available option to help minimize territorial behaviors and aggression as each cat can access necessities without confrontation [33].

Cats require personal space and may exhibit stress when their living area is too confined. In densely populated environments, such as urban settings or homes with multiple indoor cats, the availability of and access to personal space becomes even more crucial [10]. In multi-cat households, it is crucial to provide sufficient space, both horizontally and vertically, to allow each cat to maintain a comfortable social distance.

Cats benefit greatly from vertical spaces, which satisfy their need to climb and survey their surroundings from a safe height. Structures such as cat trees, shelves, and wall-mounted perches allow for these natural behaviors. Furthermore, these structures help in establishing territories within a vertical dimension, effectively enlarging the living space [31]. Similarly, ensuring ample horizontal space with clear pathways can prevent ambushes and reduce stress during movement around the home. Providing hiding spots such as covered beds, boxes, or even dedicated rooms where cats can retreat when stressed is crucial. These safe zones should be accessible to all cats without them having to pass through another cat's territory. The sense of security these safe havens provide can greatly reduce anxiety and the potential for conflict [33]. While some cats may form close bonds and share spaces harmoniously, others might prefer to use communal areas at different times, highlighting the importance of offering multiple safe and comfortable space [34].

Because cats naturally hunt alone for small prey, they may be more comfortable eating from individual bowls placed out of sight from each other in multi-cat households. Placing food bowls in quiet areas away from noisy appliances can prevent disturbances while eating and avoid stress-induced abnormal behaviors. Cats typically prefer multiple small meals rather than fewer large ones [34].

Proper litter box setup is crucial for a cat's well-being, emphasizing the need for large, open boxes to accommodate natural behaviors like digging and covering. While self-cleaning litter boxes maintain cleanliness, their noise might deter some cats. Covered boxes can trap odors and block views, potentially making them undesirable. Litter boxes should be placed away from noisy areas and food sources, with one per cat plus an extra, all out of sight from each other. Unscented, clumping litter is preferred, and boxes should be cleaned regularly to maintain hygiene [34]. Cats generally prefer clean litter boxes and are not influenced by the odor or identity of the previous user, but physical or visual obstructions do affect their preferences. Regular cleaning and ensuring unobstructed litter boxes are highlighted as important for preventing out-of-box elimination, a common reason cats are relinquished to shelters [35].

Sensory and cognitive enrichment

Engaging the cats' senses and minds can significantly reduce boredom and associated stress behaviors. This includes the provision of toys that encourage hunting behaviors, puzzle feeders that stimulate their problem-solving skills, and safe outdoor enclosures that allow them to experience the outdoors safely [36]. A statement from the American Association of Feline Practitioners discusses the behavioral needs of cats in relation to feeding. It emphasizes creating feeding programs that offer to a cat's natural behaviors such as hunting and foraging, which improves their health and well-being. The consensus statement suggests using puzzle feeders, providing multiple small meals, and setting up separate feeding areas in multi-cat households to reduce stress and prevent overeating. The aim is to mimic natural feeding behaviors, thereby reducing behavioral problems and enhancing the cat's quality of life [37]. As an additional cognitive enrichment, cats can learn specific behaviors like targeting and sitting through brief, structured training sessions. Regular clicker training can improve shelter cats' welfare and potentially increase their chances of adoption by teaching them desirable behaviors [38]. Different types of environmental enrichment can address the various sensory needs of domestic cats [39]:

- Visual stimulation is crucial for keeping indoor cats engaged and can be facilitated through the strategic placement of perches near windows to allow cats to observe outdoor activity. Additionally, toys that mimic the appearance and movements of prey can capture a cat's attention and encourage playful behavior. Incorporating moving elements, such as fluttering feathers or rolling balls, can provide continual visual interest.
- Gustatory enrichment involves stimulating a cat's taste senses by providing a variety of food flavors and textures. This can be achieved through a mix of wet and dry foods, treats, or food supplements that offer new and interesting tastes. Engaging cats in food puzzles or hiding small amounts of food around the house makes mealtime both mentally stimulating and physically engaging.
- Tactile experiences are essential for cats, which use touch to explore their environment and communicate. Providing a range of textures in bedding, scratching posts, and play areas can satisfy this need. Materials like corrugated cardboard, sisal, soft fleece, or rugs offer different sensations. Additionally, grooming and petting by the owner provide comforting tactile interactions that strengthen the human–animal bond and contribute to the cat's tactile enrichment.
- Olfactory enrichment, cats have a highly developed sense of smell, making olfactory enrichment a vital

component of their environment. Introducing different scents such as catnip, silver vine, essential oils, or the scent of dried herbs can stimulate a cat's interest and curiosity [40].

Cats detect a variety of smells with their nose and chemical signals through the VNO, an auxiliary olfactory apparatus sensitive to pheromones—chemicals that transmit information among members of the same species. Cats emit olfactory and pheromonal signals by marking their territory with facial and body rubbing. This marks the boundaries of their core living area, a space where they feel secure and safe. Humans should avoid disrupting a cat's olfactory and chemical signals and scent profile whenever possible [36]. Synthetic pheromones can also be used to create a sense of calm and familiarity in the home, reducing stress and promoting feelings of safety [39]. These synthetic pheromones mimic the natural scents that cats use to mark their territory as safe, which can be particularly effective in multi-cat homes [33].

Social enrichment and stress reduction

When exposed to a variety of stimuli categorized into human social interaction, food, toys, and scents, adult cats showed notable individual differences in preferences. However, across both the pet and shelter populations, social interaction with humans emerged as the most favored category, closely followed by food [41]. However, not all cats in a household will have the same social preferences and therefore providing hiding spots and quiet retreats where cats can escape when overwhelmed is crucial [31].

Interactive play and training

Scheduled playtimes not only help in reducing potential aggression by using up excess energy but also strengthen the bond between cats and their owners. Cats should engage in naturalistic predatory play and feeding behaviors. Providing toys, play opportunities with the owner or other compatible cats, and feeding mechanisms that require active engagement can facilitate this. Encouraging cats to express their predatory instincts through play and feeding activities is beneficial as such activities not only provide exercise but also reduce boredom and behavioral issues [31]. To keep the environment stimulating and prevent habituation, it is beneficial to rotate toys, scratching posts, and even rearrange furniture occasionally. This rotation helps maintain the cats' interest in their environment and provides new and interesting challenges that keep their minds active [33].

Behavioral interventions and modifications

Regularly observing and adjusting the living environment based on the cats' interactions and behavior changes are critical. This proactive approach allows for timely interventions that can prevent stress accumulation and behavioral issues, promoting a healthier environment for all cats involved. Understanding each cat's unique preferences and behavioral patterns is vital. For instance, some cats might prefer solitary play, while others thrive on social interaction with fellow cats or humans. Tailoring the environment to meet these individual needs can significantly enhance their well-being and reduce inter-cat tensions. Successfully managing a multi-cat household requires a nuanced understanding of feline behavior coupled with strategic environmental modifications. Understanding cat behavior and signs of stress can help in early identification of resource-related issues. For example, changes in eating habits or litter box usage can indicate that a cat feels its resources are threatened or inadequate. Proactive monitoring of these behaviors is essential for early intervention and preventing escalation.

Veterinarians and cat behaviorists play a vital role in educating owners about the needs of their cats, particularly in multi-cat households. They can provide valuable advice on how to structure the living environment and distribute resources effectively to minimize competition and stress among cats [10].

BEHAVIORAL PROBLEMS RELATED TO MULTI-CAT HOUSEHOLDS
Social compatibility and cat interactions

As previously mentioned, some of the most common undesirable behaviors are presented in multi-cat houses (scratching furniture, spraying, increased vocalizations, or aggression between cats) [3]. It is sometimes hard to cope with more than one cat at home: cohabitation can become problematic, because of cats' ethological, social preferences and needs [10]. Opportunities for educating the client before adoption and before the introduction of a new cat must be considered the first tool to minimize the risk in having cohabitation-related problems in multi-cat households [8]. It is important to highlight the complexity of cat social structures, and suggesting that while providing sufficient resources is essential. It is also crucial to consider the quality of the interactions and profiling the individual personalities of the cats [10].

Indoor aggression

Usually, first contacts during a new cat introduction are problematic. In cats, first contacts outside the social group are rare and minimal. Lacking a clear, linear hierarchy or complex social structures, a key strategy for cats is to first attempt escape and manage intimidation to minimize the risk of aggression [42]. Signs of conflict are often evident from the very beginning of an introduction (video 2). If the relationship starts well, affiliative behaviors are more frequent and signs of conflict less common compared to introductions that do not go well [8].

Scent profile is fundamental in cats to identify themselves and is often correlated with a high rate of tactile communication, rubbing, and sniffing between cats belonging to the same colony or social group [20]. Scent also provides a self-directed form of communication increasing a perception of security. Unfamiliar scents have been known to elicit stress and anxiety, increasing conflicts and aggression [43]. Tactile behaviors help to confirm and maintain social relationships and provide social group stability, but importantly allogrooming permits the creation of a common scent and bonding relationships [44]. Interestingly, some authors [8] suggested that it could be counterintuitive that providing an adequate quantity of resources like food, litter boxes, and scratching posts would not correlate with a reduction in conflict behaviors among cats. Typically, it is thought that having enough resources would prevent competition and reduce stress, thereby lowering the chances of conflict. This research suggests that while conflict signs were not reduced, affiliative behaviors such as allogrooming, sleeping or sharing the same room, and sleep-touching were less frequent in households with an adequate number of litter boxes and food stations [8]. This could imply that with more resources, cats have less need to interact with each other for survival, leading to fewer positive interactions as well. Moreover, the perception of proactive, social, and physical contact between cats is often observed at least daily in approximately half of the multi-cat households [8]. Possible differences could be related to the age of the resident cats: younger (adult) ones are more involved in more active conflicts that include chasing and stalking, whereas these behaviors are less common in aged cat households [8]. More active forms of aggression are evident if there are no means of escape [34].

Furthermore, rapidly increasing the quantity of resources in a cat's environment should be paired with giving the resident cat a specific period to adjust to these changes before introducing a new cat. This adaptation period can vary depending on the cat's profile, the original level of environmental enrichment, mood responses, or any preexisting behavioral issues.

Indoor redirected aggression

If a cat is highly aroused by an outdoor neighbor cat, fearful triggers, or another animal, the cat may redirect that aggression toward another cat (or humans) in the household. It could be easily involved a cat with which there had been no previous problems or any showed aggression.

More than that, cats that never learned as kittens to adapt their behavioral response, to have good self-control, and to temper their responses may play too aggressively with the other cats [3]. It could arouse some interactions and let the introduction of a new cat be complicated. Moreover, play-related aggressions could interrupt good existing relationships through resident cats. Some behavioral protocols, interesting for the introduction of a new cat, would help to cope with possible conflicts and restoring shared contacts.

Repetitive or self-directed behaviors

Different scientific studies tried to focus on compulsive or redirected cat behaviors. Triggers as possible changes in the social environment (eg, the introduction of a new cat) would often produce some mood imbalance potentially correlated to excessive self-licking and over-grooming, potentially exiting in a psychogenic alopecia [45]. The behavior would be usually directed to the posterior ventral abdomen and/or between the thighs [46]. As social stress can be a trigger for recurrent cystitis [44,47], there has been some suggestion that bladder pain can result in licking the caudal abdomen, so this should be considered a possible behavioral outcome. Pica, the act of ingesting various materials such as wool, plastic, and other materials, has been related to stress, and redirected ingestive behavior could be easily associated with social triggers [9].

Feline hyperesthesia syndrome is characterized by repetitive licking and biting of the back and tail, often leading to self-mutilation. Other signs include skin rippling, dilated pupils, drooling, intensive scratching, and chasing one's own tails. Some cats may vocalize or urinate during these episodes. During an episode of hyperesthesia, the affected area becomes sensitive (particularly on the back from the shoulders to the tail). The cat responds by violently biting and licking itself, attempting to escape the perceived harassment or irritation. This behavioral syndrome has also been associated with a stressful social environment [48].

Elimination problems and urine-marking behaviors

Cat spraying/elimination can indeed be a complex issue to treat, not only because of potential pathologic causes but also because it is often influenced by stress, cat density, and social dynamics within their environment [35,49]. Considering feline communication, confident cats might spray more openly as a form of territorial marking or social challenge, while less confident cats may choose more discreet forms of marking (squatting) or avoid spraying altogether [46]. Social stress can also be associated with feline idiopathic cystitis, a common diagnosis of feline lower urinary tract disease [50]. Less common "maddening" is the act of feline fecal marking in an exposed and prominent location, and it could be an obvious sign of socially related communication during conflicts or general stress-related responses [20]. Social stress (directly or indirectly related to the environment) could be linked to any differential approach to cat elimination problems [35,43].

The connection between stress and feline interstitial cystitis is well documented. Stressors such as moving, conflicts with other household animals, and restricted access to litter trays can increase the risk of this pain-related behavior. The introduction of a new cat could easily modify all these variables [44,47]. It is assumed today from different studies that an increased risk of cystitis is correlated with the time that cats spend indoors [51–53]. Increased plasma norepinephrine levels [54], associated with stress, can indeed affect bladder permeability, potentially leading to conditions like interstitial cystitis. Managing a cat's stress through environmental modifications, providing safe access to litter trays, and ensuring positive interactions within the household can help mitigate these risks [54]. Some studies found that behaviorally normal cats and from households that including a urine sprayer had elevated fecal glucocorticoids (an indicator of chronic arousal), compared with individuals from homes with a cat that was failing to use the litter tray, suggesting that urine spraying is a more common behavioral outcome of chronic stress than failure to use the litter tray [55].

SUMMARY

The management of cohabitation among multiple cats is a sensitive process and is not always successful. Many factors influence their living style, including aspects related to the cats themselves (including their personality, physical characteristics, and behavioral traits), as well as environmental factors. Effective environmental enrichment can positively influence coexistence. Owners need to be guided by veterinarians and receive information aimed to increase their knowledge of feline ethology and communication, as well as preventive strategies to

implement in multi-cat households. By addressing these factors thoughtfully, cat owners can increase the likelihood of peaceful coexistence within multi-cat households, enhancing the welfare and harmony of their feline companions.

CLINICS CARE POINTS

- The stress caused by cohabitation and an inadequate environment can be predisposing factors to behavioral disorders.
- Environmental enrichment measures are essential for the well-being of felines and in preventing conflicts in multi-cats households.
- Positive experiences of living with other cats during the socialization period are important for future interactions.
- Introducing a new cat into the household should be approached by considering factors related to both the new and resident cats, environmental conditions, and resource management. Effective management of these factors is crucial for minimizing stress in the animals and promoting positive interactions between them.

DISCLOSURE

The authors have nothing to disclose.

SUPPLEMENTARY DATA

Supplementary data to this article can be found online at https://doi.org/10.1016/j.yasa.2024.06.014.

REFERENCES

[1] Abinpet abinpet folder dados mercado, in https://abinpet.org.br. 2024. Available at: https://abinpet.org.br/wp-content/uploads/2024/03/abinpet_folder_dados_mercado_2024_draft2_web.pdf. Accessed April 4, 2024.
[2] Driscoll CA, Menotti-Raymond M, Roca AL, et al. The near eastern origin of cat domestication. Science 2007;317(5837):519–23.
[3] International Cat Care (n.d. a) Indoor vs Outdoor. Advice. Available at: https://icatcare.org/advice/keeping-your-cat-happy/indoors-versus-outdoors. [Accessed 4 April 2019].
[4] Worsley RF, Farnworth MJ. A systematic review of social and environmental factors and their implications for indoor cat welfare. App Anim Behav Sci 2019;220.

[5] Broom DM. Indicators of poor welfare. Br Vet J 1986; 142(6):524–6.

[6] Foreman-Worsley Rachel, Farnworth Mark J. App Anim Behav Sci 2019. https://doi.org/10.1016/j.applanim.2019. 104841.

[7] Levine E, Perry P, Scarlett J, et al. Intercat aggression in households following the introduction of a new cat. App Anim Behav Sci 2005;90(3–4):325–36, ISSN 0168-1591.

[8] Elzerman AL, DePorter TL, Beck A, et al. Conflict and affiliative behavior frequency between cats in multi-cat households: a survey-based study. J Feline Med Surg 2020;22(8):705–17.

[9] Bradshaw J. Normal feline behaviour: … and why problem behaviours develop. J Feline Med Surg 2018;20(5): 411–21.

[10] Clark C. Dealing with multi-cat households: understanding how problems develop. Companion Animal 2016; 21:8–14.

[11] Da Graça Pereira G, Fragoso S, Morais D, et al. Comparison of interpretation of cat's behavioral needs between veterinarians, veterinary nurses, and cat owners. J Vet Behav 2014;9(6):324–8, ISSN 1558-7878.

[12] Levine E, Perry P, Scarlett J, et al. Intercat aggression in households following the introduction of a new cat. App Anim Behav Sci 2005;90(3–4):325–36, ISSN 0168-1591.

[13] Lowe SE, Bradshaw JWS. Ontogeny of individuality in the domestic cat in the home environment. Anim Behav 2001;61(1):231–7.

[14] Finka LR. Conspecific and Human Sociality in the Domestic Cat: Consideration of Proximate Mechanisms, Human Selection and Implications for Cat Welfare. Animals 2022;12:298.

[15] McCune S. The impact of paternity and early socialisation on the development of cats' behaviour to people and novel objects. Appl Anim Behav Sci 1995;45(1–2): 109–24, ISSN 0168-1591.

[16] Mikkola S, Salonen M, Hakanen E, et al. Fearfulness associates with problematic behaviors and poor socialization in cats. iScience 2022;25(10):105265:ISSN 2589-0042.

[17] Bennett PC, Rutter NJ, Woodhead JK, et al. Assessment of domestic cat personality, as perceived by 416 owners, suggests six dimensions. Behav Process 2017 S03766357 16303308.

[18] Fukimoto N, Melo D, Palme R, et al. Are cats less stressed in homes than in shelters? A study of personality and faecal cortisol metabolites levels. Appl Anim Behav Sci 2020;224:104919.

[19] Cecchetti M, Crowley SL, McDonald J, et al. Owner-ascribed personality profiles distinguish domestic cats that capture and bring home wild animal prey. Appl Anim Behav Sci 2022;256:105774:ISSN 0168-1591.

[20] Crowell-Davis SL, Curtis TM, Knowles RJ. Social organization in the cat: a modern understanding. J Feline Med Surg 2004;6(1):19–28, PMID: 15123163.

[21] Natoli E, Litchfield C, Pontier D. Coexistence between Humans and 'Misunderstood' Domestic Cats in the Anthropocene: Exploring Behavioural Plasticity as a Gatekeeper of Evolution. Animals (Basel) 2022;12(13):1717.

[22] Martínez-Byer S, Hudson R, Bánszegi O, et al. Effects of early social separation on the behaviour of kittens of the domestic cat. Appl Anim Behav Sci 2023;259: 105849:ISSN 0168-1591.

[23] Denenberg S, Machin KL, Landsberg GM. Behavior and Cognition of the Senior Cat and Its Interaction with Physical Disease. Vet Clin North Am Small Anim Pract 2024; 54(1):153–68, Epub 2023 Oct 19. PMID: 37865588.

[24] Piotti P, Pierantoni L, Albertini M, et al. Inflammation and Behavior Changes in Dogs and Cats. Vet Clin Small Anim Pract 2024;54(1):1–16, ISSN 0195-5616.

[25] Camps T, Amat M, Manteca X. A Review of Medical Conditions and Behavioral Problems in Dogs and Cats. Animals 2019;9(12):1133.

[26] Stella JL, Buffington CAT. Individual and environmental effects on health and welfare. In: Turner DC, Bateson P, editors. The domestic cat: the biology of its behaviour. 3rd edition. Cambridge: Cambridge University Press. © Cambridge University Press; 2014. p. 185–200.

[27] Hemsworth PH, Barnett JL, Hansen C. The influence of inconsistent handling by humans on the behaviour, growth and corticosteroids of young pigs. Appl Anim Behav Sci 1987;17(3–4):245–52.

[28] Finka LR, Ward J, Farnworth MJ, et al. Owner personality and the wellbeing of their cats share parallels with the parent-child relationship. PLoS One 2019;14(2):e0211862.

[29] Bouma EMC, Reijgwart ML, Dijkstra A. Family Member, Best Friend, Child or 'Just' a Pet, Owners' Relationship Perceptions and Consequences for Their Cats. Int J Environ Res Publ Health 2022;19:193.

[30] Vitale KR, Behnke AC, Udell MAR. Attachment bonds between domestic cats and humans. Curr Biol 2019; 29(18):R864–5, PMID: 31550468.

[31] Ellis SLH, Rodan I, Carney HC, et al. AAFP and ISFM Feline Environmental Needs Guidelines. J Feline Med Surg 2013;15:219–30.

[32] Haywood C, Ripari L, Puzzo J, et al. Providing humans with practical, best practice handling guidelines during human-cat interactions increases cats' affiliative behaviour and reduces aggression and signs of conflict. Front Vet Sci 2005;8:714143.

[33] Pachel CL. Intercat Aggression: Restoring Harmony in the Home: A Guide for Practitioners. Vet Clin Small Anim Pract 2014;44(Issue 3):565–79.

[34] Herron ME, Buffington CA. Environmental enrichment for indoor cats. Compend Contin Educ Vet 2010 Dec; 32(12):E4:PMID: 21882164; PMCID: PMC3922041.

[35] Ellis JJ, McGowan RTS, Martin F. Does previous use affect litter box appeal in multi-cat households? Behav Process 2017;141(Part 3, 2017):284–90, ISSN 0376-6357.

[36] Halls V. Inter-cat aggression issues BSAVA congress scientific proceedings: veterinary programme, 8–11 2010, Birmingham: 39.

[37] Carney HC, Sadek TP, Curtis TM, et al. AAFP and ISFM guidelines for diagnosing and solving house-soiling

behavior in cats. J Feline Med Surg 2014;16(7):579–98. https://doi.org/10.1177/1098612X14539092.

[38] Kogan L, Kolus C, Schoenfeld-Tacher R. Assessment of clicker training for shelter cats. Animals (Basel) 2017; 7(10):73, PMID: 28937608; PMCID: PMC5664032.

[39] Rochlitz I. A review of the housing requirements of domestic cats (Felis silvestris catus) kept in the home. Appl Anim Behav Sci 2005;93(1–2):97–109, ISSN 0168-1591.

[40] Uenoyama R, Ooka S, Miyazaki T, et al. Assessing the safety and suitability of using silver vine as an olfactory enrichment for cats. Science 2023;26(10):107848.

[41] Vitale Shreve KR, Mehrkam LR, Udell MA. Social interaction, food, scent or toys? A formal assessment of domestic pet and shelter cat (Felis silvestris catus) preferences. Behav Process 2017;141(Part 3):322–8.

[42] Leyhausen P. Cat behavior: the predatory and social behavior of domestic and wild cats. New York: Garland STPM Press; 1979.

[43] Bowen J, Heath S. Behavior problems in small animals: practical advice for the veterinary team. Edinburgh: Elsevier Saunders; 2006.

[44] Cameron ME, Casey RA, Bradshaw JW, et al. A study of environmental and behavioural factors that may be associated with feline idiopathic cystitis. J Small Anim Pract 2004;45:144–7.

[45] Overall KL. Manual of clinical behavioral medicine for dogs and cats. St Louis, MO: Else-vier Mosby; 2013.

[46] Bourdin DVMM. Feline psychogenic alopecia and behavioural disorders. Proceedings of the 2nd European Congress of the Federation of European Companion Animal Veterinary Associations. 27–29 October 1995, Brussels, Belgium: 241–2 Bowen J, Heath S (2006) Behaviour problems in small animals. Practical advice for the veterinary Team. London: Elsevier Saunders; 1995.

[47] Pryor PA, Hart BL, Bain MJ, et al. Causes of urine marking in cats and effects of environmental management on frequency of marking. J Am Vet Med Assoc 2001;219(12):1709–13.

[48] Luescher A, McKeown D, Halip J. Stereotypic or obsessive-compulsive disorders in dogs and cats. Vet Clin North Am Small Anim Pract 1991;21:401–41.

[49] Horwitz. House soiling by cats. In: Horwitz D, Mills D, Heath S, editors. BSAVA Manual of canine and feline Behavioural Medicine. Gloucester: BSAVA; 2002. p. 97–107.

[50] Amat M, Camps T, Manteca X. Stress in owned cats: behavioural changes and welfare implications. J Feline Med Surg 2015;(pii) 1098612X15590867.

[51] Reif JS, Bovee KC, Gaskell CJ, et al. Feline urethral obstruction: a case-control study. J Am Vet Med Assoc 1977;170:1320–4.

[52] Walker AD, Weaver AD, Anderson RS, et al. An epidemiological survey of the feline urological syndrome. J Small Anim Pract 1977;18:282–301.

[53] Willeberg P. Epidemiology of naturally-occurring feline urologic syndrome. Vet Clin North Am Small Anim Pract 1984;14:455–69.

[54] Buffington CT, Pacak K. Increased plasma norepinephrine concentration in cats with interstitial cystitis. J Urol 2001;165(6):2051–4.

[55] Ramos D, Reche-Junior A, Mills D, et al. Are cats with housesoiling problems stressed? A case-controlled comparison of faecal glucocorticoid levels in urine spraying and toileting cats. In: Mills, Da Graca Pereira, Jacinto, editors. Proceedings of the Ninth International Veterinary Behavioural Meeting Conference. Lisbon, Portugal; 26–28, 2013. p. 113–114.

SECTION II - DIAGNOSTIC IMAGING

Advances in Small Animal Care 5 (2024) 31–49

ADVANCES IN SMALL ANIMAL CARE

Computed Tomographic Imaging of the Gastrointestinal Tract in Small Animals

Jia Wen Siow, BSc(VB) DVM GradCert(SAUA) MVetStud MVetClinStud FANZCVS(Veterinary Radiology)

Department of Diagnostic Imaging, Small Animal Specialist Hospital, Kent Town, SA, Australia

KEYWORDS

- Computed tomography • Contrast-enhanced • Canine • Feline • Stomach • Small intestine • Colon

KEY POINTS

- Compared to other imaging modalities, computed tomography (CT) allows the evaluation of the entire gastrointestinal tract regardless of patient size, gastrointestinal content, and operator experience.
- Gastrointestinal tract distension with fluid or gas improves wall conspicuity and assessment of mural changes.
- Use of appropriate contrast-enhanced CT protocols further optimizes evaluation of the wall, particularly wall layering.
- CT can aid surgical planning.
- CT is better for the evaluation of gastrointestinal ulceration, similar to ultrasound for detecting mechanical obstruction, and superior for the evaluation of gastric neoplasia.

INTRODUCTION

Gastrointestinal disease is a common cause for presentation to veterinary hospitals [1,2]. Traditionally, survey radiography is frequently used for investigation because of its wide availability in veterinary practice and low cost. Unlike other modalities, specific affected sites, such as location of foreign body obstruction or intussusception, may not be identifiable, and radiographs may appear normal in the presence of disease [3,4]. Assessment of wall thickness is also unreliable, but it can be improved with positive contrast gastroenterography. This is time consuming and has largely been superseded by other imaging modalities.

Ultrasound can distinguish intraluminal, intramural, and extramural gastrointestinal disease, and wall layering and thickness measurements correlate well with histology [5,6]. The modality is dependent on operator experience and the patient, with gastrointestinal tract visualization limited by patient size and demeanor, and the presence

of gas and food [7]. Image acquisition also tends to be longer than other modalities [8]. Its utility is variable, with low-to-moderate utility reported for the evaluation of canine diarrhea and prediction of the site of histologic lesions in cats with gastrointestinal disorders [9–12].

Endoscopy is often used complementarily as it is superior for the evaluation of the mucosa and facilitates biopsy of the superficial gastrointestinal layers for histopathology [13,14]. However, it cannot evaluate the entire intestinal tract, all gastrointestinal wall layers, or extramural pathology.

CT has superior contrast resolution to radiography. Compared to ultrasonography, it may be more useful for evaluating patients over 25 kg, obese animals, and aerophagic patients [15]. It allows the evaluation of the intrapelvic portions of the gastrointestinal tract, which cannot be seen with ultrasound. Image acquisition is also much faster [8,16]. In one study of dogs with acute abdominal signs, CT was more useful for

E-mail address: jiawensiow@gmail.com

https://doi.org/10.1016/j.yasa.2024.06.003

detecting clinically important pneumoperitoneum compared to ultrasonography and was more accurate than radiography and ultrasonography for identifying surgical conditions [16]. Disadvantages of CT include higher radiation exposure and a need for heavier sedation or anesthesia for patient positioning and image acquisition. Unlike ultrasonography, gastrointestinal motility cannot be evaluated, and the evaluation of the gastrointestinal wall is limited. Presumed mucosal layer enhancement has been reported, but other layers are not generally distinguishable, and there are few references regarding normal wall thickness measurements, which also have not been correlated with histology [17–22]. Evaluation of the gastrointestinal wall is optimized by distending the gastrointestinal tract and by using appropriate contrast medium administration protocols. This has rarely been investigated in previous veterinary studies [17–27].

Canine and feline studies describing gastrointestinal disease use widely variable contrast protocols and few concurrently consider both gastrointestinal distension and contrast protocols [22,28–31]. Despite this, there are common features of specific disease processes. This review will include normal and abnormal gastrointestinal studies utilizing CT imaging.

DISCUSSION
Normal gastrointestinal tract
Few canine CT studies evaluate the normal gastrointestinal tract [17–21], and only one is reported in cats [23]. Table 1 provides a summary of these CT protocols.

Using the CT protocol by Hoey and colleagues [18], 62.8% of gastrointestinal segments could be distinguished from serosa to serosa, while 77.7% could be distinguished from mucosa to serosa [18] and 21.8% had postcontrast wall layering [18]. Subsequently, Fitzgerald and colleagues [17] found that an early phase scan acquired at 30 seconds from the start of contrast administration improved gastrointestinal wall conspicuity with visualization of 84.5% of segments compared to 56.7% precontrast [17]. At 30 seconds, small intestinal mucosal enhancement could be seen, and the addition of a late postcontrast phase improved the detection of gastric mucosal enhancement [17]. Lee and colleagues [20] used a test bolus technique to evaluate the canine small intestine. Using this technique, mucosal enhancement was more common in the arterial and intestinal phases compared to the venous phase, and intestinal wall enhancement was higher in the intestinal phase than the arterial phase [20]. Kim and colleagues

[19] evaluated the use of a spit-bolus contrast administration technique to evaluate the canine small intestine combined with enterography. Arterial and venous phase enhancement are acquired in a single postcontrast CT scan acquisition, reducing radiation exposure, image acquisition time, and the number of images to be interpreted [19]. Using this technique, most intestinal sites had transmural enhancement rather than mucosal enhancement [19]. The duodenal and ileal walls enhanced less than the traditional dual-phase technique [19]. Most recently in dogs, Siow and colleagues [21] evaluated a fixed injection duration technique to evaluate the canine stomach and small intestine. Like others, intestinal mucosal enhancement was more common in earlier phase imaging and gastric mucosal enhancement was more common in the later phase [21]. At a 10 second scan delay, there was optimal intestinal mucosal enhancement; at 15 second scan delay, there was peak intestinal wall enhancement; and at 40 second scan delay, there was peak gastric mucosal and overall wall enhancement [21]. Compared to other administration techniques, a fixed injection duration technique has been said to be an easily reproducible protocol across CT scanners [32].

One feline study has evaluated the normal gastrointestinal tract with CT [23]. Contrast administration techniques were markedly varied, potentially limiting the relevance of the described contrast enhancement characteristics [23]. Unlike in dogs, contrast administration had a lesser impact on improving gastrointestinal wall conspicuity [23]. Presumed mucosal enhancement was commonly seen in the gastric cardia and fundus in early phase images [23]. Transmural enhancement was more common in other segments in both postcontrast phases. If mucosal enhancement was seen, it was more likely in the early phase images [23]. Fig. 1 illustrates examples of presumed mucosal enhancement.

In dogs, gastrointestinal wall thickness generally increases with body weight [18,33]. Like in humans, wall thickness decreases with increasing luminal distension [18,33]. Therefore, the assessment of the gastrointestinal wall will be most accurate in distended segments. Procedures to distend the gastrointestinal tract should be considered to more accurately assess wall thickness, which is the standard of care in human medicine [34–38]. Comparisons of CT wall thickness measurements with ultrasonographic reference values are found in Tables 2 and 3, though it should be noted that direct comparisons cannot be made as different bodyweight categories are used. In cats, CT measurements of wall thickness were similar to or slightly below ultrasonographic reference values [23].

TABLE 1
Comparison of computed tomography acquisition protocols for the gastrointestinal tract in dogs and cats

Authors	Hoey et al, [18] 2013	Fitzgerald et al, [17] 2017	Lee et al, [20] 2019	Kim et al, [19] 2020	Siow, et al, [21] 2023	Holle et al, [23] 2023
Species	Canine	Canine	Canine	Canine	Canine	Feline
kV	—	120	120	120	120	120
mA/mAs	—	150	120	120	<5 kg: 100, 5–10 kg: 150, >10 kg: 250	100–130
Tube rotation (s)	—	0.5	0.6	0.6	<10 kg: 0.5, >10 kg: 0.75	—
Pitch	—	—	0.8	0.8	0.938	—
Slice thickness (mm)	2–5	3	1	1	Up to 10 kg: 1.5, >10 kg: 2	2–3
Contrast medium administration technique	—	Power injector (unspecified rate)	Test bolus and power injector (3 mL/s)	Split bolus with test bolus and power injector (3 mL/s): 60% of total dose at 0 s, 40% at 13 s. Split-bolus tracking with power injector (3 mL/s)	Bolus tracking and power injector (fixed injection duration [20 s])	Manual injection, unspecified, or power injector (4 mL/s)
Contrast dose (mg I/kg)	300	600	Test bolus: 150, Diagnostic scan: 600 (ok)	Test bolus: 150, Diagnostic scan: 600, Split-bolus tracking: 750	700	600
Postcontrast scan timings	—	Early phase: 30 s from start of contrast injection, Late phase: 60–180 s	Arterial phase: 2 s after aortic arrival. Intestinal phase: time to peak enhancement of intestinal wall. Venous phase: time to peak enhancement of cranial mesenteric vein	Split bolus: 20 s after first contrast injection. Split bolus-tracking: Aorta at the level of the cranial mesenteric artery reached 100 HU	Early phase: 10–15 s after abdominal aorta reached 150 HU. Late phase: 40 s after abdominal aorta reached 150 HU	Early phase: 30 s from start of contrast injection. Late phase: 60–176 s

Data from Refs[17–21,23].

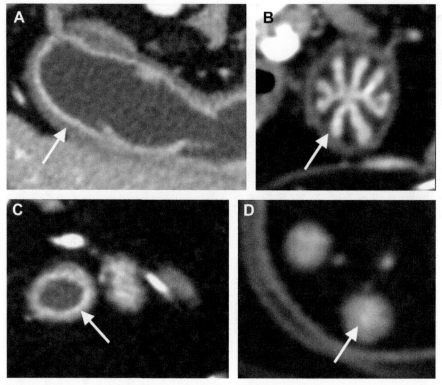

FIG. 1 Transverse plane images of the stomach (*A, B*) and small intestine (*C, D*) acquired using a 20 second fixed injection duration technique. The inner layer of hyperenhancement (*arrows*) represents presumed mucosal enhancement in the stomach in dogs (*A, C*) and cats (*B, D*).

Gastric distension

The stomach can be distended with gas or fluid (Fig. 2). Terragni and colleagues [22] determined that 30 mL/kg warm tap water administered via gastric tube in anesthetized dogs and cats provided adequate distension. Yamada and colleagues [27] used 500 to 700 cm^3 of air via orogastric catheter in dogs for virtual endoscopy. Most recently, a clinical study used an unspecified volume of air for the evaluation of canine gastric neoplasia [30]. No adverse effects were reported in these studies.

Small intestinal distension

CT enterography has been evaluated in 2 studies of healthy dogs [19,24]. These used 60 mL/kg of 1.34 g/mL lactulose diluted 1:4 with warm water followed by 0.4 mg/kg butylscopolamine bromide intravenously [19,24]. Keh and colleagues [24] administered this via nasoesophageal tube over 45 minutes, or via orogastric tube as a bolus under general anesthesia, followed by butylscopolamine bromide. Continuous administration provided better distension of the small intestine,

and CT scan acquisition was recommended beginning 15 minutes after the end of lactulose administration [24]. Self-resolving adverse effects included nausea, vomiting, and diarrhea [24]. Safety has not been evaluated in diseased dogs. Anecdotally, the bolus administration protocol was used by the current author and the patient regurgitated on recovery from anesthesia. Postprocedure suction of gastric contents is, therefore, suggested. An example of fluid distended small intestine is seen in Fig. 3.

Large intestinal distension

Appropriate patient preparation minimizes residual fecal volume prior to CT colonography or pneumocolonography. In one study, the protocol resulting in the least residual fecal volume comprised 36 hours of fasting and 4 doses of 6 g sodium phosphate monobasic monohydrate/sodium phosphate dibasic anhydrous tablet colonic cleansing agent orally every 8 hours [26].

To then distend the large intestine, a balloon-tipped Foley catheter is passed into the rectum [25,26,46].

TABLE 2
Comparison of reported gastrointestinal wall thicknesses (millimeters) in dogs using computed tomography compared to ultrasound

Author(s)	Hoey et al, [18] 2013	Siow [33] 2023	Penninck et al, [39] 1989	Gladwin et al, [40] 2014	Delaney et al, [41] 2003
Modality	CT	CT	Ultrasound	Ultrasound	Ultrasound
Gastric fundus	0–9 kg: 0.98–1.3 >9 kg: 2–3.08	<10 kg: 0.85–14.77 10–25 kg: 1.35–11.47 >25 kg: 1.2–30.73	Stomach: 3–5	—	—
Gastric body	0–9 kg: 1.27–1.59 >9 kg: 2.7–4.1	<10 kg: 1.67–8.75 10–25 kg: 2.73–8.92 >25 kg: 3–15.1	—	—	—
Gastric pylorus	0–9 kg: 1.43–2.13 >9 kg: 1.92–3.55	<10 kg: 2.62–9.6 10–25 kg: 2.7–6.54 >25 kg: 2.93–12.33	—	—	—
Duodenum	0–9 kg: 2.59–3.3 >9 kg: 4.61–5.26	<10 kg: 3.33–8.68 10–25 kg: 1.89–7.05 >25 kg: 1.9–8.94	—	<15 kg: 2.9–4.7 15–30 kg: 3–5.5 >30 kg: 3.1–5.7	—
Jejunum	0–9 kg: 2–2.93 >9 kg: 3.31–3.87	<10 kg: 1.03–6.26 10–25 kg: 1.8–7.75 >25 kg: 1.07–7.02	—	<15 kg: 2.2–4.1 15–30 kg: 2.4–4.8 >30 kg: 2.7–4.7	—
Ileum	—	<10 kg: 1.38–6.05 10–25 kg: 1.29–6.28 >25 kg: 1.18–6.2	—	—	<15 kg: 3 15–30 kg: 3.5 >30 kg: 3.8
Colon	0–9 kg: 1.05–1.45 >9 kg: 1.78–2.35	—	—	<15 kg: 1–2 15–30 kg: 1.1–1.9 >30 kg: 1.1–2.6	—

Data from Refs [18,33–36].

TABLE 3
Comparison of reported gastrointestinal wall thicknesses (millimeters) in cats using computed tomography compared to ultrasound

Author(s)	Holle et al, [23] 2023	Couturier et al, [42] 2012	Di Donato et al, [43] 2013	Besso et al, [44] 2004	Newell et al, [45] 1999
Modality	CT	US	Ultrasound	Ultrasound	Ultrasound
Gastric cardia	4.8	4.1–4.5	—	—	1.1–3.6 (stomach)
Duodenum	0.6–3.9	—	1.78–2.51	—	1.6–3.5
Jejunum	0.8–3.0	—	1.96–2.67	—	1.5–2.5 (small intestine)
Ileum	1.1–2.5	—	1.66–2.27	—	—
Caecum	0.3–2.3	—	—	0.7–1.4	—
Colon	0.2–3.4	—	—	—	1.1–2.5
Rectum	0.5–2.5	—	—	—	—

Data from Refs [23,37–40].

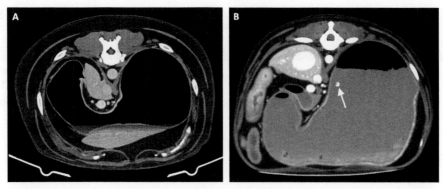

FIG. 2 Transverse plane postcontrast images of gas-distended (*A*) and fluid-distended (*B*) canine stomachs. The tip of a gastric tube is seen in B (*arrow*). Note how the large degree of distension affects gastric wall thickness compared to the appearance in Fig. 1A. In theory, this will aid in detection of subtle or early changes in the gastric wall.

Some authors also place a temporary purse string suture [25,26]. In one study, gas distension using an insufflation pressure of 20 mm Hg was recommended, with CT imaging initiated 2 minutes after the initiation of insufflation [25]. Another study compared distension with 20 mL/kg water, barium, or room air and found that water with intravenous iodinated contrast yielded a greater conspicuity score and lower artifact scores than the other methods [46]. An example of a gas-distended colon is seen in Fig. 3.

Abnormal gastrointestinal tract

The CT features of multiple gastrointestinal diseases have been described in retrospective studies, case reports, and case series. These will be categorized into congenital, obstructive, inflammatory/infectious, neoplasia, and miscellaneous. This section summarizes these findings.

Congenital

Duplication cyst. Duplication cysts have been reported in the feline and canine duodenum and feline rectum [47–49]. They appeared as a smoothly margined, round, rim-enhancing cyst-like mass associated with the intestinal wall and may be associated with mechanical obstruction [47–49]. In one case, contrast-enhanced CT demonstrated a shared vascular supply

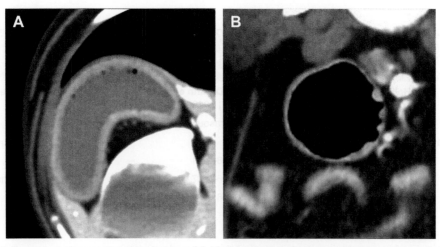

FIG. 3 Transverse plane postcontrast images of fluid-distended small intestine (*A*) and gas-distended large intestine (*B*) in dogs. Note the appearance of the small intestinal wall compared to Fig. 1C. Like with the stomach, increasing luminal distension may aid in earlier detection of mural changes.

with the normal intestine [47]. CT was useful to plan the surgical approach [47–49].

Colonic duplication. Pneumocolonography identified a band-like soft tissue structure dividing the descending colon into a blind ending ventral compartment and dorsal compartment in one case [28]. In another case, there was a focal area of mineral density surrounded by gas within the lumen of the colon close to the ileococcolic junction [50]. Histologically, this corresponded with a discrete colonic duplication impacted with fecal material and protruding into the main colonic lumen through a small stoma [50]. In both cases, CT was helpful for surgical planning.

Duodenocolic fistula. CT identified a communication between the caudal duodenal flexure and descending colon where ultrasound only identified mild diffuse intestinal wall thickening [51].

Obstruction
Foreign body/mechanical obstruction. In one study, an intestinal diameter/L5 height ratio 2.5 or greater had 79.1% sensitivity and 72.2% specificity for the diagnosis of mechanical obstruction [52].

CT may be superior for diagnosing mechanical obstructions and determining surgical conditions. An older study of dogs with acute abdominal signs found CT had 100% agreement with the recommendation for surgery, compared to 89% agreement with the

recommendation for radiography and ultrasonography [16]. More recently, CT had 100% agreement with surgical findings for mechanical intestinal obstructions and was able to distinguish obstructive and nonobstructive foreign material [53]. Studies comparing imaging modalities for diagnosing mechanical intestinal obstructions have small sample sizes, limiting statistical comparisons. One study comparing CT and radiography found no statistically significant differences for the diagnosis of mechanical obstruction or recommendation for surgery [52]. A study comparing ultrasound and CT could not perform statistical analysis due to the small sample size [8]. In this study, CT had 100% positive predictive value for mechanical obstruction and ultrasonography 93%. One case was ultrasonographically misdiagnosed as a partial mechanical obstruction where a functional ileus was diagnosed via CT and surgery [8]. CT also correctly identified intestinal adhesions where ultrasound identified a mesenteric mass and identified adhesions as a cause of mechanical obstruction where ultrasound could not [8].

Examples of various gastric and intestinal foreign body obstructions are seen in Fig. 4.

Gastrogastric intussusception. In a postmortem CT case, the greater curvature of the stomach, associated mesenteric fat and a blood vessel invaginated into the lumen of the gastric fundus and body with heterogeneously hypoattenuating thickening [54]. In an

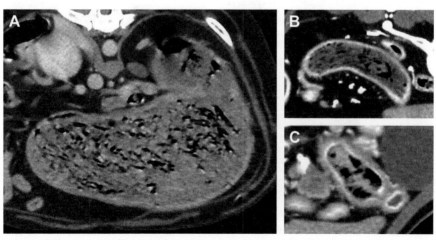

FIG. 4 Several examples of foreign body mechanical obstructions in the stomach (A) and small intestine (B, C). The foreign material in A and B are fabric. Note the linear to irregular, streaky gas pattern within the noncontrast enhancing soft tissue attenuating material. The foreign body in C is a corn cob. This foreign body is more focal and cylindrical with a central noncontrast enhancing soft tissue attenuating component and peripheral round to triangular gas foci.

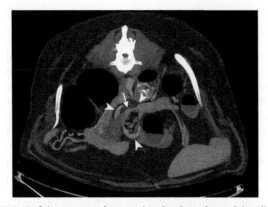

FIG. 5 A transverse plane postcontrast maximum intensity projection reconstruction image of a dog with a colonic torsion. A mixed, soft-tissue, and fat attenuating "whirl" is present, composed of the colonic vessels (*arrowheads*), surrounding the collapsed descending colon (*arrow*). (*Adapted from* Barge P, Fina CJ, Mortier JR, et al. CT findings in five dogs with surgically confirmed colonic torsion. Vet Radiol Ultrasound 2020;61(2):190–96.)

antemortem case, a markedly thickened pyloric antrum invaginated into the gastric body with additional gastric foreign bodies, perigastric fat stranding, peritoneal fluid, and gastric lymphadenomegaly [55].

Cecal inversion/cecocolic intussusception. The caecum ± mesenteric fat invaginates into the ascending colon [56]. There may be concurrent cecal wall thickening and associated mesenteric lymphadenomegaly, peritonitis, and pneumoperitoneum [56].

Volvulus/torsion

Major advantages of CT are the ability to identify a whirl sign (Fig. 5) and easier identification of organ or intestinal displacement, which are characteristic of volvulus and torsion. However, torsion can be dynamic and the absence of a whirl sign does not exclude a diagnosis [57].

Mesenteric volvulus

In a canine case report, the CT findings of mesenteric volvulus included a whirl sign, left-sided displacement

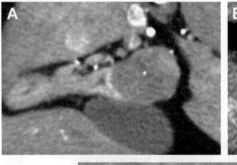
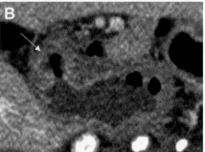
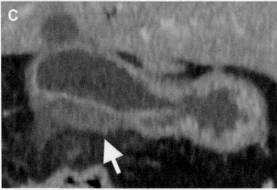

FIG. 6 Postcontrast transverse or dorsal plane CT images of a gastroduodenal hyperplastic polyp (*A*, *asterisk*), perforated gastric ulcer (*B*, *white arrow*), and gastric wall edema (*C*, thick *arrow*). The polyp is a smoothly margined soft tissue mass with relatively homogeneous contrast enhancement. The perforated gastric ulcer is a focal gastric wall thickening with mural defect, pneumoperitoneum, and peritonitis. The gastric wall edema in C is a segmental asymmetric gastric wall thickening with only 2 wall layers appreciated (inner enhancing mucosal layer and outer nonenhancing, fluid attenuating layer) compared to the reported 3 layer appearance.

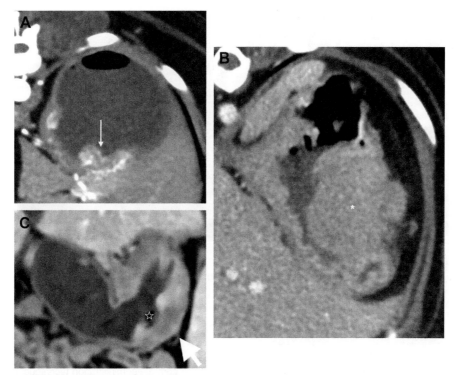

FIG. 7 Postcontrast CT images obtained using a 20 second fixed injection duration technique, illustrating cases of canine gastric adenocarcinoma in an arterial phase (A, *arrow*), canine gastric adenocarcinoma in a venous phase (B, *asterisk*) and feline gastric lymphoma in a venous phase (C, large *arrow*). A and B demonstrate the variable appearance of gastric adenocarcinoma. In A, it is a focal small lobulated endophytic gastric wall thickening with mildly heterogeneous contrast enhancement. In this particular case, an arterial blood supply could be identified. In B, the adenocarcinoma is a large rounded, irregularly margined, heterogeneously enhancing soft tissue mass. In C, the gastric lymphoma is a large ovoid homogeneously enhancing exophytic wall thickening. There is also a focal concave mucosal defect with a small, interposed gas attenuation and thinning to absence of the presumed mucosal layer suggestive of a concurrent mucosal erosion/ulcer (star).

of the cecum and ascending colon, small intestinal enhancement and fluid distension, and engorgement of and thrombi within jejunal vein and peritoneal effusion [58].

Ileocecocolic volvulus

Ileocecocolic volvulus has been associated with a whirl sign, distended ileum with gravel sign, dilated and tortuous mesenteric veins, and mesenteric edema, steatitis, and/or peritoneal fluid [59].

Colonic torsion

In a case series in dogs, the descending colon was most frequently affected [57]. Common CT features included a whirl sign, segmental distension and focal narrowing of the colon, cecal and colonic displacement, distended

colonic and mesenteric vasculature, mild jejunal lymphadenomegaly, and peritoneal effusion and peritonitis [57]. Other findings may include pneumatosis coli, small intestinal distension, or portal vein thrombosis [57].

A case of colonic entrapment with dynamic torsion had CT features of colonic torsion and an oblique thin soft tissue band at the most narrowed point of the affected colon and the absence of a whirl sign [60].

Inflammatory/infectious

Examples of various inflammatory gastric conditions are seen in Fig. 6.

Gastrointestinal ulceration. Imaging features of gastrointestinal ulceration include a gastrointestinal

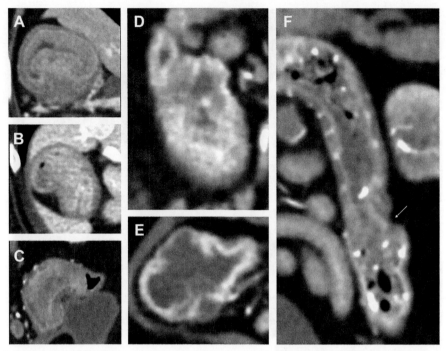

FIG. 8 Postcontrast CT images of canine intestinal adenocarcinoma (*A–C*) and feline intestinal adenocarcinoma (*D–F*) obtained using a 20 second fixed injection contrast administration technique. Images A and E are portal venous phase images, while all others are arterial phase. Images A, B, and D are transverse plane images while the others are dorsal plane images. These demonstrate the variable appearance of intestinal adenocarcinoma. All cases have endophytic components. Most cases are circumferential intestinal wall thickenings (*A, C–F*), while B is eccentric. More specifically, in A, the duodenal adenocarcinoma was associated with mucosal ± submucosal thickening and hypoattenuation of the outer wall layer. In B, the proximal descending duodenal adenocarcinoma is heterogeneously enhancing with partial loss of mucosal layering. In C, the colonic adenocarcinoma involves inner wall layer/mucosal thickening. In D, the jejunal lesion is heterogeneously enhancing. In E, the jejunal lesion is endophytic with small nodular exophytic components, is hypoattenuating, and has preserved outer wall layering/enhancement. In F, the colonic adenocarcinoma has predominantly preserved wall layering and attenuation except caudally, where there is more marked mucosal thickening and hyperenhancement (*arrow*).

mural lesion, mucosal defect or ulcer, peritoneal fluid, and pneumoperitoneum when perforated [61]. The underlying cause of gastrointestinal ulceration may only be identified in 50% of patients [61]. In this canine study, the most common underlying diagnoses were primary gastrointestinal neoplasia, inflammatory gastrointestinal disease, and intestinal foreign body [61]. For nonperforated ulcers, sensitivity was poor for all evaluated modalities: 17%, 30%, 65%, and 67% for Focused Assessment with Sonography in Trauma (FAST), radiography, ultrasonography, and CT, respectively [61]. Sensitivity greatly increased when ulcers were perforated, increasing to 79%, 79%, 86% and 93% for FAST, radiography, ultrasonography, and CT, respectively [61]. CT had the highest sensitivity for nonperforated and perforated gastrointestinal ulcers.

Gastric wall edema. Gastric wall edema often appears as a focal concentric or asymmetric gastric wall thickening with a 3 layer appearance (thin inner and outer enhancing layer with intervening thick nonenhancing fluid-attenuating middle layer) [62]. Thin, tortuous, tubular blood vessels may also be visible within the affected wall [62]. The average wall thickness was 11.1 mm [62]. The most commonly affected regions are the pyloric portion and gastric body [62].

Gastric wall edema has been associated with hypoalbuminemia, cerebral hemorrhage, urinary obstruction, gastric ulcer, pancreatitis, or coagulopathy [62].

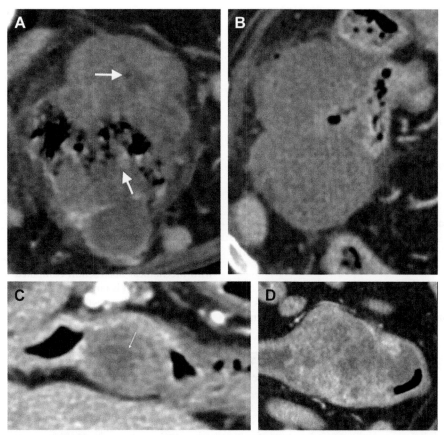

FIG. 9 Arterial phase CT images of cecal gastrointestinal stromal tumors (*A*, sagittal plane; *B*), intestinal leiomyosarcoma (*C*), and nonangiogenic, nonlymphogenic gastrointestinal stromal tumor (*D*) obtained using a 20 second fixed injection duration technique. The cecal masses are large, multilobulated or bilobed, concentric, exophytic, and endophytic heterogeneously enhancing soft tissue masses containing variable small gas and fluid attenuating foci (thick *arrows*). These masses are much larger than the small intestinal spindle cell tumors in C and D, possibly associated with their cecal origin. In C and D, the small intestinal lesions are asymmetric/eccentric endophytic and exophytic heterogeneously enhancing soft tissue masses. In C, the mass originates from the outer portion of the intestinal wall and has fluid attenuating areas (*arrow*).

Inflammatory/hyperplastic polyp. Polyps have been reported as a focal soft tissue lesion/mass that may be localized to the mucosal layer and has a polypoid attachment and homogeneous or heterogeneous enhancement [30,31,63]. Inflammatory polyps and gastric hyperplasia appear similar and have been reported in the pylorus or pyloric antrum [30,31,63].

Pyogenic granuloma. Pyogenic granuloma has been reported in a dog affecting the pylorus, pyloric antrum, and greater and lesser curvatures of the stomach [31]. This appeared as a symmetric segmental wall thickening with homogeneous enhancement and retained wall layering [31].

Focal lipogranulomatous lymphangitis. Focal lipogranulomatous lymphangitis often appears as a segment of circumferential intestinal wall thickening of the distal ileum and ileocolic junction and can resemble neoplasia [64]. A case report identified circumferential thickening of the distal ileum with stratified enhancement (strongly enhancing inner layer, hypoattenuating thickened middle layer, and mildly enhancing outer layer) with suspected small intramural nodules [65]. Importantly, these authors noted that stratified wall enhancement is more commonly seen with benign lesions [65].

Eosinophilic sclerosing fibroplasia. CT features have been reported in the feline rectum. Findings were a large eccentric, asymmetric, heterogeneously enhancing soft tissue mass causing marked luminal narrowing/compression, mild thickening of the distal descending colonic and rectal wall, caudal mesenteric lymphadenomegaly, and minimal peritoneal effusion [66].

Neoplasia

Most CT studies describing gastrointestinal neoplasia are in dogs. In a study comparing CT with ultrasound, CT more successfully correctly identified the presence and location of gastric tumors and identified more locations of lymphadenopathy [67]. An important benefit of CT over other imaging modalities is increased detection of lymph nodes, which can affect tumor staging and prognostication [67]. Examples of gastric neoplasia, intestinal epithelial tumors, intestinal spindle cell tumors, and intestinal round cell tumors are seen in Figs. 7–10, respectively.

Epithelial. Most reported CT features of epithelial gastrointestinal neoplasms are in dogs, with features of intestinal adenocarcinoma also described in cats (Table 4).

Adenoma

Gastric adenoma has been reported in the pylorus as a focal mucosal mass with early-phase and late-phase heterogeneous enhancement [31].

Adenocarcinoma

Gastric adenocarcinoma often affects multiple regions, most commonly the gastric body and pylorus [22,29–31,67].

Adenocarcinoma may be smoothly or irregularly margined [29]. The gastric form usually has focal or segmental mural thickening, but diffuse thickening is also reported [22,31,67].

Importantly, many adenocarcinomas are associated with mechanical obstruction compared to lymphoma, where obstruction is rare [29,68,70]. This may be attributed to endophytic growth or the epithelial origin of the neoplasm [30].

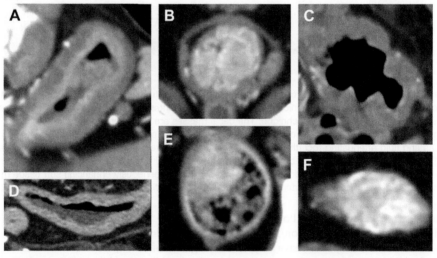

FIG. 10 Postcontrast CT images of canine intestinal lymphoma (*A, D*) and rectal plasmacytoma (*B, E*), and feline intestinal lymphoma (*C, F*). B is a venous phase image; all others are in various early-to-late arterial phases. A and D were obtained using a 20 second fixed injection duration technique. B, C, and E were obtained using a fixed injection rate technique. F was obtained using a hand injection technique. In general, the lymphoma cases appear as a circumferential intestinal wall thickening, whereas the plasmacytoma cases are endophytic nodules. In A and D, the lymphoma is relatively isoattenuation to the more normal intestine, and in A, there is retained mucosal enhancement. Mucosal enhancement is not evident in D, likely associated with acquisition of an early arterial phase. In C, the ileal lymphoma is homogeneously hypoattenuating with loss of wall layering. In F, the lymphoma is endophytic and exophytic and associated with loss of mucosal layering/enhancement. In B, the rectal plasmacytoma appears as 2 round smoothly margined homogeneously enhancing soft tissue nodules that involve the inner/mucosal layer and are isoattenuating to the rectal mucosa. In E, the nodule is heterogeneously enhancing with loss of wall layering.

TABLE 4
Collated computed tomography imaging features of epithelial gastrointestinal neoplasms in dogs and cats

Tumor type	Adenoma (n = 5)	Adenocarcinoma (n = 48)	Carcinoid tumor (n = 1)
Location	Pylorus (5)	Cardia (1), fundus (1), body (14), and pylorus (8) Duodenum (1), jejunum (5), and ileocecal (3) Cecum/ceocolic junction (1), colon (3), and colorectal (3)	Caecum
Growth pattern	Focal mass (5)	Concentric (9) Concentric and eccentric (4) Endophytic (11) Asymmetric/symmetric circumferential (19) Focal broad-based thickening (6)	Focal mass
Enhancement	Heterogeneous in early and late phases (5)	Heterogeneous (43) 5/9 early phase, 7/9 late phase	Strong arterial enhancement
Layer involvement	Mucosal (5)	Mucosal enhancement (24) Transmural enhancement (3) Outer layer (3)	—
Mineralization	—	2	—
Cystic portion	—	6	—
Obstruction/stenosis	—	23	—
Ulceration	—	3	—
Fat stranding	—	2	—
Lymphadenomegaly	3	22	1

Data from Refs [18,22,29–31,67–70].

In a canine study, gastric adenocarcinoma ranged from 1 to 2.5 cm thickness and intestinal adenocarcinoma 1 to 6.5 cm [29]. In a feline study, the mean thickness of intestinal adenocarcinoma was 6.4 mm [68].

Mucosal enhancement may be seen, which may reflect its epithelial origin, though transmural enhancement and loss of layering are also reported [18,22,29,31,67,70]. In feline intestinal cases, gradual increasing mucosal enhancement occurred [68].

Approximately 60% have an associated regional lymphadenopathy [29–31,67,68,70]. Affected lymph nodes included gastric, hepatic, splenic, pancreaticoduodenal, jejunal, and sternal lymph nodes [30,68]. Other metastatic sites included the lungs and liver [30,67].

Carcinoid tumor

The CT features of a cecal carcinoid tumor were reported in a dog with concurrent cecal inversion. It was a smoothly margined mass displaying strong arterial enhancement that decreased in the venous phase and had regional mesenteric lymphadenomegaly [69].

Mesenchymal. Gastrointestinal mesenchymal tumors mainly comprise leiomyoma, leiomyosarcoma, and gastrointestinal stromal tumor (GIST). CT descriptions are reported in dogs with variable differentiation of the tumors (ie, reported as spindle cell tumours/sarcomas" or "leiomyoma, leiomyosarcoma and GIST" or "leiomyoma and leimyosarcoma/GIST are not differentiated; Table 5).

GISTs are more common in the cecum and large intestine, whereas leiomyomas and leiomyosarcomas are more common in the stomach and small intestine [29].

In one study, small intestinal spindle cell sarcomas were significantly larger than adenocarcinomas and lymphomas [70]. A minimum diameter/L5 vertebral body height ratio cutoff of 5.8 or greater had an 85.71% sensitivity and 100% specificity to distinguish intestinal spindle cell sarcoma from adenocarcinoma and lymphoma

TABLE 5
Collated computed tomography imaging features of spindle cell gastrointestinal neoplasms in dogs and cats

Tumor type	Spindle cell tumors (n = 35)	Leiomyoma (n = 13)	Leiomyosarcoma/ GIST (n = 23)	PNST (n = 1)
Location	—	Cardia (7), fundus (1), body (1), pylorus (2) Colorectal (3)	Cardia (1), fundus (1), body (1), pylorus (9) Cecum/cecocolic junction (3) and colorectal (3)	Colon
Growth pattern	Spherical/ellipsoidal, lobulated, and eccentric (35)	Focal mass (6) Eccentric (7) Smoothly margined (10)	Eccentric (14), multilobular, irregularly/smoothly margined Focal (8) Polypoid mass (1) Exophytic (1)	Focal mass
Enhancement	Heterogeneous (14/14)	Homogeneous to moderately heterogeneous (6) Heterogeneous (4) Heterogeneous in early and late phases (1)	Heterogeneous (19) Heterogeneous in early and late phases (1)	Heterogeneous
Layer involvement	Outer layer (22)	—	Outer layer (2)	—
Mineralization	10	—	1	—
Cystic portion	14	1	3	—
Obstruction/stenosis	8	—	7	—
Perforation	—	—	2	—
Fat stranding	17	—	—	—
Lymphadenomegaly	6	2	7	—

Abbreviation: PNST, peripheral nerve sheath tumor.
 Data from Refs [29–31,67,70,71].

[70]. Masses may be detected at a later stage than other neoplasms due to their exophytic growth and lack of association with obstruction [70]. Masses have ranged between 1.5 and 20 cm [29]. Mechanical obstruction has occurred in colorectal and gastric locations, likely associated with limited anatomic space [29].

Cystic areas are not uncommon and multiloculated cystic jejunal leiomyosarcoma has also been reported [67,70,72]. Related to this, a minimum Hounsfield unit (HU_{min})/Hounsfield unit in the aorta (HU_{Aorta}) ratio of 0.26 or greater had 92.86% sensitivity and 82.61% specificity for differentiating intestinal spindle cell sarcoma from adenocarcinoma or lymphoma [70]. Unlike other neoplastic types, mucosal enhancement has not been reported [70]. This could be attributable to its origin typically in the muscularis layer of the gastrointestinal wall.

Less than 50% of spindle cell tumors are associated with lymphadenopathy. Affected lymph nodes included axillary, pancreaticoduodenal, splenic, hepatic/periportal, mesenteric, and colic lymph nodes [72].

Leiomyosarcoma
Size may be a negative prognostic indicator for leiomyosarcoma [72]. Potential metastatic sites included lymph nodes, liver, spleen, adrenal glands, large intestine, and peritoneum [29,67].

Gastrointestinal stromal tumor
Gastric GISTs are usually in the pylorus and/or pyloric antrum and did not have lymphadenopathy [31,67]. Possible metastatic sites included liver, spleen, and adrenal glands [31,67].

Peripheral nerve sheath tumor

A PNST has been reported in the feline colon as a hypo-attenuating, predominantly peripherally, and heterogeneously enhancing mass [71].

Round cell. CT descriptions of gastrointestinal lymphoma have been reported in dogs and cats, and a duodenal plasmacytoma in a cat (Table 6).

Lymphoma

Multifocal lesions can occur, with reported combinations including stomach and ileocolic junction; ileum/jejunum, colon, and rectum; and ileum/jejunum, caecum, and colon [29,68].

Lymphoma most commonly has a mixed concentric and eccentric wall thickening [29]. In the intestine, the majority have exophytic growth [70]. In the stomach, diffuse, segmental, and multifocal involvements are reported [30,67]. Secondary mechanical obstruction is much less common than with adenocarcinoma [29,70]. In one canine study, wall thickness ranged from 1 to 10 cm [29]. In a feline study, the mean thickness of intestinal lymphoma was 12.1 mm [68].

Unlike other gastrointestinal neoplasms, gastrointestinal lymphoma is typically homogeneously enhancing [29,30,67,70]. However, gastric lymphomas may have heterogeneous enhancement in late phase postcontrast images [30]. Mucosal enhancement was common in canine intestinal tumors but not in cats [68,70]. In some studies, gastric lymphoma is hypoattenuating compared to other neoplasms in all phases [30,67]. This may relate to lymphoma cell density or its origins in the submucosa and lamina propria [30].

Almost all cases have a diffuse rather than regional lymphadenopathy [29,30,67,68,70]. Affected lymph nodes included gastric, hepatic, splenic, pancreaticoduodenal, jejunal, ileocecal, and sternal lymph nodes [30,68].

Plasmacytoma

A duodenal plasmacytoma has been reported in a cat as a mass associated with perforation and jejunal lymphadenomegaly [73].

Miscellaneous

Gastric malposition. A recent case series of dogs with chronic or intermittent gastrointestinal signs

TABLE 6
Collated computed tomography imaging features of round cell gastrointestinal neoplasms in dogs and cats

Tumor type	Lymphoma/Round cell neoplasia (n = 43)	Plasmacytoma (n = 1)
Location	Cardia (3), fundus (2), body (7), pylorus (4), and "Stomach" (1) Duodenum (4), jejunum/ileum (15), and ileococolic junction (4) Caecum (1), colon (2), and rectum (1)	Duodenum (1)
Growth pattern	Concentric and eccentric (7) Exophytic (10) Endophytic (2) Diffuse/segmental (9) Circumferential (6)	—
Enhancement	Homogeneous (25) 4/5 early phase, 2/5 late phase Heterogeneous (8)	—
Layer involvement	Mucosal enhancement (15)	—
Cystic portion	1	—
Obstruction/stenosis	5	—
Ulceration	1	—
Perforation	—	1
Fat stranding	7	—
Lymphadenomegaly	39; generally diffuse	1

Data from Refs [22,29,30,68,70,73].

(≥3 weeks) identified CT and surgical features of gastric malposition suggestive of chronic gastric instability [74]. The most common findings were that the pyloric canal was in the left cranial abdomen close to the gastric cardia, the pyloric antrum left or ventral to the fundus, duodenum and pancreas left of midline, and the proximal extremity of the spleen was caudoventral or ventral to the left kidney [74].

Gastropexy can result in a gastric position that is significantly different to the natural anatomic location. After gastropexy, the pylorus is typically located in the right cranioventral abdominal quadrant in the 9 to 10 o'clock position at the level of the ninth intercostal space [75]. These authors suggested that recurrent gastric dilatation after a gastric dilatation and volvulus episode could be a consequence of the gastropexy procedure or represent persistence of factors contributing to the initial volvulus episode [75].

Pneumatosis. Pneumatosis appears as gas within the gastrointestinal wall [76,77]. There may be concurrent peritonitis and pneumoperitoneum [77]. Pneumatosis has been reported in a cat with severe gastric ulceration and pancreatitis and a dog with clostridial overgrowth [76,77].

Hematoma. CT features of a feline colonic intramural hematoma have been reported, causing mechanical obstruction, constipation, and anorexia [78]. It was a nonenhancing fluid-to-soft tissue attenuating mass between the submucosal and serosal layers of the colonic wall [78]. In the dependent portion, the material measured 40 to 60 HU, and in the upper portion, the content measured 30 to 40 HU [78].

SUMMARY AND FUTURE AVENUES

When disease of the gastrointestinal tract is suspected prior to performing a CT examination, gastrointestinal distension and contrast protocols should be considered to optimize evaluation of the gastrointestinal wall and maximize the probability of detecting gastrointestinal disease.

In large dogs, CT may be preferred to other modalities to ensure visualization of the entire gastrointestinal tract.

Gas distension of the gastrointestinal tract is easy and possibly safer to perform than fluid distension. Further studies should be considered to evaluate the safety of fluid distension protocols in diseased animals.

At the minimum, dual-phase CT should be used to evaluate the gastrointestinal tract because the small intestine tends to enhance earlier than the stomach. A fixed-injection-duration technique has been suggested to be more easily reproducible than other contrast administration techniques. This has been evaluated in dogs. In cats, ideal postcontrast scan timings have not been determined. Using standardized CT protocols in clinical cases will provide more robust data for describing abnormal imaging findings and identifying features that may aid in prioritizing differential diagnoses.

CT features have been described for many diseases. Benign diseases may be more likely to retain a layered wall appearance. Few studies have evaluated the utility of CT compared to other imaging modalities. CT may be more accurate for the detection of gastrointestinal ulceration, mechanical obstruction and surgical conditions, and is superior to ultrasound for staging and evaluation of gastric neoplasia. Some morphologic features may allow the differentiation of gastrointestinal neoplasms, such as mucosal versus outer wall layer involvement, size, and CT attenuation value.

CLINICS CARE POINTS

- CT allows visualization and evaluation of the entire gastrointestinal tract regardless of patient size, gastrointestinal content, and operator experience.
- Appropriate postcontrast scan timings, which are affected by the contrast administration technique, maximize wall conspicuity and wall layering. Dual-phase imaging is recommended, as the small intestine tends to enhance earlier than the stomach.
- Fluid or gas distension of the gastrointestinal tract further improves wall conspicuity, which may allow earlier detection of changes in wall thickness seen with disease. Only one study evaluated a gastric fluid distension protocol in cats.
- CT is often useful to aid surgical planning.
- CT is superior to ultrasound for the evaluation of canine gastric neoplasia and may be better for the evaluation of large dogs and patients with mechanical obstruction or gastrointestinal ulceration.
- Spindle cell tumors tend to be larger, heterogeneous, and involve the outer gastrointestinal wall compared to epithelial and round cell neoplasms. Adenocarcinomas are more commonly associated with gastrointestinal obstruction. Gastric lymphoma may be hypoattenuating to other gastric neoplasms.
- There is limited published literature in cats.

DISCLOSURE

The author has nothing to disclose.

REFERENCES

[1] Rakha GM, Abdl-Haleem MM, Farghali HA, et al. Prevalence of common canine digestive problems compared with other health problems in teaching veterinary hospital, Faculty of Veterinary Medicine, Cairo University, Egypt. Vet World 2015;8(3):403–11.

[2] Kim E, Choe C, Yoo JG, et al. Major medical causes by breed and life stage for dogs presented at veterinary clinics in the Republic of Korea: a survey of electronic medical records. PeerJ 2018;6:e5161.

[3] Riedesel EA. Small Bowel. In: Thrall DE, editor. Textbook of veterinary diagnostic radiology. 7th edition. St Louis, Missouri: Elsevier; 2018. p. 926–54.

[4] Riedesel EA. Stomach. In: Thrall DE, editor. Textbook of veterinary diagnostic radiology. 7th edition. St Louis, Missouri: Elsevier; 2018. p. 894–925.

[5] Martinez M, Pallares FJ, Soler M, et al. Relationship between ultrasonographic and histopathological measurements of small intestinal wall layers in fresh cat cadavers. Vet J 2018;237:1–8.

[6] Le Roux AB, Granger LA, Wakamatsu N, et al. Ex Vivo Correlation of Ultrasonographic Small Intestinal Wall Layering with Histology in Dogs. Vet Radiol Ultrasound 2016;57(5):534–45.

[7] Penninck DG, Moore AS, Gliatto J. Ultrasonography of canine gastric epithelial neoplasia. Vet Radiol Ultrasound 1998;39(4):342–8.

[8] Winter MD, Barry KS, Johnson MD, et al. Ultrasonographic and computed tomographic characterization and localization of suspected mechanical gastrointestinal obstruction in dogs. J Am Vet Med Assoc 2017;251(3):315–21.

[9] Freiche V, Faucher MR, German AJ. Can clinical signs, clinicopathological findings and abdominal ultrasonography predict the site of histopathological abnormalities of the alimentary tract in cats? J Feline Med Surg 2015; 18(2):118–28 [published Online First: Epub Date]].

[10] Guttin T, Walsh A, Durham AC, et al. Ability of ultrasonography to predict the presence and location of histologic lesions in the small intestine of cats. J Vet Intern Med 2019;33(3):1278–85.

[11] Leib MS, Larson MM, Grant DC, et al. Diagnostic Utility of Abdominal Ultrasonography in Dogs with Chronic Diarrhea. J Vet Intern Med 2012;26(6):1288–94.

[12] Mapletoft EK, Allenspach K, Lamb CR. How useful is abdominal ultrasonography in dogs with diarrhoea? J Small Anim Pract 2018;59(1):32–7.

[13] Moore LE. The advantages and disadvantages of endoscopy. Clin Tech Small Anim Pract 2003;18(4):250–3.

[14] Weston PJ, Maddox TW, Hõim S-E, et al. Diagnostic utility of abdominal ultrasound for detecting non-perforated gastroduodenal ulcers in dogs. Vet Rec 2022;190(1): e199.

[15] Fields EL, Robertson ID, Osborne JA, et al. Comparison of abdominal computed tomography and abdominal ultrasound in sedated dogs. Vet Radiol Ultrasound 2012; 53(5):513–7.

[16] Shanaman MM, Schwarz T, Gal A, et al. Comparison between survey radiography, b-mode ultrasonography, contrast-enhanced ultrasonography and contrast-enhanced multi-detector computed tomography findings in dogs with acute abdominal signs. Vet Radiol Ultrasound 2013;54(6):591–604.

[17] Fitzgerald E, Lam R, Drees R. Improving conspicuity of the canine gastrointestinal wall using dual phase contrast-enhanced computed tomography: a retrospective cross-sectional study. Vet Radiol Ultrasound 2017; 58(2):151–62.

[18] Hoey S, Drees R, Hetzel S. Evaluation of the gastrointestinal tract in dogs using computed tomography. Vet Radiol Ultrasound 2013;54(1):25–30.

[19] Kim C, Lee S-K, Je H, et al. Assessment of a split-bolus computed tomographic enterography technique for simultaneous evaluation of the intestinal wall and mesenteric vasculature of dogs. Am J Vet Res 2020; 81(2):122–30.

[20] Lee S-K, Yoon S, Kim C, et al. Triple-phased mesenteric CT angiography using a test bolus technique for evaluation of the mesenteric vasculature and small intestinal wall contrast enhancement in dogs. Vet Radiol Ultrasound 2019;60(5):493–501.

[21] Siow JW, Chau J, Podadera JM, et al. Investigation of scan delays for CT evaluation of inner wall layering and peak enhancement of the canine stomach and small intestine using a 20 second fixed-injection-duration and bolus tracking technique. Vet Radiol Ultrasound 2023;64(1): 42–52.

[22] Terragni R, Vignoli M, Rossi F, et al. Stomach wall evaluation using helical hydro-computed tomography. Vet Radiol Ultrasound 2012;53(4):402–5.

[23] Holle HM, Ghilagaber G, Drees R. Evaluation of the normal gastrointestinal tract in cats using dual-phase computed tomography. J Small Anim Pract 2023;64(7): 463–76.

[24] Keh S, Sohn J, Choi M, et al. Evaluation of computed tomographic enterography with an orally administered lactulose solution in clinically normal dogs. Am J Vet Res 2016;77(4):367–73.

[25] Steffey MA, Daniel L, Taylor SL, et al. Computed tomographic pneumocolonography in normal dogs. Vet Radiol Ultrasound 2015;56(3):278–85.

[26] Steffey MA, Zwingenberger AL, Daniel L, et al. Assessment of 3 Bowel Preparation Protocols for Computed Tomography Pneumocolonography in Normal Dogs. Vet Surg 2016;45(7):929–35.

[27] Yamada K, Morimoto M, Kishimoto M, et al. Virtual endoscopy of dogs using multi-detector row CT. Vet Radiol Ultrasound 2007;48(4):318–22.

[28] de Battisti A, Harran N, Chanoit G, et al. Use of negative contrast computed tomography for diagnosis of a

colonic duplication in a dog. J Small Anim Pract 2013;54(10):547–50.

[29] De Magistris AV, Rossi F, Valenti P, et al. CT features of gastrointestinal spindle cell, epithelial, and round cell tumors in 41 dogs. Vet Radiol Ultrasound 2023;64(2):271–82.

[30] Tanaka T, Akiyoshi H, Mie K, et al. Contrast-enhanced computed tomography may be helpful for characterizing and staging canine gastric tumors. Vet Radiol Ultrasound 2019;60(1):7–18.

[31] Tanaka T, Wada Y, Noguchi S, et al. Contrast-enhanced CT features of pyloric lesions in 17 dogs: Case series. Vet Radiol Ultrasound 2023;64(2):262–70.

[32] Thierry F, Chau J, Makara M, et al. Vascular conspicuity differs among injection protocols and scanner types for canine multiphasic abdominal computed tomographic angiography. Vet Radiol Ultrasound 2018;59(6):677–86.

[33] Siow JW. Multi-phase computed tomography of the canine stomach and small intestine [master]. Sydney, Australia: University of Sydney; 2023.

[34] Ba-Ssalamah A, Prokop M, Uffmann M, et al. Dedicated multidetector CT of the stomach: spectrum of diseases. Radiographics 2003;23(3):625–44.

[35] Insko EK, Levine MS, Birnbaum BA, et al. Benign and malignant lesions of the stomach: evaluation of CT criteria for differentiation. Radiology 2003;228(1):166–71.

[36] Tsurumaru D, Miyasaka M, Muraki T, et al. Histopathologic diversity of gastric cancers: Relationship between enhancement pattern on dynamic contrast-enhanced CT and histological type. Eur J Radiol 2017;97:90–5.

[37] Balthazar EJ. CT of the gastrointestinal tract: principles and interpretation. AJR Am J Roentgenol 1991;156(1):23–32.

[38] Murphy KP, McLaughlin PD, O'Connor OJ, et al. Imaging the small bowel. Curr Opin Gastroenterol 2014;30(2):134–40.

[39] Penninck DG, Nyland TG, Fisher PE, et al. Ultrasonography of the normal canine gastrointestinal tract. Vet Radiol Ultrasound 1989;30(6):272–6.

[40] Gladwin NE, Penninck DG, Webster CRL. Ultrasonographic evaluation of the thickness of the wall layers in the intestinal tract of dogs. Am J Vet Res 2014;75(4):349–53.

[41] Delaney F, O'Brien RT, Waller K. Ultrasound evaluation of small bowel thickness compared to weight in normal dogs. Vet Radiol Ultrasound 2003;44(5):577–80.

[42] Couturier L, Rault D, Gatel L, et al. Ultrasonographic characterization of the feline cardia and pylorus in 34 healthy cats and three abnormal cats. Vet Radiol Ultrasound 2012;53(3):342–7.

[43] Di Donato P, Penninck D, Pietra M, et al. Ultrasonographic measurement of the relative thickness of intestinal wall layers in clinically healthy cats. J Feline Med Surg 2013;16(4):333–9.

[44] Besso J, Rault D, Begon D. Feline cecum and ileocecolic junction: normal ultrasonographic features and clinical applications. Vet Radiol Ultrasound 2004;45:599.

[45] Newell SM, Graham JP, Roberts GD, et al. Sonography of the normal feline gastrointestinal tract. Vet Radiol Ultrasound 1999;40(1):40–3.

[46] Cheon B, Moon S, Park S, et al. Comparison of contrast media for visualization of the colon of healthy dogs during computed tomography and ultrasonography. Am J Vet Res 2016;77(11):1220–6.

[47] Agut A, Carrillo JD, Martínez M, et al. Imaging diagnosis—radiographic, ultrasonographic, and computed tomographic characteristics of a duodenal duplication cyst in a young cat. Vet Radiol Ultrasound 2018;59(3):E22–7.

[48] Kook PH, Hagen R, Willi B, et al. Rectal duplication cyst in a cat. J Feline Med Surg 2010;12(12):978–81.

[49] Mutascio L, Vilaplana Grosso F, Ramos-Vara J, et al. Multimodality characterization of a noncommunicating congenital duodenal duplication cyst causing pyloric outflow obstruction in a young dog. Vet Radiol Ultrasound 2019;60(2):E10–4.

[50] Fernandez N, Morrison L, Liuti T, et al. Type Ia (spherical) communicating colonic duplication in a dog treated with colectomy. J Small Anim Pract 2017;58(5):298–300.

[51] Lecoindre A, Saade D, Barthez P, et al. Congenital duodenocolic fistula in a dog. J Small Anim Pract 2018;59(5):311–4.

[52] Drost WT, Green EM, Zekas LJ, et al. Comparison of computed tomography and abdominal radiography for detection of canine mechanical intestinal obstruction. Vet Radiol Ultrasound 2016;57(4):366–75.

[53] Miniter BM, Gonçalves Arruda A, Zuckerman J, et al. Use of computed tomography (CT) for the diagnosis of mechanical gastrointestinal obstruction in canines and felines. PLoS One 2019;14(8):e0219748.

[54] Graham LT, Auger M, Watson AM, et al. Imaging and clinical features of a true gastrogastric intussusception in a dog. Can Vet J 2020;61(7):715–8.

[55] Bruwier A, Fouhety A, Boursier JF, et al. Ultrasonographic and computed tomographic features of a true gastrogastric intussusception with concurrent foreign bodies in a dog. Can Vet J 2022;63(4):407–10.

[56] Phipps WB, Mortier JR, Booth M, et al. Use of computed tomography in the diagnosis of caecal inversion in a dog and a cat. Vet Rec Case Reports 2019;7(2):e000839.

[57] Barge P, Fina CJ, Mortier JR, et al. CT findings in five dogs with surgically confirmed colonic torsion. Vet Radiol Ultrasound 2020;61(2):190–6.

[58] Chow KE, Stent AW, Milne M. Imaging diagnosis—use of multiphasic contrast-enhanced computed tomography for diagnosis of mesenteric volvulus in a dog. Vet Radiol Ultrasound 2014;55(1):74–8.

[59] Javard R, Specchi S, Benamou J, et al. Ileocecocolic volvulus in a German shepherd dog. Can Vet J 2014;55(11):1096–9.

[60] Brand KJ, Lim CK, Cichocki BN. Radiographic and CT features of colonic entrapment due to an omental rent in a dog. Vet Radiol Ultrasound 2021;62(1):E6–10.

[61] Fitzgerald E, Barfield D, Lee KCL, et al. Clinical findings and results of diagnostic imaging in 82 dogs with gastrointestinal ulceration. J Small Anim Pract 2017;58(4):211–8.

[62] Murakami M, Heng HG, Sola M. CT features of confirmed and presumed gastric wall edema in dogs. Vet Radiol Ultrasound 2022;63(6):711–8.

[63] Kim K, Jun B, Han S, et al. Gastric Hyperplastic Polyp Causing Upper Gastrointestinal Hemorrhage and Severe Anemia in a Dog. Veterinary Sciences 2022;9(12):680.

[64] Lecoindre A, Lecoindre P, Cadoré JL, et al. Focal intestinal lipogranulomatous lymphangitis in 10 dogs. J Small Anim Pract 2016;57(9):465–71.

[65] Lee H-W, Jung J-W, Park S, et al. Computed tomographic features of focal lipogranulomatous lymphangitis for differentiating from malignant intestinal lesions in a dog. J Vet Sci 2023;24(2):e25.

[66] Goffart LM, Durand A, Dettwiler M, et al. Feline gastrointestinal eosinophilic sclerosing fibroplasia presenting as a rectal mass. J Feline Med Surg Open Reports 2022;8(2):20551169221114330.

[67] Zuercher M, Vilaplana Grosso F, Lejeune A. Comparison of the clinical, ultrasound, and CT findings in 13 dogs with gastric neoplasia. Vet Radiol Ultrasound 2021;62(5):525–32.

[68] Tanaka T, Noguchi S, Wada Y, et al. Preliminary study of CT features of intermediate- and high-grade alimentary lymphoma and adenocarcinoma in cats. J Feline Med Surg 2021;24(10):1065–71.

[69] Yoon S, Lee S-K, Lee J, et al. Dual-phase computed tomography angiography of intestinal carcinoid tumor as a lead point for cecocolic intussusception in a dog. J Vet Med Sci 2019;81(6):928–32.

[70] Lee S, Hwang J, Kim H, et al. Computed tomographic findings may be useful for differentiating small intestinal adenocarcinomas, lymphomas, and spindle cell sarcomas in dogs. Vet Radiol Ultrasound 2023;64(2):233–42.

[71] Boland L, Setyo L, Sangster C, et al. Colonic malignant peripheral nerve sheath tumour in a cat. J Feline Med Surg Open Reports 2019;5(1):2055116919849979.

[72] Kim M-Y, Lee JK, Mietelka KA, et al. Case Report: Giant Multiloculated Pseudocystic Jejunal Leiomyosarcoma in a Dog: Atypical Morphologic Features of Canine Intestinal Leiomyosarcoma. Front Vet Sci 2022;9:791133.

[73] Tamura Y, Chambers JK, Neo S, et al. Primary duodenal plasmacytoma with associated primary (amyloid light-chain) amyloidosis in a cat. J Feline Med Surg Open Reports 2020;6(2):2055116920957194.

[74] White C, Dirrig H, Fitzgerald E. CT findings in dogs with gastric malposition: 6 cases (2016-2019). J Small Anim Pract 2020;61(12):766–71.

[75] Tomlinson AW, Lillis SM, German AJ, et al. Pyloric localisation in 57 dogs of breeds susceptible to gastric dilatation-volvulus using computed tomography. Vet Rec 2016;179(24):626.

[76] Hwang TS, Yoon YM, Noh SA, et al. Pneumatosis coli in a dog - a serial radiographic study: a case report. Vet Med-Czech 2016;61(7):404–8.

[77] Silveira C, Benigni L, Gugich K, et al. Feline gastric pneumatosis. J Feline Med Surg Open Reports 2018;4(2):2055116918782779.

[78] Hsu T-C, Lin L-S, Chung C-S, et al. Colonic Intramural Hematoma in a Cat: A Case Report. Front Vet Sci 2022;9:913862.

Advances in Small Animal Care 5 (2024) 51–65

ADVANCES IN SMALL ANIMAL CARE

Advanced Imaging of Small Mammals

Lauren von Stade, DVM, DACVR[a],*, Miranda J. Sadar, DVM, DACZM[b]

[a]Veterinary Teaching Hospital, Colorado State University, 300 West Drake Road, Fort Collins, CO 80523, USA; [b]Department of Clinical Sciences, Veterinary Teaching Hospital, Colorado State University, 300 West Drake Road, Fort Collins, CO 80523, USA

KEYWORDS
- Chinchilla • Computed tomography • Ferret • Guinea pig • MRI • Rabbit

KEY POINTS
- Cone beam computed tomography (CT) is superior to conventional multidetector CT for evaluation of dental disease and osseous maxillofacial changes in small mammals due to its increased spatial resolution.
- Conventional multidetector CT is superior to cone beam CT for evaluation of soft tissues due to improved contrast resolution, and should be preferentially chosen if a clinical question involves soft tissues or if intravenous contrast is administered.
- Emphasis on CT acquisition parameters and post-processing reconstruction is recommended in small mammals for improved spatial resolution. Multiplanar and 3 dimensional reconstructions aid in study evaluation.
- MRI provides superior contrast resolution to CT and is particularly useful for evaluating neurologic and musculoskeletal conditions.

INTRODUCTION

Computed tomography (CT) and MRI are increasingly being used for diagnostic imaging of small mammals, as availability within both the private practice and academic sectors increases. Benefits of these cross-sectional modalities relative to other diagnostic modalities, such as ultrasound and radiography, include the ability to evaluate anatomic structures without interference from superimposition of other structures and the ability to use multiplanar reconstruction [1].

The use of CT is increasing due to the relative decreased cost compared to MRI, as well as its speed of acquisition. It provides excellent anatomic detail of osseous structures and dental anatomy. Due to this, one of the most common uses for CT in zoologic companion animals is for evaluation of the skull, including the dentition for presence of dental disease. However, CT is additionally useful for evaluation of soft tissues, and reconstruction algorithms allow for targeted evaluation of differing tissue densities, such as bone, lung, or soft tissue.

Preparation of the patient is equally important for both CT and MRI. Positioning is commonly performed in sternal recumbency [2–6]. When evaluating the skull, the head may be elevated to position the hard palate parallel with the table [4]. Anesthesia is necessary for optimal imaging using MRI in small mammals to minimize motion artifact, and to promote patient safety during the procedure, including ventilation control. It also has a longer procedure time relative to CT. Given the shorter scan times needed for CT, sedation may be preferred over anesthesia, given other patient factors or emergent presentations. Conscious restraint may also be possible in certain species with the aid of devices such as the VetMouseTrap plexiglass tube (Universal Medical Systems, Solon, OH USA) [2,7].

The ability to secure vascular access in small mammals may dictate the use of contrast for the procedure. Vascular access is necessary for the ability to acquire contrast-enhanced CT or MRI, which improves identification of vascular structures, and adds information

---

*Corresponding author, E-mail address: lauren.von_stade@colostate.edu

https://doi.org/10.1016/j.yasa.2024.06.004
2666-450X/24/

regarding parenchymal features of both normal and diseased organs. Contrast administration is not necessary when the clinical question is focused on skeletal or dental anatomy. However, contrast is a preferred component of cross-sectional studies evaluating soft tissues, as its use aids in differentiation and detailed evaluation of both normal and abnormal structures, as well as features that may not be possible without the use of contrast media. Despite its significant utility for interpretation of studies, potential risks of contrast media administration should always be considered and its use avoided when contraindicated for patient safety.

Regarding CT acquisition, special attention should be given to the selection of specific parameters to achieve high quality studies, especially given the small size of small mammal patients. Parameters to prioritize when configuring the acquisition of the CT include a narrow field of view around the region of interest and small slice thicknesses [5]. Keeping both of these factors low will increase spatial resolution and image quality at the expense of slightly higher noise, which in the authors' experience is a negligible drawback.

Post-processing reconstruction of the acquired CT can be exceptionally useful in small mammals to improve the quality of the acquired study. It is the authors' experience that whole body CTs are commonly obtained in small mammals, despite a clinical question focused on a particular body cavity, such as the thorax or abdomen. In these cases, small field of view reconstructions collimated to the region of interest should be created for each body region of interest (Fig. 1). If acquisition of the CT is performed with larger slice thicknesses on a multidetector CT, selection of thinner, ideally sub-millimeter, slice thicknesses can be chosen during post-processing to improve spatial resolution. Reconstruction algorithms in various spatial frequencies for optimal evaluation of bone, lung, and soft tissues are recommended. Additionally, as images are typically acquired in a transverse or axial plane, dorsal and sagittal reconstructions are useful for evaluation of many structures, and additional multiplanar and 3 dimensional reconstructions may be used depending on the clinical question [8,9].

Various CT technologies are currently used for small mammals, with the most common being conventional multidetector and cone beam. Conventional multidetector CT involves the rotation of a fan-shaped x-ray beam around a patient onto multiple rows of linear detector arrays. The rotation of the x-ray beam occurs in a helical fashion as a patient is moved through a gantry. This is the most employed CT technology in the clinical setting, and allows for improved contrast resolution and evaluation of soft tissues relative to cone beam CT [8]. Cone beam CT involves the rotation of a cone-shaped x-ray beam and area detector around a patient, allowing imaging of a large volume with a single rotation. Benefits compared to other systems include a higher spatial resolution and typically lower cost, at the expense of greater artifacts and poorer contrast resolution, limiting evaluation of soft tissues [10]. It is commonly used in small mammals for evaluation of dental anatomy due to the high spatial resolution, and for radiation oncology planning [8,10,11]. In a prior study evaluating dental disease in rabbits, cone beam CT was considered superior to multidetector for evaluating dentition and osseous maxillofacial structures, including the periodontal ligament space (Fig. 2) [8].

Additional CT technology that is used sparingly at this time for use in clinical patients includes both micro-CT and PET-CT, with both technologies predominantly limited to academic settings. Micro-CT is most commonly used for research applications, however it has been sporadically used for clinical purposes [9,12–14]. It can acquire the highest resolution images, with resolution up to 0.077 cm reported in one study; however, scan time is variable, ranging from very fast to up to an hour, and reconstruction algorithms may be complex in order to reduce artifact and noise to improve image quality [12,13,15]. Additionally, this technology may be an excellent option for very small patients, but is not practical in larger animals due to its small field of view [12,15]. The feasibility of PET-CT has been described in ferrets, and its technology used in experimental research studies involving mice, rabbits, and guinea pigs; however, to the authors' knowledge its use in clinical patients has not yet been employed [16–18].

Finally, MRI provides superior contrast resolution relative to other diagnostic modalities and is generally considered the gold standard modality for evaluation of neurologic disease involving the brain and spinal cord [1]. However, its superior contrast resolution may also be useful for evaluation of thoracic, abdominal, and musculoskeletal disease. Factors to consider when determining the use of MRI in small mammals include the available magnet strength, as lower magnet field strengths will have decreased resolution particularly in small patients, and length of scan time, which is longer than CT [19]. The use of MRI in veterinary medicine is increasing; however, additional major limitations to more widespread use include cost and availability.

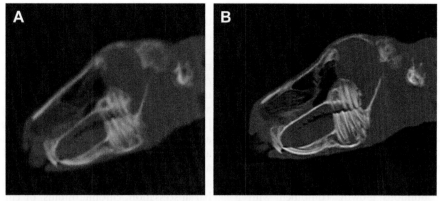

FIG. 1 Multiplanar parasagittal reconstructions of a rabbit skull, illustrating the importance of reconstruction techniques on evaluating anatomy. Note the improved clarity in (**B**) relative to (**A**) achieved by selecting a small field of view around the region of interest and decreased slice thickness during post-acquisition reconstruction of the head in a performed whole body computed tomography (CT). The nasal turbinates and dental anatomy can be better evaluated in (**B**). For both images, window width = 4000, window level = 1000, kVP 110, current 250, matrix 512 x 512. (**A**) Zoomed in parasagittal evaluation of the head of the initial entire acquired whole body CT with 2 mm slice thickness and a field of view of 18.5 cm (**B**) Additional parasagittal reconstruction performed with field of view changed to view only the head anatomy and slice thickness decreased to 1 mm slice thickness and a field of view of 9.9 cm.

Descriptions and images of normal CT imaging are available for numerous small mammal species including ferrets [16], chinchillas [20–22], rabbits [15,22–31], and guinea pigs [1,22,32], and resources regarding MRI in small mammals [1,33], primarily for research, have been published and are beyond the scope of this review. Larger retrospective studies evaluating the use of CT imaging in clinical patients are limited, with most resources limited to case reports and series. The use of MRI in the clinical setting is even more sporadically reported. This review will focus on consolidating the currently known available research in small mammal advanced imaging as a resource for guiding application of CT and MRI in the clinical setting for

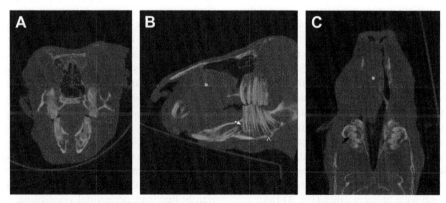

FIG. 2 Transverse (**A**), sagittal (**B**), and dorsal (**C**) reconstructions of the skull of a rabbit presenting for epistaxis. Note the improved spatial resolution of the dentition with the cone beam CT relative to the images from the multidetector CT in Fig. 3. There is good visibility of the periodontal ligaments (*white arrow*), germinal centers (*open white bracket*), and pulp cavities (*black arrow*) of the included teeth on these images. Additionally, there is a large soft tissue attenuating mass occupying the right nasal cavity and causing leftward deviation of the nasal septum (*white asterisk*). CT parameters: kVP 84, current 4, WW/WL 5000/1000, Slice thickness 0.2 mm.

these species and for exposing gaps in knowledge to guide further research.

SIGNIFICANCE
Computed Tomographic Imaging of Dental Disease in Small Mammals

Chinchillas, rabbits, and guinea pigs all have long-crowned incisors, premolars, and molars with enamel that extends past the alveolar bone and lack true roots, allowing for continued tooth growth throughout life, termed hypsodont, aradicular, and elodont dentition [5,34]. This continuous growth, combined with a poorly abrasive diet, can lead to malocclusion, coronal and apical elongation, sharp dental points, and periodontal disease, which in many cases occurs before clinical detection is possible and can lead to further dental issues and sequela including mucosal ulceration, facial abscessation, and osteomyelitis [5,10,34]. CT is superior in detecting many dental lesions compared to oral examination and conventional radiography in chinchillas, rabbits, and guinea pigs [4,5,34]. This is partly due to the difficulty of performing oral examinations in these species, and the ability to provide excellent detail of the oral cavity, superior contrast resolution, and lack of superimposition of skull bones that occurs with conventional radiography [34]. However, CT should be used in combination with oral examination as detection of certain findings, such as fractures at the tip of the clinical crown, may only be identified by clinical examination [4].

Due to these patient factors, evaluation of dental disease is one of the most used applications of CT in small mammals, with multiple larger retrospective studies describing its application in clinically affected patients. In a study comparing clinical examination, conventional radiography, and CT imaging for the detection and assessment of dental lesions in chinchillas, CT was superior in identifying the presence and extent of early and moderate apical tooth elongation, extensive apical maxillary and mandibular elongation and deformities, remodeling of cortical bone around, or penetration of cortical bone by, apical portions of teeth, moderate coronal elongation, caries, mineralization defects, and occlusal wear abnormalities (Fig. 3) [34].

In rabbits, CT is useful in identifying multiple pathologies not visible with oral examination including, but not limited to, periodontal ligament space widening, periapical lucencies, alveolar bone lysis, tooth resorption, mandibular or lacrimal canal deformation, and apical tooth growth [5,10]. Compared to skull radiography in rabbits, CT provides more subtle detail of dental and bony changes, as well as evaluation of secondary changes [35]. It may provide additional, or more diagnostic information, compared to skull radiography in up to 80% of cases with dental disease [36]. Additionally, multiple studies have found increased utility in the use of dorsal multiplanar reformatted images for evaluation of the periodontal ligament space [5,10]. Widening of the periodontal ligament space and interproximal space are both correlated with periapical abscess formation in rabbits [5]. Finally, it can aid in identification of sequela to dental disease, such as osteomyelitis of the mandible and maxilla, retrobulbar abscessation, chronic rhinitis, or empyema of the bony cavities of the skull [14,31].

In a study evaluating 66 guinea pigs with dental disease receiving oral examination and subsequent evaluation with advanced imaging, a cause for the dental disease was identified by CT in 80% of patients [4]. In 10 guinea pigs with unilateral exophthalmos, 8 animals were diagnosed with periapical disease of the upper cheek tooth region as the causative reason for eye protrusion, with no causative cause in 2 patients, using CT [4]. CT was useful in identifying tooth fracture, macrodontia, and periapical disease in 12/13 patients with mandibular swelling on examination [4]. Macrodontia was detected in incisor teeth in some animals on clinical examination, however only identified on premolars and molars using CT [4]. A combination of clinical examination and CT may be necessary to identify all tooth fractures, as few cases in this study were detected only by clinical examination (typically at the very tip of the clinical crown) whereas all fractures of incisors, premolars, and molars below the gingival line required CT for diagnosis [4]. Finally, CT was useful for detection of multiple tooth abnormalities, evaluation of periapical disease of incisor, premolar, and molar teeth, and detecting concurrent abnormalities, such as the presence of otitis media [4].

Computed Tomographic Imaging of Other Head and Neck Diseases in Small Mammals

Various other conditions, aside from dental disease, affecting the head and neck in small mammals can be evaluated with CT, including otitis media and externa, retrobulbar and periorbital conditions, upper respiratory disease, and oral, nasal, skull, and cervical masses.

Otitis media is a common disease affecting small mammal species, and early diagnosis is considered important to prevent progression of infection to the inner ear, causing otitis interna, and in some cases, to the brain [6]. Neurologic signs such as peripheral vestibular

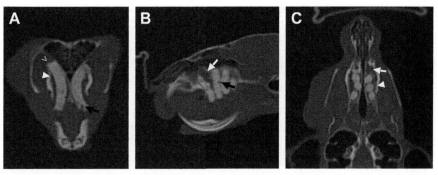

FIG. 3 Transverse (**A**), sagittal (**B**), and dorsal (**C**) reconstructions of the skull of a chinchilla presenting for dental disease. (**A**) Is at the level of the first maxillary molar teeth. Note the apical elongation of the first right maxillary molar tooth (*open white bracket*), periodontal ligament space widening (*white arrowhead*), and tooth resorptive lesions (*black arrow*). (**B**) Parasagittal reconstruction at the level of the left maxillary premolar and molars. Note the large periapical lucency of the left maxillary premolar tooth (*white arrow*) and resorptive lesions along the first molar tooth (*black arrow*). (**C**) Dorsal reconstruction of the maxilla. Note the same large periapical lucency of the left maxillary premolar tooth denoted in (**B**) (*white arrow*) as well as the normal periodontal ligament adjacent to the second left maxillary molar tooth (*white arrowhead*). CT parameters: kVP 90, current 83, WW/WL 7000/1800, slice thickness 0.75 mm.

disease, facial nerve paralysis, or Horner's syndrome may occur with otitis interna, and central vestibular disease may occur with intracranial infection [6]. However, it is common for otitis media to initially be subclinical [2,6]. Compared to skull radiographs in rabbits, CT provides superior detection of lesions in the nasal cavities, maxillary recesses, and tympanic bullae [36]. In a retrospective study evaluating the differences in CT findings between rabbits with clinical and subclinical middle ear disease, the presence of bulla lysis in clinical disease was significantly higher, and rabbits with subclinical disease and bulla lysis had a higher prevalence of developing vestibular signs [6]. In patients with vestibular signs, CT changes to the middle ear, including soft tissue attenuating material within the tympanic bullae, bulla lysis, and/or bulla thickening were commonly ipsilateral to the side with vestibular signs, or in the case of bilateral disease, more severe on the ipsilateral side (Fig. 4) [6]. A separate study similarly used CT findings including tympanic bulla soft tissue material and changes to the tympanic bulla shape to create a grading scale of CT diagnosed otitis media [2]. 66% of rabbits with otitis media had a lop ear conformation, unilateral was more common than bilateral disease, and grade was strongly correlated with the volume of material within the external ear canal [2]. CT was additionally useful in several case reports of chinchillas with otitis media, both for surgical planning and post-surgical evaluation of a total ear canal ablation and temporary bulla fenestration, and for diagnosis of a soft tissue

attenuating mass within the external ear canal on investigation of a lack of response to treatment for otitis media [37,38].

The retrobulbar and periorbital regions are challenging to image with radiographs and ultrasound, particularly in small mammals, due to their proximity to the skull and the small size of the regions. CT can be beneficial for further anatomic information. Ideally, contrast administration is used; however, non-contrast CT has proven useful for diagnosis and surgical planning of retrobulbar disease in several species [39,40]. CT findings of an orbital cyst in a chinchilla caused by a parasitic (*Taenia coenurus*) infection included a soft tissue mass in the periorbital region with central fluid attenuation, consistent with a cyst, and small mineral attenuating foci within the periphery and lumen of the structure [39]. Non-contrast CT was useful in identifying the presence of a retrobulbar lacrimal ductal carcinoma in a European hedgehog, tracking the mass' size over time, and guiding surgical planning for its removal [40]. On CT examination, a soft tissue attenuating mass with a capsule and necrotic center and dorsolateral displacement of the globe was noted [40].

Several small mammal species, including guinea pigs and rabbits, are obligate nasal breathers, and diseases of the upper respiratory tract can significantly impact quality of life and lead to considerable dyspnea [3,31]. CT has been diagnostic for nasopharyngeal stenosis in 4 guinea pigs presenting with respiratory distress [3]. Findings included concentric thickened

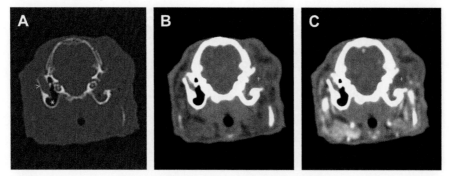

FIG. 4 Transverse images in a bone (**A**) and soft tissue algorithm pre-(**B**) and post-(**C**) contrast of the head of a lop rabbit presenting with left-sided vestibular signs and facial paralysis diagnosed on CT with bilateral otitis externa and unilateral left-sided otitis media. The right side of the rabbit is to the left in each of these images. Note the air-filled right-sided tympanic bulla (*white asterisk*) compared to the soft tissue attenuating, non-contrast enhancing material filling the left-sided tympanic bulla (*black asterisk*). There is mild expansion of the bony margins of the left tympanic bulla relative to the right. Also note the soft tissue attenuating, non-enhancing material filling the right external ear canal with preservation of the bony margins of the distal, vertical portion (*open white bracket*) compared to the soft tissue attenuating, non-enhancing material (*white plus signs*) filling the left external ear canal and causing expansile lysis and lateral pouching of the left external ear canal (*open black brackets*). The lack of enhancement of this material helps to diagnose this left-sided external ear canal material as caseous/non-vascular versus a neoplastic mass.

soft tissue attenuating material at the rostral aspect of the nasopharynx at the level of the choana resulting in incomplete narrowing of the lumen, and additional findings of otitis media and rhinitis [3]. Multiplanar reconstruction of the head and use of a bone algorithm for reviewing this region may prove useful in diagnosis (Fig. 5).

CT is also valuable for the evaluation of skull and cervical masses in small mammals, including abscessation and salivary gland pathology. In a small case series of 2 ferrets, the identification of soft tissue and fluid attenuating, rim contrast-enhancing masses on CT guided diagnosis of abscessation secondary to *Pseudomonas luteola* [41]. Differentiation of abscessation from salivary mucoceles may be difficult in similar cases given the proximity to the regional salivary glands. Other cervical pathology may similarly be difficult to differentiate from salivary mucoceles [42]. In a rabbit diagnosed with sialectasis, in the cervical region, CT identified a large, tubular to multicameral, fluid-filled and rim contrast-enhancing mass in the submandibular region [42]. Given the location, this mass was initially thought to represent a sialocele of the left mandibular salivary gland and histopathology was required to differentiate these processes [42]. At the authors' institution, contrast-enhanced CT has been useful for the diagnosis of multiple cases of facial and cervical region abscessation, including the diagnosis of mandibular lymph node abscessation secondary to *Streptococcus*

zooepidemicus in the case of a chinchilla presenting for cervical swelling (Fig. 6).

CT has proven useful in multiple species for determining the extent of neoplastic disease, metastatic screening, and aiding in clinical decision making regarding medical or surgical intervention versus radiation therapy [43–48]. CT features of several neoplastic masses affecting the skull and cervical region in small mammals have been described. In a case series evaluating cervical chordomas in ferrets, CT identified hypo-attenuating and poorly enhancing soft tissue masses with multiple foci of mineralization in the region of C1-C2, with 1 ferret having a mass that caused expansion of the occipital bone and thickening of the ipsilateral bulla [43]. Skull-associated osteomas involving the temporal bone, parietal bone, and tympanic bulla in ferrets have also been described, with imaging identifying the bone of origin [46–48].

Elodontomas are hamartomatous, odontoma-like, benign neoplasms affecting the elodont dentition of species, such as the guinea pig and rabbit. CT features of elodontomas in 2 guinea pigs included mineralized masses associated with the apex and reserve crowns of incisor and premolar teeth with adjacent osseous expansion and/or lysis [49]. Radiographs in one case underestimated lesion size relative to that identified on CT, which was integral for surgical planning of the lesion [49]. Lastly, CT features of an ectopic elodontoma in a rabbit included a well-circumscribed, round, mixed soft tissue

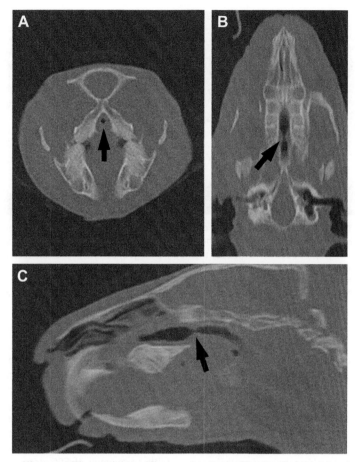

FIG. 5 Transverse (**A**), dorsal (**B**), and sagittal (**C**) reconstructions of the head of a guinea pig diagnosed with nasopharyngeal stenosis. The use of a bone algorithm to evaluate the soft tissues of the nasopharynx was useful to decrease the artifact from adjacent bony structures, which may limit detailed evaluation of the soft tissues of the head in a soft tissue algorithm. In all figures, note the circumferential soft tissue thickening of the nasopharynx, creating a stenotic lesion within the mid aspect of the nasopharynx (*black arrows*).

and mineral attenuating mass with mild contrast-enhancement within the buccal mucosa [50].

Computed Tomographic Imaging of Thoracic Disease in Small Mammals

CT evaluation of the thoracic cavity in small mammals can be particularly useful given the ability to specifically evaluate the lung parenchyma and intrathoracic soft tissue structures. It is considered superior in rabbits for diagnosis of intrapulmonary disease, and has been instrumental in the diagnosis of pulmonary emphysema and bullae, spontaneous pneumothorax, multifocal granulomas, pulmonary abscessation, and characterization of extrapulmonary intrathoracic neoplastic disease (Fig. 7) [19,51,52].

In a retrospective evaluation of thoracic CT in rabbits, pulmonary emphysema was identified in 10.7% of the population, with approximately half being asymptomatic and the other half presenting with upper respiratory signs, including dyspnea or nasal discharge [51]. The most common feature of pulmonary emphysema in rabbits was focal, multifocal, or diffuse hypoattenuation of the pulmonary parenchyma, most commonly affecting the cranial lung lobes [51]. In a separate study of 4 rabbits with pneumothorax, details including the laterality and severity of gas accumulation, regions of interstitial or alveolar parenchymal infiltrate, cavitary lesions suggestive of bullae, soft tissue attenuating pulmonary nodules and masses, and concomitant abdominal and orthopedic changes were

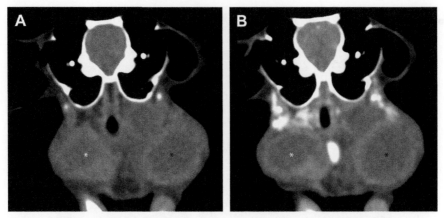

FIG. 6 Transverse pre (**A**) and post (**B**) images of the head and neck of a chinchilla evaluated for submandibular swelling. The patient's left is on the right of the images. The right (*white asterisk*) and left (*black asterisk*) mandibular lymph nodes are bilaterally markedly enlarged, centrally fluid-attenuating, and peripherally hyperattenuating in the pre-contrast sequence and moderately rim contrast-enhancing following contrast administration, consistent with abscessation of the mandibular lymph nodes. This patient was diagnosed with *Streptococcus equi*, subspecies *zooepidemicus* following culture of fine needle aspiration samples of these lymph nodes.

identified (Fig. 8) [52]. CT identified more lesions in these cases than did radiography, and was additionally useful in characterizing pulmonary changes over time [52].

Computed Tomographic Imaging of Abdominal Disease in Small Mammals

Liver lobe torsions in rabbits are a common emergency, with clinical signs often mimicking those of gastrointestinal hypomotility syndrome. Most commonly, ultrasonography is used for diagnosis, but a recent study evaluated CT features of liver lobe torsion in 6 rabbits using this modality [53]. Features included an enlarged, rounded, and heterogeneous caudate liver lobe with scant volume of regional peritoneal effusion [53]. Visual inspection of attenuation and the use of Hounsfield units were also useful for diagnosis [53]. The torsed lobes were consistently hypoattenuating precontrast to normal liver, with lower measured Hounsfield units (mean 39.3 HU) compared to normal (mean 55.1 HU), and minimally to non-contrast enhancing, with an average of 50% less contrast enhancement of the torsed lobe (mean 38.4 HU) compared to normal liver (mean 108.4) (Fig. 9) [53].

CT may also be useful in identification of sacculitis and appendicitis in rabbits presenting with signs of

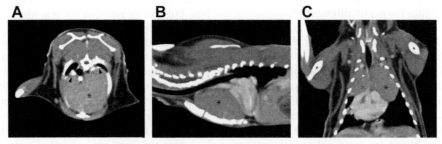

FIG. 7 Transverse (**A**), sagittal (**B**), and dorsal (**C**) reconstructions in a post-contrast soft tissue algorithm of the thorax of a rabbit diagnosed with a thymoma. Note the large, homogeneously contrast enhancing mass within the cranioventral mediastinum (*black asterisk*) causing caudal and mild rightward displacement of the heart and dorsal displacement of the aorta (*open black bracket*), right and left cranial vena cava (*black arrowheads*), and right common carotid artery (*white arrowhead*).

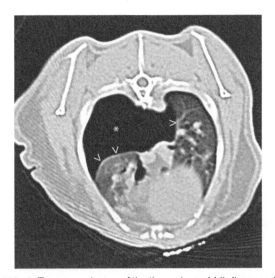

FIG. 8 Transverse image of the thorax in a rabbit diagnosed with spontaneous pneumothorax. Note the asymmetry of the gas accumulation within the right hemithorax (*white asterisk*) with secondary retraction of the lung lobes (*open white brackets*). This rabbit had a consolidated contrast-enhancing lesion within the right cranial lung lobe with a gas-filled interior component (not pictured), considered to be the most likely cause of the identified pneumothorax.

gastrointestinal hypomotility syndrome [7]. Features reported for this condition include thickening of the sacculus rotundus, identified as a rounded structure in the right caudoventral abdomen, as well as rounding and elongation of the appendix, a blind-ended structure at the distal aspect of the cecum, with concurrent mesenteric lymph node enlargement and mild peritoneal effusion [7]. As the sacculus rotundus and appendix are commonly not identified on CT in normal rabbits due to compression from gas and food distension of other gastrointestinal segments, clear identification and thickening of these structures may help support a diagnosis of sacculitis and appendicitis [7,24].

CT has been used in several ferrets for the evaluation of urinary conditions, including diagnosis of a circumcaval ureter with hydronephrosis and hydroureter, an extramural ectopic ureter, and a large urinoma in one with hydronephrosis and hydroureter [54–56]. In the ferret with the diagnosed urinoma, CT excretory urography showed lack of contrast enhancement within the distal ureter or within the cystic structure, helping to diagnose the urinoma, presumed secondary to ureteral transection during a previous ovariohysterectomy procedure, and aided in surgical planning [54].

CT may be useful in evaluation of extent of disease with abdominal neoplasia [57,58]. Limited reports

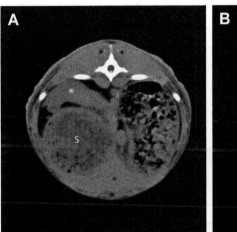
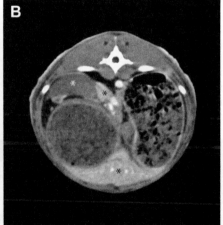

FIG. 9 Transverse pre-contrast (**A**) and post-contrast (**B**) images of the abdomen in a rabbit diagnosed with a chronic liver lobe torsion. (**A**) The caudate liver lobe (*white asterisk*) is visible in the right, cranial abdomen dorsal to the stomach (S), which contains a moderate volume of heterogeneous mixed soft tissue and gas attenuating material consistent with normal ingesta. Additional liver is identified in the ventral abdomen (*black asterisk*). Although the caudate lobe is mildly hypoattenuating relative to normal liver, this is difficult to visibly identify without the use of measured Hounsfield units. (**B**) Post-contrast administration, note that the torsed caudate lobe (*white asterisk*) is non-enhancing relative to normal liver (*black asterisks*).

include the CT description of a ferret with an adrenal neuroblastoma and hedgehog with a fused bilateral malignant ovarian teratoma and peritoneal metastasis [57,58]. This multi-lobulated, mineralized mass was identified as connecting to 2 tubular structures extending into the pelvic cavity, consistent with uterine horns [58]. A smaller metastatic peritoneal mass with internal mineralization was also identified [58]. At the authors' institution, CT has been used in several ferrets diagnosed with lymphoma for radiation therapy planning (Fig. 10).

Finally, functional CT techniques, such as evaluation of glomerular filtration rate, have been performed in rabbits to guide surgical decision making regarding unilateral nephrectomy in the case of both a unilateral renal nephroblastoma and obstructive ureterolithiasis [59]. This technique was considered useful for evaluation of renal function and determination of surgical intervention; however, caution is advised when applying this technique to additional cases as reference values for rabbits are still necessary [59].

Neurologic and Musculoskeletal Applications of Computed Tomography in Small Mammals

CT may be used as a first line diagnostic in investigating neurologic signs as MRI is not as widely available and may be cost limiting. In a ferret with a T3-L3 myelopathy and multiple osseous lesions identified on radiographs, CT allowed for identification and characterization of spinal cord compression associated with contrast-enhancing, osteolytic, and expansile spinal masses, identified on cytology as multicentric lymphoma [60]. In another ferret with non-ambulatory paraparesis, CT was useful as a first-line diagnostic in determining the presence of compressive myelopathy, articular process fracture, and bony lysis secondary to an osseous plasmacytoma [61]. In this case, MRI was useful as an adjunct diagnostic for better definition of

the regional soft tissue changes, including evaluation of intervertebral discs and extent of spinal cord compression [61]. In a ferret with acute onset of seizures and other neurologic signs, CT revealed the presence of a contrast-enhancing intracalvarial mass, a pyogranulomatous meningitis secondary to systemic coronavirus infection [62]. Finally, in a ferret with central vestibular signs, CT diagnosed a hyperattenuating, contrast-enhancing mass lesion in the region of the right cerebellopontine angle, a choroid plexus papilloma in the fourth ventricle [63].

CT has additionally been used to evaluate neurologic signs in rabbits. Contrast CT was useful in the identification of a peripheral nerve sheath tumor of the brachial plexus in a rabbit with right thoracic lameness; imaging features included a homogeneously contrast enhancing, lobular to rounded mass within the ventral vertebral canal with extension into multiple intervertebral foramina and secondary thoracic limb muscle atrophy [64]. In a rabbit with pelvic limb paresis, mineralized uteromegaly, and multifocal osteolytic lesions identified on radiographs, CT identified additional osteolytic lesions and characterized the presence of a heterogeneously contrast-enhancing mass extending into the thoracic vertebral canal, which was diagnosed as metastatic uterine adenocarcinoma [65].

CT provides excellent detail of osseous abnormalities; however, its use in musculoskeletal applications in small mammals is minimally reported. A retrospective study of 210 rabbits used micro-CT to characterize fractures caused by trauma from accidental drops, and pathologic neoplastic fractures both from primary bone tumors and metastatic lesions [13]. CT was superior to radiography for both maxillary and lumbar fractures due to improved visualization of detail of structures and lack of superimposition [13]. It was also useful in the identification of bilateral traumatic temporomandibular joint fractures and dislocations in

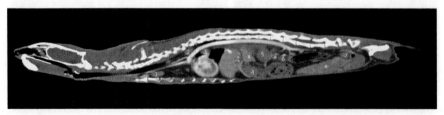

FIG. 10 Parasagittal reconstruction whole body post-contrast CT in a soft tissue algorithm of a ferret with multicentric lymphoma performed for radiation planning purposes. Note the marked multifocal thoracic and abdominal lymphadenopathy, and heterogeneous splenic enhancement. Labeled intrathoracic lymph nodes include the sternal (1), tracheal (2), and middle tracheobronchial (3), with several additional smaller enlarged nodes present within the mediastinal fat. Labeled intraabdominal lymph nodes include a gastric (4), hepatic (5), jejunal (6), and left colic (7). The splenic head and tail are denoted with white asterisks.

a rabbit with prior head trauma and subsequent anorexia [66].

Finally, CT was used in a case of a distal tibial chondrosarcoma, where described features included cavitation and mineralization of a mass arising from the articular surface of the tibial epiphysis, which extended caudolaterally with suspected involvement of the tibiotarsal joint [67].

MRI in Small Mammals

MRI is the gold standard for evaluation of soft tissues due to its excellent contrast resolution; however, its use in small mammals remains limited due to cost, availability, prolonged scanning time, and greater necessity for significant sedation or general anesthesia [14,19]. Although larger scale studies are not present, multiple case reports of its use in small mammals are present and can provide insight into its future use.

MRI was useful in a ferret to diagnose unilateral adrenomegaly diagnosed on histopathology as an adrenal adenoma. Features included an ovoid to circular mass with increased T1w signal intensity relative to the contralateral, presumed normal, adrenal gland [68]. The MRI

appearance of chordomas within the cranial cervical spine in 2 ferrets, and in the thoracic vertebra in 1, have been described [43,69]. Features included multilobulated and invasive extra-axial and extradural masses causing osteolysis of vertebrae and compression of adjacent neural tissue [43,69]. They were isointense to muscle and mildly hypointense to gray matter on T1w sequences, moderately hyperintense to gray matter on T2w, and moderately heterogeneously to faintly rim-contrast enhancing [43,69]. MRI was particularly useful in these cases to identify spinal cord and brainstem compression, which would have been challenging to fully evaluate on CT due to the presence of artifact from surrounding bone. Finally, MRI was superior to radiographs and CT in the identification of atlantoaxial subluxation in a ferret with associated T2w hyperintensity within the spinal cord, presumed to be gliosis from chronic instability [70]. At the authors' institution, MRI has been used to evaluate a ferret with pelvic limb paresis suspected to have either neurologic trauma or an insulinoma. In this case, excellent contrast resolution of the abdomen and detailed evaluation of the lumbar spine helped to rule out grossly visible neurologic or pancreatic disease (Fig. 11).

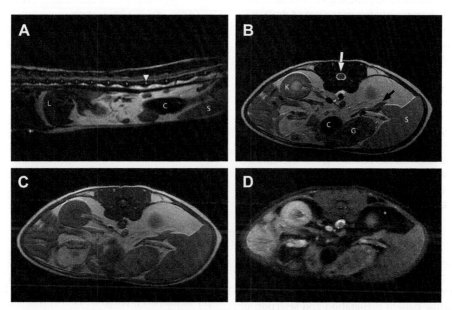

FIG. 11 Sagittal T2w (**A**), transverse T2w (**B**), T1w (**C**), and post-contrast fat saturated T1w (**D**) magnetic resonance images of a ferret for evaluation of pelvic limb paresis. Note the healthy hydrated nuclei pulposi (*white arrowhead* in **A**) and lack of observable dorsal protrusion of the intervertebral discs of the lumbar spine. Evaluation of the hyperintense epidural space/subarachnoid space surrounding the spinal cord is visible in transverse T2w images (*white arrow* in [**B**]). The left limb of the pancreas is visible on transverse images (*black arrow* in [**B**]) and shows slight homogeneous contrast enhancement in (**D**) relative to (**C**). The white asterisk in (**D**) shows the saturation of fat relative to (**C**). Other labels included: C, colon; G, gastric lumen; K, kidney; L, liver; S, spleen.

MRI has also been used to evaluate the size and extent of disease in rabbits with thymomas, and may be considered optimal in these cases relative to CT due to the excellent soft tissue resolution, particularly at higher magnetic field strengths [19]. Additionally, MRI can provide detail including size, location, and extent of retrobulbar or odontogenic abscessation in small mammals, and be used to identify rhinitis and empyema of the nasal cavity or to investigate vestibular signs [14,19,31,71,72]. It can aid in planning surgical approaches using multiplanar reconstructions in cases of retrobulbar abscessation by identifying proximity to structures such as the optic nerve and identifying focal disease that may otherwise be missed in surgery [14,71]. Given the proximity to osseous and gas-filled structures, and potential for bony changes in the skull with local abscessation such as adjacent osteomyelitis, CT may be a useful adjunct diagnostic test in these cases.

Present Relevance and Future Avenues to Consider or to Investigate

Many future avenues remain to be investigated regarding the utility of CT and MRI in the diagnosis of a wide range of diseases and pathologies in small mammals. Large retrospective studies of the use of these modalities in investigating common pathologies would be useful, such as an evaluation of CT findings in ferrets with lymphoma or MRI features of the brain and spinal cord of rabbits diagnosed with *Encephalitozoon cuniculi*. To the authors' knowledge, no CT studies investigating thoracic disease in ferrets have been published, and no literature on CT use in sugar gliders was identified. Further evaluation of additional technology such as the use of PET-CT in clinical small mammal patients could also be considered. Finally, given the limited case reports of MRI in small mammals, future avenues for research using this modality for the diagnosis of disease in clinical patients are widespread.

SUMMARY

CT and MRI are widely increasing in use in clinical small mammal practice for diagnosis of a range of diseases. Particular attention to details of the acquisition of studies, including patient preparation and selection of technologic parameters is particularly important in small mammals due to their size to optimize spatial and contrast resolution. Although CT is commonly used for the evaluation of dental disease in small mammals, many additional uses of CT and MRI have been described, from evaluation of otitis and respiratory difficulty to uses in neoplasia staging, and surgical and

radiation therapy planning. Further research, particularly larger scale retrospective studies, on CT and MRI features of common and uncommon small mammal diseases are broadly needed to further the field of diagnostic cross-sectional imaging and improve the diagnostic capability of veterinarians regarding these species.

CLINICS CARE POINTS

- CT and MRI are useful for evaluation of a wide range of disease processes due to the high level of detail, lack of superimposition, and use of multiplanar reformatting.
- CT is superior to conventional radiography and oral examination in small mammals for the detection of dental disease abnormalities including tooth elongation and associated alveolar bone lysis, periodontal ligament widening, and resorptive tooth lesions.
- Use of intravenous contrast and multidetector CT is preferred for small mammal skulls when evaluating soft tissue structures including the detection and assessment of facial abscessation, retrobulbar disease, and cervical masses.
- MRI has superior contrast resolution relative to CT; it is the modality of choice for evaluation of changes to neurologic tissues, including assessment of spinal cord changes and/or compression, and may be useful for surgical planning for abscessation and/or empyema of the facial region.

DISCLOSURE

The authors have no conflicts of interest or funding sources to disclose.

REFERENCES

[1] Mahdy MAA. Correlation between computed tomography, magnetic resonance imaging and cross-sectional anatomy of the head of the guinea pig (*Cavia porcellus, Linnaeus 1758*). Anat Histol Embryol 2022;51(1):51–61.

[2] Richardson J, Longo M, Liuti T, et al. Computed tomographic grading of middle ear disease in domestic rabbits (*Oryctolagus cuniculi*). Vet Rec 2019;184(22):679.

[3] Knutson KA, Petritz OA, Sadar MJ, et al. Diagnosis and management of nasopharyngeal stenosis in four guinea pigs (*Cavia porcellus*). J Exot Pet Med 2022;40:21–8.

[4] Schweda MC, Hassan J, Böhler A, et al. Paper: The role of computed tomography in the assessment of dental disease in 66 guinea pigs. Vet Rec 2014;175(21):538.

[5] Artiles CA, Sanchez-Migallon Guzman D, Beaufrère H, et al. Computed tomographic findings of dental disease in domestic rabbits (*Oryctolagus cuniculus*): 100 cases (2009–2017). J Am Vet Med Assoc 2020;257(3):313–27.

[6] De Matos R, Ruby J, Van Hatten RA, et al. Computed tomographic features of clinical and subclinical middle ear disease in domestic rabbits (*Oryctolagus cuniculus*): 88 cases (2007–2014). J Am Vet Med Assoc 2015; 246(3):336–43.

[7] Longo M, Thierry F, Eatwell K, et al. Ultrasound and computed tomography of sacculitis and appendicitis in a rabbit. Vet Radiol Ultrasound 2018;59(5):E56–60.

[8] Riggs GG, Arzi B, Cissell DD, et al. Clinical Application of Cone-Beam Computed Tomography of the Rabbit Head: Part 1 – Normal Dentition. Front Vet Sci 2016;3. https://doi.org/10.3389/fvets.2016.00093.

[9] Sasai H, Iwai H, Fujita D, et al. The use of micro-computed tomography in the diagnosis of dental and oral disease in rabbits. BMC Vet Res 2014;10(1):209.

[10] Riggs GG, Cissell DD, Arzi B, et al. Clinical Application of Cone Beam Computed Tomography of the Rabbit Head: Part 2 - Dental Disease. Front Vet Sci 2017;4. https://doi.org/10.3389/fvets.2017.00005.

[11] Sangiorgi ZV, Boss MK, Leary D, et al. Hypofractionated radiation therapy for treatment of an adrenal mass in a ferret. J Exot Pet Med 2021;38:5–8.

[12] Souza MJ, Greenacre CB, Avenell JS, et al. Diagnosing a Tooth Root Abscess in a Guinea Pig (*Cavia porcellus*) Using Micro Computed Tomography Imaging. J Exot Pet Med 2006;15(4):274–7.

[13] Sasai. Characteristics of bone fractures and usefulness of micro CT for fracture detection in rabbits 210 cases. JAVMA 2015;246(12):1339–44.

[14] Capello V. Diagnostic Imaging of Dental Disease in Pet Rabbits and Rodents. Vet Clin Exot Anim Pract 2016; 19(3):757–82.

[15] De Rycke LM, Boone MN, Van Caelenberg AI, et al. Micro-computed tomography of the head and dentition in cadavers of clinically normal rabbits. Am J Vet Res 2012;73(2):227–32.

[16] Wu A, Zheng H, Kraenzle J, et al. Ferret Thoracic Anatomy by 2-Deoxy-2-(18F)Fluoro-D-Glucose (18F-FDG) Positron Emission Tomography/Computed Tomography (18F-FDG PET/CT) Imaging. Available at: https://academic.oup.com/ilarjournal/article/53/1/E9/656111.

[17] Hag AMF, Ripa RS, Pedersen SF, et al. Small animal positron emission tomography imaging and in vivo studies of atherosclerosis. Clin Physiol Funct Imag 2013;33(3): 173–85.

[18] Dyke JP, Synan M, Ezell P, et al. Characterization of bone perfusion by dynamic contrast-enhanced magnetic resonance imaging and positron emission tomography in the Dunkin–Hartley guinea pig model of advanced osteoarthritis. J Orthop Res 2015;33(3):366–72.

[19] Capello V, Lennox AM. Diagnostic Imaging of the Respiratory System in Exotic Companion Mammals. Vet Clin Exot Anim Pract 2011;14(2):369–89.

[20] Karakurum E, Dimitrov R, Stamatova-Yovcheva K, et al. Anatomical Computed Tomography and Magnetic Resonance Imaging Architecture of the Kidneys in the Chinchilla (*Chinchilla lanigera*). IJAR 2022.

[21] Doss GA, Mans C, Hoey S, et al. Vertebral heart size in chinchillas (*Chinchilla lanigera*) using radiography and CT: Heart measurements in chinchillas. J Small Anim Pract 2017;58(12):714–9.

[22] Capello V, Cauduro A. Clinical Technique: Application of Computed Tomography for Diagnosis of Dental Disease in the Rabbit, Guinea Pig, and Chinchilla. J Exot Pet Med 2008;17(2):93–101.

[23] Buch D, Saldanha A, Muehlbauer E, et al. Computed tomographic findings of the urinary tract in rabbits (*Oryctolagus cuniculus*). J Exot Pet Med 2022;40:1–7.

[24] Buch D, Saldanha A, Santos I de A, et al. Computed tomographic findings of the gastrointestinal tract in rabbits (*Oryctolagus cuniculus*). J Exot Pet Med 2022;42(March):11–9.

[25] Chernev C, Procter T, Isaac I, et al. Computed tomographic features of the normal spleen in rabbits (*Oryctolagus cuniculus domesticus*). Vet Radiol Ultrasound 2023; 64(5):844–50.

[26] Van Caelenberg AI, De Rycke LM, Hermans K, et al. Computed tomography and cross-sectional anatomy of the head in healthy rabbits. Am J Vet Res 2010;71(3): 293–303.

[27] Müllhaupt D, Wenger S, Kircher P, et al. Computed tomography of the thorax in rabbits: a prospective study in ten clinically healthy New Zealand White rabbits. Acta Vet Scand 2017;59(1):72.

[28] Dimitrov RS. Computed tomography imaging of the prostate gland in the rabbit (Oryctolagus cuniculus). Vet Arhiv 2010;8(6):771–8.

[29] Zotti A, Banzato T, Cozzi B. Cross-sectional anatomy of the rabbit neck and trunk: Comparison of computed tomography and cadaver anatomy. Res Vet Sci 2009;87(2): 171–6.

[30] Kwan V, Quesenberry K, Le Roux AB. Mensuration of the rabbit pituitary gland from computed tomography. Vet Radiol Ultrasound 2020;61(3):322–8.

[31] Capello V. Rhinostomy as Surgical Treatment of Odontogenic Rhinitis in Three Pet Rabbits. J Exot Pet Med 2014; 23(2):172–87.

[32] Zehtabvar O, Masoudifard M, Rostami A, et al. CT anatomy of the lungs, bronchi and trachea in the Mature Guinea pig (*Cavia porcellus*). Veterinary Medicine & Sci 2023;9(3):1179–93.

[33] Abd El-Hameed ZS, El-Shafey AAE, Metwally MA, et al. Anatomy of the rabbit inner ear using computed tomography and magnetic resonance imaging. Anat Histol Embryol 2023;52(3):403–10.

[34] Crossley DA, Jackson A, Yates J, et al. Use of computed tomography to investigate cheek tooth abnormalities in chinchillas (*Chinchilla lanigera*). J Small Anim Pract 1998;39(8):385–9.

[35] Van Caelenberg A, De Rycke L, Hermans K, et al. Comparison of Radiography and CT to Identify Changes in

the Skulls of Four Rabbits with Dental Disease. J Vet Dent 2011;28(3):172–81.

[36] Capello V, Cauduro A. Comparison of Diagnostic Consistency and Diagnostic Accuracy Between Survey Radiography and Computed Tomography of the Skull in 30 Rabbits With Dental Disease. J Exot Pet Med 2016; 25(2):115–27.

[37] Bertram CA, Klopfleisch R, Erickson NA, et al. Leiomyosarcoma of the external ear canal as a cause of otitis externa, media, interna in a chinchilla (*Chinchilla lanigera*). J Exot Pet Med 2019;31:13–6.

[38] Rockwell K, Wells A, Dearmin M. Total Ear Canal Ablation and Temporary Bulla Fenestration for Treatment of Otitis Media in a Chinchilla (*Chinchilla lanigera*). J Exot Pet Med 2019;29:173–7.

[39] Holmberg BJ, Hollingsworth SR, Osofsky A, et al. Taenia coenurus in the orbit of a chinchilla. Vet Ophthalmol 2007;10(1):53–9.

[40] Kuonen VJ, Wilkie DA, Morreale RJ, et al. Unilateral exophthalmia in a European hedgehog (*Erinaceus europaeus*) caused by a lacrimal ductal carcinoma. Vet Ophthalmol 2002;5(3):161–5.

[41] Schmidt L, Doss G, Hawkins S, et al. Cranial cervical abscessation and sialadenitis due to Pseudomonas luteola in two domestic ferrets (Mustela putorius furo). J Exot Pet Med 2019;31:120–6.

[42] Gardhouse S, Guzman DSM, Petritz OA, et al. Diagnosis and Treatment of Sialectasis in a Domestic Rabbit (*Oryctolagus cuniculus*). J Exot Pet Med 2016;25(1):72–9.

[43] Yarto-Jaramillo E, Graham J, McEntee MC, et al. Diagnosis of cervical chordoma in domestic ferrets (*Mustela putorius furo*): 3 cases. J Exot Pet Med 2022;41:48–53.

[44] Lacqua A, Dreizen R, Helmer P. Surgical and medical management of an oral spindle cell sarcoma in an African hedgehog (*Atelerix albiventris*). Veterinary Medicine & Sci 2022;8(3):1079–84.

[45] Harrison TM, Dominguez P, Hanzlik K, et al. Treatment of an Amelanotic Melanoma Using Radiation Therapy in a Lesser Madagascar Hedgehog Tenrec (*Echinops telfairi*). J Zoo Wildl Med 2010;41(1):152–7.

[46] De Voe RS, Pack LA, Greenacre CB. Radiographic and CT imaging of a skull associated osteoma in a ferret. Vet Radiol Ultrasound 2002;43(4):346–8.

[47] Paushter A, Early P, Perkins T, et al. Surgical Resection of a Parietal Osteoma in a Domestic Ferret Using Advanced Neurosurgical Techniques. J Am Anim Hosp Assoc 2021; 57(2):91–5.

[48] Johnson JG, Brandão J, Fowlkes N, et al. Calvarial Osteoma with Cranial Vault Invasion in the Skull of a Ferret (*Mustela putorius furo*). J Exot Pet Med 2014;23(3): 266–9.

[49] Capello V, Lennox A, Ghisleni G. Elodontoma in Two Guinea Pigs. J Vet Dent 2015;32(2):111–9.

[50] Zaheer OA, Ludwig L, Gardhouse S, et al. Diagnosis, treatment, and characterization with advanced diagnostic imaging of an oral ectopic elodontoma in a pet rabbit (*Oryctolagus cuniculus*). J Exot Pet Med 2021;37:28–31.

[51] Athinodorou A., Richardson J., Schwarz T., et al., Clinical and computed tomographic findings of rabbits with pulmonary emphysema. In: Proceedings in the 2022 EVDI Annual Conference. 2022.

[52] Guillerit F, Gros L, Touzet C, et al. Spontaneous pneumothorax pet rabbits (*Oryctolagus cuniculus*): four cases (2017–2022). J Exot Pet Med 2023;45:30–7.

[53] Daggett A, Loeber S, Le Roux AB, et al. Computed tomography with Hounsfield unit assessment is useful in the diagnosis of liver lobe torsion in pet rabbits (*Oryctolagus cuniculus*). Vet Radiol Ultrasound 2021;62(2):210–7.

[54] Sailler A, Risi E, Magrans J, et al. Surgical management of a pararenal pseudocyst in a ferret (Mustela Putorius Furo). J Exot Pet Med 2019;30:60–4.

[55] Bernhard C, Linsart A, Mentré V. Circumcaval ureter in two ferrets. J Exot Pet Med 2022;42:42–6.

[56] Vekšins A, Makarovs A, Sandersen C, et al. Extramural ectopic ureter diagnosed by computed tomography in a domestic ferret. Veterinary Record Case Reports 2022; 10(3). https://doi.org/10.1002/vrc2.413.

[57] Miwa Y, Uchida K, Nakayama H, et al. Neuroblastoma of the Adrenal Gland in a Ferret. J Vet Med Sci 2010;72(9): 1229–32.

[58] Song SH, Park NW, Jung SK, et al. Bilateral Malignant Ovarian Teratoma With Peritoneal Metastasis in a Captive African Pygmy Hedgehog (*Atelerix albiventris*). J Exot Pet Med 2014;23(4):403–8.

[59] Zoller G, Langlois I, Alexander K. Glomerular filtration rate determination by computed tomography in two pet rabbits with renal disease. J Am Vet Med Assoc 2017;250(6):681–7.

[60] Suran JN, Wyre NR. Imaging findings in 14 domestic ferrets (mustela putorius furo) with lymphoma. Vet Radiol Ultrasound 2013;54(5):522–31.

[61] Liatis T, Gardini A, Marçal VC, et al. Surgical Treatment of a Vertebral Fracture Caused by Osseous Plasmacytoma in a Domestic Ferret (Mustela Putorius Furo). J Exot Pet Med 2019;29:202–6.

[62] Gnirs K, Quinton JF, Dally C, et al. Cerebral pyogranuloma associated with systemic coronavirus infection in a ferret. J Small Anim Pract 2016;57(1):36–9.

[63] Van Zeeland Y, Schoemaker N, Passon-Vastenburg M, et al. Vestibular Syndrome Due to a Choroid Plexus Papilloma in a Ferret. J Am Vet Med Assoc 2009;45(2): 97–101.

[64] Stern H, Sanchez-Migallon Guzman D, Gleeson M, et al. Cervical spinal nerve and brachial plexus schwannoma in a rabbit (*Oryctolagus cuniculus*). J Exot Pet Med 2019; 31:75–8.

[65] Browning GR, Carpenter JW, Tucker-Mohl K, et al. Skeletal metastasis and spinal cord compression due to uterine adenocarcinoma in a domestic rabbit (*Oryctolagus cuniculus*). J Exot Pet Med 2021;36:60–1.

[66] Monge E, Loc'h GL, Pignon C. Successful conservative management of a bilateral temporomandibular joint dislocation in a pet rabbit (*Oryctolagus cuniculus*). J Exot Pet Med 2022;40:76–9.

[67] Maguire R, Reavill DR, Maguire P, et al. Chondrosarcoma associated with the appendicular skeleton of 2 domestic ferrets. J Exot Pet Med 2014;23(2):165–71.

[68] Neuwirth L, Isaza R, Bellah J, et al. Adrenal neoplasia in seven ferrets. Vet Radiol Ultrasound 1993;34(5):340–6.

[69] Pye G, Bennett R, Roberts G, et al. Thoracic vertebral chordoma in a domestic ferret (*Mustela putorius furo*). J Zoo Wildl Med 2000;31(1):107–11.

[70] Jayson SL, Dennis R, Mateo I, et al. Atlantoaxial subluxation with complex occipitoatlantoaxial malformation in two domestic ferrets (*Mustela putorius furo*). Vet Record Case Reports 2018;6(1):e000530.

[71] Capello V, Lennox A. Advanced diagnostic imaging and surgical treatment of an odontogenic retromasseteric abscess in a guinea pig. J Small Anim Pract 2015;56(2):134–7.

[72] Boncea AM, Măcinic M, Ifteme CV, et al. Inflammatory polyp in the middle ear of a chinchilla: A case report. J Exot Pet Med 2019;31:79–81.

Advances in Small Animal Care 5 (2024) 67–77

ADVANCES IN SMALL ANIMAL CARE

Artificial Intelligence in Diagnostic Imaging

Ryan B. Appleby, DVM, DACVR[a],*, Parminder S. Basran, PhD, FCCPM[b]

[a]Department of Clinical Studies, Ontario Veterinary College, University of Guelph, 50 Stone Road East, Guelph, Ontario, Canada N1G 2W1; [b]Section of Medical Oncology, Department of Clinical Sciences, Cornell University College of Veterinary Medicine, 930 Campus Road, Box 31, Ithaca, NY, USA

KEYWORDS

- Artificial intelligence • Machine learning • Deep learning • Convolutional neural networks
- Computer-aided diagnosis • Radiomics

KEY POINTS

- Artificial intelligence (AI) is the branch of computer science aimed at performing tasks ordinarily requiring human intelligence.
- This field can be applied to veterinary diagnostic imaging to improve efficiency, image quality, and diagnosis.
- Uses include image acquisition optimization and improvement, computer-aided diagnosis, radiomic analysis, and workflow optimization.
- While there is enormous potential for AI in veterinary imaging, current uses are limited by a lack of evidence and lack of transparency.
- Further work in this field should involve establishing evidence-based practices to ensure appropriate and ethical use of the technology.

INTRODUCTION

Artificial intelligence (AI) represents a potentially revolutionary shift in the landscape of diagnostic imaging. Through leveraging large digital imaging datasets, AI adoption in this space is one of the first in veterinary medicine. In veterinary medicine, AI promises to enhance diagnostic accuracy, efficiency, and overall patient care, offering advancements over traditional diagnostic methods. By leveraging algorithms that can learn from vast datasets, AI has the potential to identify patterns and anomalies that might elude the human eye, facilitating early detection of conditions that were previously challenging to diagnose.

Despite its potential, the adoption of AI in veterinary imaging is met with several challenges [1]. Infrastructure limitations, such as the lack of digital integration in many veterinary practices, the lack of AI-enabled picture archiving and communications software (PACS), and the need for significant investment in technology, pose considerable barriers. Furthermore, the development and implementation of AI technologies require a solid evidence base, underscoring the need for rigorous research and validation to ensure these tools are both effective and reliable. Critical evaluation of AI tools is essential, requiring not only technical assessments but also considerations of their practicality, usability, and impact on veterinary workflows.

Another layer of complexity is introduced by the ethical considerations [2] surrounding AI's use in veterinary medicine. Questions of data privacy, informed consent, the potential for bias in AI algorithms, and the untested legal landscape necessitate careful

---

*Corresponding author, E-mail address: rappleby@uoguelph.ca

https://doi.org/10.1016/j.yasa.2024.06.005
2666-450X/24/

attention to ensure that these technologies benefit patients and support veterinarians and specialists as humans in the loop. There is an ongoing need for collaboration among technologists, clinicians, computing, and data scientists, and regulatory bodies to establish standards and guidelines for the ethical use of AI in veterinary settings.

The benefits of AI in veterinary diagnostic imaging, however, are compelling. For one, AI can significantly enhance the quality of diagnostic images and improve the efficiency and accuracy of interpretation. Through AI-based techniques, we can improve image quality or the speed of acquisition. Additionally, AI-driven tools have the potential to automate aspects of the diagnostic process, from optimizing imaging parameters in real time to providing preliminary assessments, thereby speeding up diagnosis. In theory, this may allow veterinarians and veterinary radiologists to focus on other aspects of their job, including patient care and client communication.

AI algorithms have shown promise in aiding diagnosis by identifying and classifying a wide range of conditions. This capability could lead to more precise diagnoses, better informed treatment decisions, and improved patient outcomes. However, these systems are unproven, with very few internal performance metrics provided by developers and even fewer external validation studies. No studies to date have evaluated the clinical effect of AI tools in veterinary imaging.

The success of AI in transforming veterinary diagnostic imaging depends not only on technological advancements but also on addressing the challenges that currently impede its adoption. This includes developing a clear understanding of AI's potential and limitations, ensuring the availability of high-quality data for training AI models, and fostering collaboration across disciplines to drive innovation. Importantly, developing technologies in adherence to good machine learning (ML) practices [3] and based on use cases developed by domain experts [2], which will foster improvements in veterinary practice, are important parts of ensuring the success of imaging AI. Professional and public trust in AI algorithms should be fostered with transparency [4] to engender trust from both professionals and the public.

This article aims to explore the current state of AI in veterinary diagnostic imaging comprehensively. It discusses the technological underpinnings of AI, its applications in enhancing diagnostic workflows, and the potential benefits it offers to veterinary medicine. Simultaneously, we will critically examine the barriers to AI's adoption, including infrastructure challenges, the need for evidence-based development, and ethical considerations. By providing a balanced perspective on both the opportunities and obstacles presented by AI, this work seeks to contribute to the ongoing dialogue on how to best leverage this technology in veterinary diagnostic imaging. In doing so, it underscores the importance of evidence-based practices, interdisciplinary collaboration, and ethical frameworks in realizing the full potential of AI to improve patient care in veterinary medicine.

SIGNIFICANCE
Key Concepts in Artificial Intelligence
AI is a collection of technologies for which a single universal definition is not agreed upon [5]. The authors suggest considering AI as a branch of computer science in which computer programs are designed to perform tasks that previously would have required human-level intelligence [5,6]. At the core of AI's transformative potential in veterinary imaging are several pivotal concepts and technologies that warrant a comprehensive understanding.

Machine learning (ML) is a subfield of AI that uses algorithms trained on datasets to create models that can continually improve when new information is added [7]. Common ML techniques include neural networks, support vector machines, and decision trees (classification and regression) [7]. These techniques can be used in a supervised, unsupervised, or semi-supervised manner. In the latter 2 instances, the advantage lies in being able to discern patterns and optimize algorithms without specific direction from a statistician or a computer scientist [7].

Deep learning (DL), a subset of ML, further refines this capability through the implementation of *artificial neural networks (ANNs)*, so named because they simulate the neural architecture of the human brain [6]. DL occurs on a neural network at least 10 layers deep, but in practice, usually dozens to hundreds of layers. This allows for an even more nuanced analysis of complex data patterns, making DL especially potent in processing and interpreting diagnostic images. Another important DL architecture is a *transformer*, which is primarily used for language and text analysis but may also be used for image classification and object detection tasks. These architectures are important in *natural language processing (NLP)* and *large language models (LLMs)*, such as Chat generative pre-trained transformer (ChatGPT).

Convolutional neural networks (CNNs), a specialized form of ANNs, are particularly adept at handling image data. Through the utilization of convolutional layers, CNNs can extract hierarchical features from images, a quality that enhances their utility in identifying specific imaging markers. This precision makes CNNs an indispensable tool in the AI toolkit for veterinary diagnostic imaging. In fact, a majority of applications in diagnostic imaging use CNNs.

Transfer learning [8] represents another key concept in AI and is of particular importance for veterinary imaging. Given the challenges associated with assembling large, annotated datasets in veterinary medicine, transfer learning offers a pragmatic solution by adapting models pretrained on extensive datasets from other domains. This approach not only accelerates the development of robust diagnostic models but also circumvents the resource-intensive process of model training from scratch.

Artificial Intelligence Model Development

To understand AI systems in veterinary imaging, it may be helpful to consider how one may create an AI system (Fig. 1). First, one starts with a use case or purpose of the software. Let us take, for example, an AI algorithm to detect pulmonary nodules in dogs and cats. Once this use case is established, diagnostic images must be collected to form a dataset. In this example, the dataset should consist of thoracic radiographs and ideally be diverse based on the source (multi-institutional) as well as diverse in quality to support adoption in a real-world clinical setting. Once the dataset is established, labeling of the images should be performed, and the images should be labeled by domain experts (radiologists in this example). Labeling could include segmentation of nodules within an image (outlining and delineating the location of the nodules), labeling each image as having nodules or no nodules, or analyzing radiology reports associated with the images

for sentiment analysis. Data labeling is one of the most time-consuming and challenging aspects of AI algorithm development.

Once the labeled dataset is available, it can be divided into subsegments for training and testing. Aspects of the dataset involved in training should not overlap with those involved in testing. Overlap of these segments can result in an artificial increase in model performance. Typically, transfer learning will then be used using pretrained models adapted to the specific use case. In the case of nodule identification, a DL classification model using a CNN would be applied.

Once the model's performance is optimized, the system could be tested in a clinical environment to determine its efficacy and effect. For nodule identification, this would involve comparing detection rates prospectively in a clinical setting between primary practitioners and the model, and between veterinary radiologists and the model. This last step is often lacking from current iterations of AI in veterinary diagnostic imaging, which will be discussed later in this manuscript. Additionally, once a model is deployed in a clinical setting, ongoing error monitoring assessing the performance of the AI to ensure it maintains a high level of performance is necessary for ongoing use. This process, if it is occurring with current iterations of AI systems, is opaque and end users of AI products are not provided clear error monitoring assessments.

Transparency and Ethics

Navigating the intricacies of transparency and ethics within the domain of AI in veterinary diagnostic imaging is complex and representative of the broader dialogue on the responsible integration of technology in health care. As AI technologies become increasingly

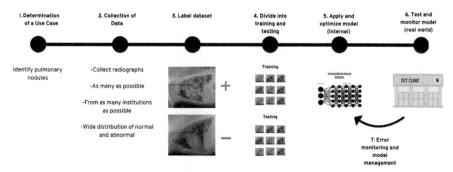

FIG. 1 A simplified 7 step process of AI model development. Following the determination of a use case, data are collected and labeled by domain experts. The data are then divided into training and testing sets without overlap. A model is trained and then tested on the appropriate datasets. Once the model is sufficient for its intended application, the model is deployed and tested in a real-world setting. Error monitoring of the model in practice allows continued improvement of the model and prevents data shift.

embedded in veterinary medicine's diagnostic processes, the imperative for ethical considerations and transparency becomes paramount, ensuring these advancements serve the best interests of patients, practitioners, and the field at large.

Transparency, in the context of AI in veterinary diagnostic imaging, pertains to the clarity and openness with which the development, functionalities, and decision-making processes of AI tools are communicated to the stakeholders. It is crucial for veterinary professionals to understand how AI models are trained, the data they are trained on, and the rationale behind their diagnostic suggestions. This transparency is foundational not only for trust but also for the effective clinical application of AI technologies, allowing practitioners to make informed decisions about incorporating AI into their diagnostic workflow. The essence of transparency extends to the disclosure of limitations and uncertainties associated with AI models. Given the complexity of ML algorithms and their reliance on data quality and quantity [6], acknowledging the potential for error and bias is vital. This acknowledgment fosters a culture of cautious optimism, where AI tools are utilized judiciously, with a clear understanding of their scope and limitations.

Transparency for AI in health care supports accountability, choice, safety, and quality [4]. While transparency in human health applications is necessitated by regulatory processes and the regulation of AI applications as "software as a medical device", the same frameworks do not apply in veterinary medicine. Therefore, additional care must be taken to ensure transparency in the deployment of AI for veterinary imaging. Kiseleva and colleagues [4] describe 3 types of transparency in health care.

Insider transparency [4] is the AI's transparency to the software developers. Developers of AI in veterinary imaging must understand the system's functionalities and decision-making. This may prove challenging as many AI systems are natively "black box" in nature, meaning that their processes and reasons for decisions are inherently opaque. Developers must take additional measures to ensure transparency and understanding of their systems.

This understanding should extend to veterinary professionals in the form of *internal transparency* [4]. In human medicine, this form of transparency remains governed by strict regulatory frameworks. However, as no such framework exists in veterinary medicine, we can instead look to the guiding principles of Good Machine Learning Practice established by the US Federal Drug Administration, Health Canada, and the UK Medical and Healthcare products Regulatory Agency [3].

These principles provide a guideline for developers that can aid in transparency and therefore support accountability, choice, safety, and quality.

Only with both *insider* and *internal* transparency should AI systems be deployed in a clinical setting for veterinary imaging. Without these forms of transparency, it is impossible to have *external transparency* [4] and obtain informed consent from owners for a diagnostic test.

Ethical considerations in this field encompass a spectrum of issues [2], from data privacy and security to algorithmic fairness and the mitigation of bias. The ethical collection, storage, and use of diagnostic images for AI training necessitate data protection measures. The ethical deployment of AI tools in veterinary practice directly ties into transparency, where use of an AI tool for which there can be no informed consent may be considered an ethical violation. As Cohen and Gordon [2] point out, ethical considerations for imaging AI in veterinary medicine are in stark contrast to human medicine given the ability to euthanize in veterinary medicine.

Accountability in the use of AI also plays a critical role in ethical considerations, with questions arising about responsibility and liability for diagnostic outcomes. Establishing clear guidelines and standards for AI in veterinary imaging, including the delineation of roles and responsibilities among AI developers, veterinary professionals, and regulatory bodies, is essential for navigating these ethical waters. No single adopted framework is used today, and no legal precedent has been set. Nonetheless, a framework for responsibility has been proposed [2] based on the level of automation in the AI system. Systems with higher automation should hold more responsibility for clinical outcomes.

AI adoption is a paradigm shift, and as the adoption into veterinary diagnostic imaging becomes more common, the principles of transparency and ethics will become increasingly important and require veterinarians to consider the integration of these technologies in a manner not often encountered with the adoption of less transformative technologies. As these systems are developed and adopted, acting from a principle of prioritizing health outcomes and supporting veterinarians is of utmost importance.

Use Cases

AI has many potential applications in veterinary imaging [9]. To date, most of these remain in the domain of research but have clear implications for clinical practice if the challenges of adoption can be overcome. One way of considering the potential use cases of AI in veterinary imaging is to consider the possible points of intervention where AI can assist by improving efficiency or diagnostic accuracy (Fig. 2).

At the point of image acquisition, AI can aid in image optimization by correcting positioning or improving the signal-to-noise ratio within imaging. Additionally, AI may improve efficiency at this level by automated aspects of the image acquisition process. Both prior to and following the acquisition, AI can aid in workflow optimization to prioritize cases for interpretation, improve image display through orientation correction and image sorting, as well as improve the scheduling of cases. Following the acquisition, workflows can be optimized through improved reporting and communications. AI systems can aid in diagnosis by identifying abnormalities in images (computeraided diagnosis [CAD]). Features of images can also be analyzed to identify patterns not visible to the human eye (radiomics). Finally, generative AI may be used in a research capacity or offer a glimpse into the possible future of imaging AI where generalist models may be deployed to perform a wide variety of interpretive tasks or improve reporting efficiency.

In this section, we will review these major use cases, providing examples from the literature.

IMAGE ACQUISITION

Radiography remains a cornerstone in veterinary diagnostics; however, the variability in radiographic quality—attributable to factors such as patient positioning, exposure settings, and motion artifacts—can significantly impede diagnostic clarity [10]. While still primarily research focused, AI can be developed to detect changes in radiographic quality [11–13] at the point of image acquisition. This can improve the quality of images interpreted by veterinarians and radiologists. This may, in turn, support more accurate diagnosis or increased confidence in diagnosis. AI systems may also be used to optimize exposure parameters and image-processing techniques. These systems are already being deployed by major vendors. However, peer-reviewed publications on their effects are lacking. Instead, subjective image quality and changes in signal-to-noise ratios are used as criteria for adoption.

Many modern MRI systems utilize AI to support improved signal-to-noise ratios [14] and faster acquisition times [15]. These technologies have shown improved imaging for both spine [16] and brain [17] MRI in dogs. Similarly, AI-based reconstruction algorithms can improve computed tomographic (CT) image quality [18,19]. This has been especially valuable in pediatric imaging for people [20] where reducing radiation dose while maintaining image quality is a top priority. This same focus is not present in veterinary imaging, though some have suggested the need to reconsider the degree of concern for ionizing radiation exposure [21]. Newer CT systems and software upgrades will likely employ AI-based reconstruction as these methods are adopted for human health care. Therefore, AI-based reconstruction of CT images may have an increasing role in veterinary imaging in the future.

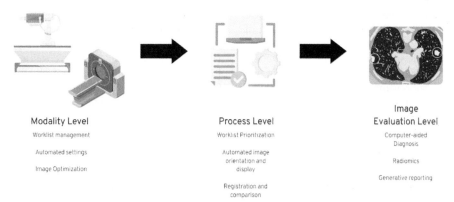

Modality Level	Process Level	Image Evaluation Level
Worklist management	Worklist Prioritization	Computer-aided Diagnosis
Automated settings	Automated image orientation and display	Radiomics
Image Optimization	Registration and comparison	Generative reporting

FIG. 2 Some examples of possible applications of AI in veterinary imaging workflows. At the imaging modality, AI can assist in worklist management, automated settings, and image quality optimization. Once images are acquired, AI can assist in worklist prioritization for radiologists, automated orientation and display, and registration of images with comparison studies. At the point of image evaluation, AI can provide CAD (for example pulmonary nodule detection in CT demonstrated by the *yellow circles* in the image evaluation level graphic), radiomic analysis, or assist in reporting through generative AI systems. These examples are not exhaustive for either the points of intervention or the possible uses at each level.

WORKFLOW OPTIMIZATION

Workflow optimization in veterinary diagnostic imaging encompasses the strategic use of AI to streamline processes, enhance efficiency, and improve the overall quality of patient care. While there are many potential applications, many remain theoretic. AI may be applied to image acquisition, segmentation and measurement, image presentation (including rotation and hanging protocols), worklist triage, and the registration and monitoring of diseases overtime [22].

As noted earlier, the initial step in diagnostic imaging, image acquisition, can benefit from AI applications. Aside from post-processing optimization of image quality, AI can also assist in optimizing case prioritization and scheduling, particularly in high-volume or emergency settings. By analyzing incoming cases based on urgency and complexity, AI algorithms can assist in prioritizing critical cases. AI algorithms can also assist technicians and veterinarians at the point of care by automatically adjusting imaging parameters. A current example of this is seen in the veterinary workflow with automatic thickness detection from MiREYE imaging where AI software detects patient thickness and selects imaging parameters without human intervention [23]. This has the potential to speed up image acquisition.

Once images have been obtained and optimized for quality, AI can help present them. An example of this is seen with IDEXX Web PACS that automatically hangs radiographs in a set orientation, reportedly saving up to 25% of time spent manipulating images according to unreleased internal data [24]. To the authors' knowledge, no published report on this application is available.

AI can also play a pivotal role in ensuring critical cases are reviewed promptly. Worklist prioritization of radiographs [25] and CT [26,27] has been demonstrated to be valuable in human health care. There is the potential for similar use cases to be explored in veterinary medicine, supporting improved reporting time by radiologists for critical cases.

The integration of AI into report generation has the potential to facilitate the creation of structured, comprehensive, and easy-to-understand reports [28,29]. NLP algorithms can be deployed to structure or annotate reports automatically. This not only speeds up the reporting process but also enhances the clarity of communication among radiologists, referring veterinarians, and pet owners, improving the decision-making process for patient care.

Despite its potential, implementing AI for workflow optimization in veterinary diagnostic imaging is not without challenges. These include the need for significant upfront investment in technology, the integration of AI tools into existing practice management systems or PACS, and staff training to use these tools effectively.

COMPUTER-AIDED DIAGNOSIS

CAD refers to software systems that provide outputs that aid clinicians in making a diagnosis. This can include detection systems, which identify regions of images that are of concern, and diagnosis systems, which identify pathology in medical images. The adoption of CAD in veterinary imaging can enhance diagnostic accuracy and efficiency. However, evidence-based practice for the adoption of this technology is currently lacking.

Currently, many commercial applications are available to veterinarians using CAD systems in thoracic, abdominal, and musculoskeletal radiography. While dozens of conditions are identified by these systems, none have released enough information to support *internal transparency* and even fewer have undergone the rigors of peer review. Veterinarians should know the current evidence for AI systems when considering adoption into clinical practice.

Antech's RapidRead system (https://info.antechimagingservices.com/rapidread/) identifies 50 radiographic findings, the majority of which are thoracic in origin. A single preprint (non-peer-reviewed publication) on the development and internal performance of this model is available [30].

Vetology AI (https://vetology.ai) does not clearly delineate the number of findings for its AI system. However, there are 3 peer-reviewed publications externally validating the performance of models for pulmonary edema (accuracy: 92%, positive predictive value (PPV): 56%, negative predictive value (NPV): 99%) [31], pleural effusion (accuracy: 88%, PPV: 90%, NPV: 81%) [32], and pulmonary nodules (accuracy: 69%, PPV: 94%, NPV: 54%) [33].

Picoxia (https://picoxia.com) similarly has 3 peer-reviewed publications on its performance, yet boasts 39 radiographic patterns identified on its Web site. The model has been shown to have a lower error rate than veterinarians for the identification of 15 thoracic findings [34]. Interestingly, the highest error rate was seen with veterinarians aided by the AI system, potentially pointing to a need for caution in primary practitioners' clinical adoption of AI systems. The Picoxia system also has a higher error rate for most findings when compared to veterinary radiologists [35] and has been shown to have good agreement with human evaluators for measurements of cardiac size [36].

Radimal (https://radimal.ai) identifies 28 conditions in dogs and 15 in cats, for which no current performance metrics have been published.

SignalPET (https://www.signalpet.com) identifies 61 abnormalities in thoracic, abdominal, and musculoskeletal radiography. No published performance metrics are currently available, though an abstract presented at the 2023 American College of Veterinary Radiology Conference showed promise for the model's accuracy. SignalPet also offers a CAD system for dental radiography for which no performance metrics are available.

While some of these systems have been externally validated, none have undergone clinical evaluation. That is, the system's effects on a veterinary workflow have not been established, and therefore, the real-life implications of such technology on patient outcomes are unknown. While strict regulations govern aspects of transparency and accountability in human health, AI systems used in human medicine also suffer from a paucity of clinical evaluation [37]. Therefore, this is a challenge across health care professions when it comes to AI adoption. One key difference between AI for veterinary and human diagnostic imaging is the targeted end user of CAD systems. In human health, the end user is a domain expert (radiologist), whereas in veterinary medicine, the end user is typically a general practitioner veterinarian without domain expertise in radiology. Whether this application will result in the best patient outcomes has not been investigated. The increased error rate of veterinarians aided by the Picoxia AI system in a nonclinical setting [34] raises some concerns for this method of adoption. CAD systems supporting radiologists to improve efficiency and accuracy offer a potential avenue of research and investigation.

RADIOMICS

Radiomics refers to the extraction and analysis of quantitative features from medical images using advanced computational methods [38]. In veterinary diagnostic imaging, radiomics offers a promising avenue to uncover patterns and information within diagnostic images that are not perceptible to the human eye. This approach transforms images into high-dimensional data, enabling the application of ML models to predict disease characteristics, treatment responses, and patient outcomes.

Radiomics begins with the extraction of a wide array of features from images, such as texture, shape, and intensity. These features can provide detailed information about a tissue's heterogeneity and architecture, which are often indicative of underlying pathologies. In veterinary medicine, radiomics can be applied to various imaging modalities, including CT, MRI, ultrasound, and radiography.

Radiomics has the potential to significantly impact several aspects of veterinary diagnostics. Tumor characterization is a primary focus of radiomics. By analyzing the textural features of tumors in diagnostic images, radiomics can help distinguish between benign and malignant masses and between types of tumors, predict tumor aggressiveness, and identify genetic mutations. Examples include the differentiation between meningiomas and gliomas [39], grades of meningioma [40–42], differentiating feline intestinal lymphoma from inflammatory bowel disease [43], differentiating types of splenic masses [44] and hepatic masses [45], as well as differentiating between inflammatory and neoplastic brain disease [46]. Nonneoplastic diseases have also been differentiated using radiomic analysis including spinal cord diseases [47] and pulmonary changes [48]. To date, these use cases remain the domain of research with no commercially available products for veterinarians or veterinary radiologists.

Disease progression and prognostication are two areas in which radiomics may be applied in the future. A lack of clinical follow-up limits the ability to develop meaningful models in veterinary medicine for progression and prognostics. Purposeful data collection may be valuable to promote the development of such models in the future.

Despite its potential, the implementation of radiomics in veterinary medicine faces several challenges [38]. The quality and consistency of diagnostic images are critical for reliable feature extraction, necessitating standardized imaging protocols. Additionally, the development of robust ML models requires large, annotated datasets, which can be difficult to obtain in veterinary practice.

Moreover, there is a need for interdisciplinary collaboration [49] to ensure the clinical relevance of radiomic features and models. Veterinary radiologists, clinicians, and data scientists must work together to validate radiomic findings in clinical settings and integrate them into diagnostic workflows.

GENERATIVE ARTIFICIAL INTELLIGENCE

Generative AI represents a subset of AI technologies that focus on generating new data that are similar to but not identical to the data on which they were trained. The most widely known generative AI model is an LLM, GPT, from OpenAI. This transformative technology has been at the forefront of a technological revolution since its launch in late 2022. Some suggest that generative AI will be a centerpiece of the future of medical imaging, with generalist models accepting multimodal data sources (non-imaging data, imaging, and clinical history) and supporting radiologists, primary practitioners, and patients/clients [50]. While this future may be realized, stepwise advancements with generative AI may also play a role by impacting both the educational and clinical aspects of the field.

One of the exciting applications of generative AI in diagnostic imaging is the generation of synthetic images [51–53]. These images can be used to augment datasets for training other AI models, particularly in situations where real-world data are scarce or difficult to obtain, the heterogeneity in the data is high, datasets are not annotated or labeled sufficiently well, large imbalances in, for example, healthy and pathologic patients, and difficulties in gathering data from highly vulnerable patients [54]. In veterinary medicine, where there are additional challenges to dataset creation, this may have additional value compared to human health care. Synthetic data can augment data sources to overcome biases. For example, synthetic overexposure and underexposure of radiographs can improve the robustness of models for a wider range of image quality [11].

Generative AI also holds potential for veterinary education. By producing high-quality, condition-specific images, these systems can offer veterinary students and professionals a resource for study. For instance, generative AI could create a series of images illustrating the progression of a particular disease, providing learners with a comprehensive view of its development and manifestations. This can enhance understanding and diagnostic skills, especially for less experienced practitioners or in the context of continuing education.

In addition to data augmentation and educational support, generative AI can enhance diagnostic capabilities directly. Techniques such as image-to-image translation can be used to convert between different imaging modalities, such as generating a synthetic CT image from an MRI [55,56]. This capability could allow veterinarians to gain the insights offered by multiple modalities from a single scan, reducing the need for multiple imaging sessions and thereby minimizing stress for the patient, radiation dose, and costs for pet owners. Generative AI can also be directly applied to radiology reporting where LLMs may assist in report generation, summarization, plain language translation, and more [57,58].

Despite its potential, the application of generative AI in veterinary diagnostic imaging comes with challenges. Ensuring the accuracy and reliability of synthetic images is paramount, as inaccuracies could lead to misdiagnosis or misinterpretation. Additionally, ethical considerations must be addressed, particularly regarding the transparency of synthetic data usage and the potential for bias in generated images.

FUTURE CONSIDERATIONS

As noted earlier, a distinction must be made between potential and reality regarding AI in veterinary imaging. While it is feasible to create accurate AI models, their real-world applications can vary. While this remains an important avenue of research and consideration in human health [59], clinical assessments of AI technologies in veterinary medicine are lacking. As we consider the impact of these technologies on both present and future applications, it is essential to address the critical distinction between internal and clinical validation of AI tools, a factor that significantly influences the transition of AI from research to real-world clinical practice.

The journey of an AI tool from development to clinical implementation should involve a rigorous validation process. Internal validation, the initial phase, assesses an AI model's performance within the dataset or environment on which it was trained. This step is pivotal for debugging and refining the AI algorithm, ensuring it performs as expected in a controlled setting. This is the key component of *insider transparency*, as described earlier. However, internal validation alone is insufficient to determine how an AI model will perform in the dynamic, variable conditions of clinical practice.

Clinical validation extends beyond the controlled conditions of internal validation, testing the AI tool in real-world clinical settings. This phase evaluates the model's accuracy, usability, and impact on diagnostic and therapeutic outcomes across a diverse range of cases, including variations in breeds, patient sizes, imaging systems, and disease states not necessarily represented in the training dataset. Importantly, it also ensures appropriate human–AI interaction. Clinical validation is essential for ensuring that AI tools are robust, reliable, and truly enhance clinical practice.

Challenges with using any AI model in the clinic are influenced by the quality of data used to develop that model. When the performance of a model fails to achieve the performance claimed by manufacturers or developers, a common culprit is the phenomenon of "data shift." Data shift refers to a mismatch between the distribution of data a model was developed on and the distribution of data the model observes in clinical practice. This data shift affects the model's overall performance and can also exacerbate bias. More specifically, these shifts can occur for several reasons. First, there may be a population shift, which is the difference in the distribution of the populations, such as age, sex, and breed. Second, there is the challenge of acquisition shift, where data trained on images with particular image quality specifications, such as scanner type, slice thickness, contrast, and voxel resolution, differ from those in the clinical environment. Third, there is the challenge of annotation shift, where the classifications used in the model development may differ from those used by the clinic, or the inter-observer and intra-observer variability in classifications is significant in the training or clinical datasets. Fourth, a prevalence shift may be present, where models trained in some areas where certain diseases are more prevalent may be overrepresented in the clinic. Fifth, there is the concept of manifestation shift, where the AI model data's disease manifestations differ from those observed in the clinic. These are some of the key reasons why it becomes critical to understand what data are being used in AI models. Finally, there are salient issues related to the network architecture, where performance shifts can only be corrected by recalibrating or replacing models with more sophisticated ones.

The distinction between internal and clinical validation underscores a critical pathway for the successful integration of AI into veterinary diagnostic imaging. As these tools undergo clinical validation, their potential to reshape veterinary diagnostics becomes increasingly tangible. This too allows the opportunity to investigate whether patient care is best supported by general practitioners or radiologists as end users of this technology.

SUMMARY

The continued evolution of AI in veterinary imaging hinges on several factors. First, the development of standardized protocols for both internal and clinical validation will be important to establish the credibility and efficacy of AI tools. Second, as more AI applications undergo successful clinical validation, regulatory bodies and veterinary practices must navigate the challenges of integrating these technologies into existing diagnostic workflows, ensuring they complement rather than complicate the diagnostic process.

Building interdisciplinary partnerships among veterinarians, AI researchers, and industry stakeholders will be crucial in driving scientifically sound and clinically relevant innovation. Together, these efforts will pave the way for AI to fulfill its potential in veterinary medicine, enhancing diagnostic precision, optimizing clinical workflows, and opening new avenues for patient care. Through further efforts toward transparency and peer-reviewed research, the veterinary community can better assess and embrace AI tools' real-world applicability and benefits.

DISCLOSURE

The authors have no commercial conflicts of interest to declare.

Both authors are members of the ACVR/ECVDI Artificial Intelligence Education and Development Committee.An AI based system (ChatGPT) was used in the writing process for improving readability of aspects of this manuscript.

CLINICS CARE POINTS

- Imaging AI is a powerful tool that can reshape veterinary care if deployed in a purposeful and ethical manner.
- It is possible to create accurate AI models for a variety of use cases for small animal care.
- Data shift refers to a mismatch between the data distribution on which a model was developed and the data distribution the model observes in clinical practice. This can affect the model's performance and exacerbate bias.
- Current commercial AI products lack transparency, disclosure of performance metrics, and multi-institutional validation.
- Interdisciplinary teams that include veterinarians, technicians, data scientists, and information technologists can improve the success of the adoption of AI technologies in the veterinary setting.

REFERENCES

[1] Basran PS, Appleby RB. The unmet potential of artificial intelligence in veterinary medicine. Am J Vet Res 2022; 83(5):385–92.

[2] Cohen EB, Gordon IK. First, do no harm. Ethical and legal issues of artificial intelligence and machine learning in veterinary radiology and radiation oncology. Vet Radiol Ultrasound 2022;63(S1):840–50.

[3] U.S. Food and Drug Administration (FDA). Canada H, Medicines & Healthcare products Regulatory agency. Good Machine Learning Practice for Medical Device Development: Guiding Principles. FdaGov. 2021. Available at: https://www.fda.gov/medical-devices/software-medical-device-samd/good-machine-learning-practice-medical-device-development-guiding-principles.

[4] Kiseleva A, Kotzinos D, De Hert P. Transparency of AI in Healthcare as a Multilayered System of Accountabilities: Between Legal Requirements and Technical Limitations. Front Artif Intell 2022;5(May). https://doi.org/10.3389/frai.2022.879603.

[5] Tran BX, Vu GT, Ha GH, et al. Global evolution of research in artificial intelligence in health and medicine: A bibliometric study. J Clin Med 2019;8(3). https://doi.org/10.3390/jcm8030360.

[6] Appleby RB, Basran PS. Artificial intelligence in veterinary medicine. J Am Vet Med Assoc 2022;260(8):819–24.

[7] Waljee AK, Higgins PDR. Machine Learning in Medicine: A Primer for Physicians. Am J Gastroenterol 2010;105(6):1224–6.

[8] Raghu M, Zhang C, Kleinberg J, et al. Transfusion: Understanding transfer learning for medical imaging. Adv Neural Inf Process Syst 2019;32(NeurIPS).

[9] Hennessey E, DiFazio M, Hennessey R, et al. Artificial intelligence in veterinary diagnostic imaging: A literature review. Vet Radiol Ultrasound 2022;63(S1):851–70.

[10] Alexander K. Reducing error in radiographic interpretation. Can Vet J 2010;51(5):533–6.

[11] Tahghighi P, Norena N, Ukwatta E, et al. Automatic classification of symmetry of hemithoraces in canine and feline radiographs. J Med Imag 2023;10(4):44004.

[12] Tahghighi P, Appleby RB, Norena N, et al. Machine learning can appropriately classify the collimation of ventrodorsal and dorsoventral thoracic radiographic images of dogs and cats. Am J Vet Res 2023;84(7):1–8.

[13] Banzato T, Wodzinski M, Burti S, et al. An AI-based algorithm for the automatic evaluation of image quality in canine thoracic radiographs. Sci Rep 2023;13(1):1–7.

[14] Rudie JD, Gleason T, Barkovich MJ, et al. Clinical Assessment of Deep Learning–based Super-Resolution for 3D Volumetric Brain MRI. Radiol Artif Intell 2022;4(2). https://doi.org/10.1148/ryai.210059.

[15] Johnson PM, Recht MP, Knoll F. Improving the Speed of MRI with Artificial Intelligence. Semin Musculoskelet Radiol 2020;24(1):12–20.

[16] Kang H, Noh D, Lee SK, et al. Deep learning-based reconstruction can improve canine thoracolumbar magnetic resonance image quality and reduce slice thickness. Vet Radiol Ultrasound 2023;64(6):1063–70.

[17] Choi H, Lee SK, Choi H, et al. Deep learning-based reconstruction for canine brain magnetic resonance imaging could improve image quality while reducing scan time. Vet Radiol Ultrasound 2023;64(5):873–80.

[18] Tamura A, Mukaida E, Ota Y, et al. Deep learning reconstruction allows low-dose imaging while maintaining image quality: comparison of deep learning reconstruction and hybrid iterative reconstruction in contrast-enhanced abdominal CT. Quant Imaging Med Surg 2022;12(5):2977–84.

[19] Oostveen LJ, Meijer FJA, de Lange F, et al. Deep learning–based reconstruction may improve non-contrast cerebral CT imaging compared to other current reconstruction algorithms. Eur Radiol 2021;31(8):5498–506.

[20] Ng CKC. Artificial Intelligence for Radiation Dose Optimization in Pediatric Radiology: A Systematic Review. Children 2022;9(7):1–12.

[21] Taylor N, Renfrew H. Does Dose Matter? Ionizing Radiation Exposure of the Veterinary Patient From Computed Tomography: A Discussion. Top Companion Anim Med 2022;51:100697.

[22] Wilson DU, Bailey MQ, Craig J. The role of artificial intelligence in clinical imaging and workflows. Vet Radiol Ultrasound 2022;63(S1):897–902.

[23] MiREYE X-ray Imaging Quality Control System. Available at: https://www.mireyeimaging.com/. [Accessed 29 February 2024].

[24] 5 Ways IDEXX Web PACS Specialty Software Will Improve Your Specialty Practice's Workflow. Available at: https://www.idexx.com/en/veterinary/diagnostic-imaging-telemedicine-consultants/five-ways-idexx-web-pacs-specialty-software-will-improve-your-specialty-practices-workflow/. [Accessed 29 February 2024].

[25] Baltruschat I, Steinmeister L, Nickisch H, et al. Smart chest X-ray worklist prioritization using artificial intelligence: a clinical workflow simulation. Eur Radiol 2021;31(6):3837–45.

[26] Topff L, Ranschaert ER, Bartels-Rutten A, et al. Artificial Intelligence Tool for Detection and Worklist Prioritization Reduces Time to Diagnosis of Incidental Pulmonary Embolism at CT. Radiol Cardiothorac Imaging 2023;5(2). https://doi.org/10.1148/ryct.220163.

[27] Batra K, Xi Y, Bhagwat S, et al. Radiologist Worklist Reprioritization Using Artificial Intelligence: Impact on Report Turnaround Times for CTPA Examinations Positive for Acute Pulmonary Embolism. Am J Roentgenol 2023;221(3):324–33.

[28] Bizzo BC, Almeida RR, Alkasab TK. Artificial Intelligence Enabling Radiology Reporting. Radiologic Clinics 2021;59(6):1045–52.

[29] Pesapane F, Tantrige P, De Marco P, et al. Advancements in Standardizing Radiological Reports: A Comprehensive Review. Medicina (Lithuania) 2023;59(9):1–11.

[30] Fitzke M, Stack C, Dourson A, et al. RapidRead: Global Deployment of State-of-the-art Radiology AI for a Large Veterinary Teleradiology Practice. 2021. Available at: http://arxiv.org/abs/2111.08165.

[31] Kim E, Fischetti AJ, Sreetharan P, et al. Comparison of artificial intelligence to the veterinary radiologist's diagnosis of canine cardiogenic pulmonary edema. Vet Radiol Ultrasound 2022;63(3):292–7.

[32] Müller TR, Solano M, Tsunemi MH. Accuracy of artificial intelligence software for the detection of confirmed pleural effusion in thoracic radiographs in dogs. Vet Radiol Ultrasound 2022;63(5):573–9.

[33] Pomerantz LK, Solano M, Kalosa-Kenyon E. Performance of a commercially available artificial intelligence software for the detection of confirmed pulmonary nodules and masses in canine thoracic radiography. Vet Radiol Ultrasound 2023;64(5):881–9.

[34] Boissady E, de La Comble A, Zhu X, et al. Artificial intelligence evaluating primary thoracic lesions has an overall

lower error rate compared to veterinarians or veterinarians in conjunction with the artificial intelligence. Vet Radiol Ultrasound 2020;61(6):619–27.

[35] Adrien-Maxence H, Emilie B, Alois DLC, et al. Comparison of error rates between four pretrained DenseNet convolutional neural network models and 13 board-certified veterinary radiologists when evaluating 15 labels of canine thoracic radiographs. Veterinary Radiology & Ultrasound 2022;63(4):456–68.

[36] Boissady E, De La Comble A, Zhu X, et al. Comparison of a Deep Learning Algorithm vs. Humans for Vertebral Heart Scale Measurements in Cats and Dogs Shows a High Degree of Agreement Among Readers. Front Vet Sci 2021;8(December):1–6.

[37] van Leeuwen KG, Schalekamp S, Rutten MJCM, et al. Artificial intelligence in radiology: 100 commercially available products and their scientific evidence. Eur Radiol 2021;31(6):3797–804.

[38] Basran PS, Porter I. Radiomics in veterinary medicine: Overview, methods, and applications. Vet Radiol Ultrasound 2022;63(S1):828–39.

[39] Banzato T, Bernardini M, Cherubini GB, et al. A methodological approach for deep learning to distinguish between meningiomas and gliomas on canine MR-images. BMC Vet Res 2018;14(1):317.

[40] Banzato T, Cherubini GB, Atzori M, et al. Development of a deep convolutional neural network to predict grading of canine meningiomas from magnetic resonance images. Vet J 2018;235:90–2.

[41] Banzato T, Bernardini M, Cherubini GBGB, et al. Texture analysis of magnetic resonance images to predict histologic grade of meningiomas in dogs. Am J Vet Res 2017;78(10):1156–62.

[42] Banzato T, Causin F, Della Puppa A, et al. Accuracy of deep learning to differentiate the histopathological grading of meningiomas on MR images: A preliminary study. J Magn Reson Imag 2019;50(4):1152–9.

[43] Basran PS, Shcherban N, Forman M, et al. Combining ultrasound radiomics, complete blood count, and serum biochemical biomarkers for diagnosing intestinal disorders in cats using machine learning. Vet Radiol Ultrasound 2023;64(5):890–903.

[44] Choi BK, Park S, Lee G, et al. Can CT texture analysis parameters be used as imaging biomarkers for prediction of malignancy in canine splenic tumors? Veterinary. Radiology and Ultrasound 2023;64(2):224–32.

[45] Shaker R, Wilke C, Ober C, et al. Machine learning model development for quantitative analysis of CT heterogeneity in canine hepatic masses may predict histologic malignancy. Vet Radiol Ultrasound 2021;62(6):711–9.

[46] Wanamaker MW, Vernau KM, Taylor SL, et al. Classification of neoplastic and inflammatory brain disease using MRI texture analysis in 119 dogs. Vet Radiol Ultrasound 2021;62(4):445–54.

[47] Biercher A, Meller S, Wendt J, et al. Using Deep Learning to Detect Spinal Cord Diseases on Thoracolumbar Magnetic Resonance Images of Dogs. Front Vet Sci 2021; 8(November):1–9.

[48] Marschner CB, Kokla M, Amigo JM, et al. Texture analysis of pulmonary parenchymateous changes related to pulmonary thromboembolism in dogs - a novel approach using quantitative methods. BMC Vet Res 2017;13(1): 1–10.

[49] Wilson D. Interdisciplinary collaboration: Data scientists and radiologists. Vet Radiol Ultrasound 2022;63(S1): 916–9.

[50] Rajpurkar P, Lungren MP. The Current and Future State of AI Interpretation of Medical Images. N Engl J Med 2023;388(21):1981–90.

[51] Shin HC, Tenenholtz NA, Rogers JK, et al. Medical image synthesis for data augmentation and anonymization using generative adversarial networks, In: Gooya A, Goksel O, Oguz I. (Eds.), et al. Simulation and synthesis in medical imaging, Springer Nature Switzerland, 2018, pp. 1–11. https://link.springer.com/content/pdf/10.100-7/978-3-030-00536-8_1.pdf

[52] Schultheiss M, Schmette P, Bodden J, et al. Lung nodule detection in chest X-rays using synthetic ground-truth data comparing CNN-based diagnosis to human performance. Sci Rep 2021;11(1):1–10.

[53] Gao C, Killeen BD, Hu Y, et al. Synthetic data accelerates the development of generalizable learning-based algorithms for X-ray image analysis. Nat Mach Intell 2023; 5(3):294–308.

[54] Osuala R, Kushibar K, Garrucho L, et al. Data synthesis and adversarial networks: A review and meta-analysis in cancer imaging. Med Image Anal 2023;84(July 2021):102704.

[55] Boulanger M, Nunes JC, Chourak H, et al. Deep learning methods to generate synthetic CT from MRI in radiotherapy: A literature review. Phys Med 2021;89(July): 265–81.

[56] Jans LBO, Chen M, Elewaut D, et al. MRI-based Synthetic CT in the Detection of Structural Lesions in Patients with Suspected Sacroiliitis: Comparison with MRI. Radiology 2021;298(2):343–9.

[57] Elkassem AA, Smith AD. Potential Use Cases for ChatGPT in Radiology Reporting. AJR Am J Roentgenol 2023;221(3):373–6.

[58] Bhayana R. Chatbots and Large Language Models in Radiology: A Practical Primer for Clinical and Research Applications. Radiology 2024;310(1). https://doi.org/10.1148/radiol.232756.

[59] Miró CQ, Vidal-Alaball J, Fuster-Casanovas A, et al. Real-world testing of an artificial intelligence algorithm for the analysis of chest X-rays in primary care settings. Sci Rep 2024;14(1):5199.

SECTION III - GASTROENTEROLOGY

Advances in Small Animal Care 5 (2024) 79–107

ADVANCES IN SMALL ANIMAL CARE

Clinical Guidelines for Fecal Microbiota Transplantation in Companion Animals

Jenessa A. Winston, DVM, PhD, DACVIM (Small Animal Internal Medicine)[a,*],
Jan S. Suchodolski, DrMedVet, PhD, DACVM, AGAF[b],
Frederic Gaschen, DrMedVet, Drhabil, DACVIM (Small Animal Internal Medicine), DipECVIM-CA[c],
Kathrin Busch, DVM, Dr Med Vet, DECVIM[d],
Sina Marsilio, Dr med vet, PhD, DACVIM (Small Animal Internal Medicine), DipECVIM-CA[e],
Marcio C. Costa, DVM, DVSc, PhD[f], Jennifer Chaitman, VMD, DACVIM (Small Animal Internal Medicine)[g],
Emily L. Coffey, DVM, DACVIM (Small Animal Internal Medicine), PhD[h],
Julien R.S. Dandrieux, BSc, Dr Med Vet, PhD, DACVIM (Small Animal Internal Medicine)[i],
Arnon Gal, DVM, MSc, PhD, DACVIM, DACVP[j],
Tracy Hill, DVM, PhD, DACVIM (Small Animal Internal Medicine)[k], Rachel Pilla, DVM, PhD[b,l],
Fabio Procoli, DVM, MVetMed, DACVIM, DipECVIM-CA, MRCVS[m],
Silke Salavati Schmitz, Dr Med Vet, PhD, DipECVIM-CA, FHEA, FRCVS[i],
M. Katherine Tolbert, DVM, PhD, DACVIM (Small Animal Internal Medicine, Small Animal Nutrition)[b],
Linda Toresson, DVM, PhD[n], Stefan Unterer, DVM, Dr med vet, Dr habil, DECVIM-CA[o],
Érika Valverde-Altamirano, DVM[p], Guilherme G. Verocai, DVM, MSc, PhD, DACVM (Parasitology)[q],
Melanie Werner, Dr Med Vet, Dipl ECVIM-CA (Internal Medicine)[r], Anna-Lena Ziese, Dr Med Vet[s]

[a]Department of Veterinary Clinical Sciences, Comparative Hepatobiliary and Intestinal Research Program (CHIRP), Veterinary Clinical Sciences, The Ohio State University College of Veterinary Medicine, Columbus, OH, USA; [b]Department of Small Animal Clinical Sciences, Gastrointestinal Laboratory, Texas A&M University, College Station, TX, USA; [c]Department of Veterinary Clinical Sciences, School of Veterinary Medicine, Louisiana State University, Baton Rouge, LA, USA; [d]Centre for Clinical Veterinary Medicine, Ludwig-Maximilian University Munich, Munich, Germany; [e]Department of Veterinary Medicine and Epidemiology, UC Davis School of Veterinary Medicine, Davis, CA, USA; [f]Department of Veterinary Biomedical Sciences, University of Montreal, Saint-Hyacinthe, Québec, Canada; [g]Veterinary Internal Medicine and Allergy Specialists, New York, USA; [h]Department of Veterinary Clinical Sciences, University of Minnesota College of Veterinary Medicine, Saint Paul, MN, USA; [i]Hospital for Small Animals, Royal (Dick) School of Veterinary Studies and the Roslin Institute, College of Medicine and Veterinary Medicine, University of Edinburgh, Midlothian, UK; [j]Department of Veterinary Clinical Medicine, University of Illinois at Urbana-Champaign, IL, USA; [k]Veterinary Science Consultancy, Ethos Veterinary Health, USA; [l]Department of Veterinary Medicine and Animal Sciences, Università degli Studi di Milano, Lodi, Italy; [m]Anicura Ospedale Veterinario i Portoni Rossi, Via Roma 57/A, Zola Predosa, Bologna 40069, Italy; [n]Evidensia Specialist Animal Hospital, Helsingborg, Sweden; [o]Clinic for Small Animal Internal Medicine, Vetsuisse Faculty, University of Zurich, Zurich, Switzerland; [p]Nutrinac, 3000 Escazu Village, San Rafael, Escazu San José, Costa Rica; [q]Department of Veterinary Pathobiology, Parasitology Diagnostic Laboratory, Texas A&M University, College Station, TX, USA; [r]Small Animal Clinic Marigin

https://doi.org/10.1016/j.yasa.2024.06.006
2666-450X/24/

Feusisberg, Firststrasse 31, Feusisberg 8835, Switzerland; ^{S}Terra Canis GmbH, Parkring 29, 85748 Garching bei München, Germany

KEYWORDS
- Fecal microbiota transplant • Fecal transplant • Dysbiosis • Microbial-directed therapeutics
- Companion animals • Microbiome • Microbiota • Clinical guidelines

KEY POINTS
- Fecal microbiota transplantation (FMT) is the transfer of feces from a healthy donor to a diseased recipient aimed at directly modifying the recipient's gut microbial ecosystem to confer a health benefit to the recipient.
- FMT is a safe, well-tolerated, minimally invasive procedure that can be performed in any veterinary practice type.
- Establishing a fecal donor program is feasible for veterinarians, and donor screening guidelines, which can be modified on a case-by-case basis, are included herein.
- Fresh feces should be utilized for FMT whenever possible. Specific recommendations for FMT product processing and preparation provided here can be tailored to meet the availability of personnel and equipment resources for each practice.
- Currently in veterinary medicine, the Companion Animal FMT Consortium recommends FMT as an adjunctive microbial-directed therapeutic for canine parvovirus enteritis, canine acute diarrhea, and chronic enteropathy in both dogs and cats.

 Video content accompanies this article at https://www.advancesinsmallanimalcare.com/.

INTRODUCTION

Evidence is rapidly mounting that modifying the gut microbiota is important for treating diseases and maintaining health. Fecal microbiota transplantation (FMT) utilizes donor feces to modify the recipient's gut microbial ecosystem to confer a health benefit in patients suffering from gut dysbiosis. Investigation into the utility of FMT is growing in diverse fields such as infectious disease [1], gastroenterology [2], endocrinology [3], neurology [4], and oncology [5]. FMT for recurrent *Clostridioides difficile* infection represents the first successful human clinical application of directly modifying the gut microbial ecosystem to restore health [6].

Currently in veterinary medicine, microbiome research surrounding FMT is in its infancy [7,8]. Mechanistic studies related to longitudinal changes in gut microbial communities, microbial engraftment, host–microbe interactions, FMT dosing, and administration routes are limited in companion animals. The paucity of information in companion animals provides evidence that further investigation into the role gut microbes and their metabolism play in disease states and how microbial-directed therapeutics, like FMT, can be used clinically are required.

The Companion Animal FMT Consortium, a unique international group of veterinary experts, was established to develop the first clinical FMT guidelines for companion animals. The Companion Animal FMT Consortium aims to increase accessibility of FMT as a microbial-directed therapeutic for dogs and cats by simplifying and demystifying the process of performing FMT in clinical practice. The information presented in later discussion is intended to serve as a summary of the technical aspects of FMT, current small animal therapeutic indications of FMT, and important considerations for establishing a fecal donor program. These FMT clinical guidelines are intended for veterinarians in a variety of clinical practice types and can be modified and adapted as needed to align with financial and technical resources available to individual practitioners.

CLINICAL GUIDELINES DEVELOPMENT PROCESS

The Companion Animal FMT Consortium aimed to develop the first veterinary clinical guidelines for FMT in dogs and cats to provide veterinarians with evidence-based recommendations for performing FMT in a variety of clinical practice settings. Aligned with methodology utilized by human FMT consensus statements for clinical practice [9], the following steps were completed: selection of experts to serve on the Companion Animal FMT Consortium; identification of main topics for clinical guidelines and formation of working groups; development of statements germane to topics with critical evaluation of evidence available; development of consensus on clinical statements through an electronic modified Delphi process [10], and virtual meetings to develop the final version of clinical statements.

Members of the Companion Animal FMT Consortium were selected based on their expertise in FMT in dogs and cats and represent diverse backgrounds from academia and private practice. The FMT Consortium is composed of 21 global experts from 19 institutions, with each member having an active role in the development of the clinical FMT guidelines presented herein. Each member was assigned based on their expertise to one of the following working groups: (1) donor selection and screening; (2) FMT preparation; and (3) FMT clinical applications and dosing. Members of each working group assigned a lead to coordinate their group and provided the FMT Consortium chair (J. Winston) finalized clinical statements for their assigned topic. The quality of evidence for each statement was adapted from the Grading of Recommendations Assessment, Development and Evaluation system [11,12]. The definitions utilized for quality of published evidence are provided in Box 1.

Statements provided by each working group were uploaded to an online voting system (Qualtrics, Provo, Utah, USA) by the FMT Consortium chair. A modified Delphi method was used to achieve consensus on all statements [10]. Each set of topic statements underwent multiple rounds of revisions based on the group's anonymous feedback during online voting. Each time statements were uploaded and sent out for the Companion Animal FMT Consortium members to evaluate. After multiple rounds, the modified Delphi method resulted in consensus on all statements provided herein.

For each statement, experts rated their level of agreement as follows: (1) agree strongly, (2) agree with reservations, (3) undecided, (4) disagree, or (5) disagree strongly. If experts selected anything other than "agree strongly," they were asked to add comments to explain

their reservation and/or disagreement with the statement and specifically explain how to improve the statement. For each statement, a predetermined threshold of 80% or greater of experts "agreeing strongly" was required for the statement to be included in the clinical FMT guidelines. All statements not reaching 80% agreement were revised and rated again in additional rounds of online voting. Once the statements were finalized for each topic (achieving 80% or greater agreement), the working group members provided commentaries for each statement based on the available evidence. Working group leads then provided the final sections to the Companion Animal FMT Consortium chair and clinical guidelines were complied.

CLINICAL GUIDELINES FOR FECAL MICROBIOTA TRANSPLANTATION IN COMPANION ANIMALS

The clinical guidelines for FMT in companion animals are divided into 3 sections: (1) donor selection and screening; (2) FMT preparation; and (3) FMT clinical applications and dosing. Each section consists of a series of statements to provide veterinarians with general recommendations relevant to the topic. Evidence germane to the topic is also provided as commentary below each statement when available, including the quality of evidence (definitions in Box 1).

Part 1: Donor Selection and Screening

In this section, general recommendations for FMT donor selection and screening are provided. It is important to note that additional considerations depending on geographic location (ie, infectious disease screening), financial resources (ie, additional bloodwork to screen donor), and other factors should be considered on a case-by-case basis. Box 2 provides a summary of the fecal donor screening recommendations.

Health status

Statement. Donors should be clinically healthy (no abnormalities identified on comprehensive physical examination and history).

Quality of evidence: Low.

Comment. While there are no data regarding the impact of general health of the FMT donor on FMT success or safety, general clinical status is a readily identifiable indicator of overall health. It is plausible that an animal that does not appear clinically normal could pose an elevated risk for pathogen shedding or have an altered gastrointestinal (GI) microbiota, known as

BOX 1 Definition of the Quality of Evidence	
QoE	**Definition**
High	At least one properly designed RCT or equivalent
Moderate	At least one well-designed clinical trial, without randomization; evidence from cohort or case series; or equivalent
Low	Opinions of respected experts, based on clinical experience, descriptive single case reports, or reports of expert committees

Abbreviations: QoE, quality of evidence; RCT, randomized clinical trial.

BOX 2
Fecal Donor Selection and Screening

Health status

- Clinically healthy (no abnormalities on comprehensive physical examination and history)
- Acceptable BCS (4–6/9)
- No history of current (within last 4 months) or chronic GI signs
- If acute GI (<2 weeks) develop, wait 3 months and then rescreen
- Permanently exclude any donor with a history of chronic GI signs (>3 weeks)

Age, signalment, and environment

- Minimum 12 months old and younger than <75% of expected lifespan
- No exclusion of breeds
- No exclusion for farm/wildlife exposure, dog parks, boarding, and so forth; unless GI signs present
- Exclude donor if hospitalized or boarded for longer than 8 to 10 hours in previous 4 weeks
  Feline fecal donors
  - Indoor cats from single-cat-household preferred
  - Ideally 6 weeks in household prior to screening

History of drugs that induce dysbiosis

  Minimum duration to exclude donor since treatment with medications that potentially induce dysbiosis:
  - Antimicrobials (oral/parenteral): At least 6 months and rescreen donor
  - Acid suppressants (anything changing gastric pH): At least 2 weeks
  - Exclude donors that have received raw food diets/treats within last 30 days

Microbiome screening

- DI should be performed where available to exclude animals with abnormal microbiomes
- Next-generation sequencing based technologies for the assessment of the microbiome are not recommended, as they are not validated, and there is no standard interpretation of results for individual animals
- Routine bacterial culture is not an effective tool for assessing the diversity of the entire microbiome

Infectious disease screening

  It is *recommended* to test for the following infectious diseases in donors:
  - *Salmonella* (fecal culture or PCR)
  - *C. jejuni* (PCR or culture by experience laboratory with identification on a species level)
  - *Giardia* (IFA, SNAP test, coproantigen, or centrifugal flotation with zinc sulfate, PCR, or a combination of these)
  - *Cryptosporidium* (IFA or antigen testing)
  - Other intestinal parasites (centrifugal fecal flotation, coproantigen tests, Baermann, and PCR)

  Additional testing for feline fecal donors:
  - *Tritrichomonas foetus/blagburni* (PCR on fresh fecal sample)
  - Enteric coronavirus (PCR; performed once for cats if an indoor cat from a single-cat-household)
  - FIV and FeLV (SNAP Triple Test or FeLV antigen ELISA, and FIV antibody testing; Regarding FeLV testing cat should be indoor and not have contact with known infected cats for at least 6 weeks prior to testing)

  It is *optional* to test for the following infectious diseases in fecal donors:
  - *C. perfringens* netF-toxin gene (PCR; optional as occurrence is rare in clinically healthy dogs)
    - Note: It is not recommended to screen for *C. perfringens* enterotoxin and alpha toxin genes as the clinical significance is unknown in dogs and cats
  - *C. difficile* (PCR; optional as evidence of pathogenicity is weak in dogs and cats and the zoonotic potential is unclear; depending on clinician's preference)

Frequency of fecal donor screening

- Screened every 6 months, potentially more frequently based on risk/environment (endemic area)

Abbreviations: GI, gastrointestinal; PCR, polymerase chain reaction.

dysbiosis. There are few practical limitations to excluding clinically abnormal animals, given the large pool of clinically normal animals, so the precautionary principle supports a requirement that donors be clinically normal. There may be some situations where clinical abnormalities could be deemed irrelevant (eg, mild orthopedic abnormalities or dental disease) and the animal may be selected as a donor. However, the default should be for animals to be clinically normal and not receive any medications.

Statement. Donors should have an acceptable body condition score (BCS: 4–6/9).
Quality of evidence: Low.

Comment. The current scientific literature does not provide information on the impact of a fecal transplant from a donor with an abnormal BCS (Canine ideal BCS: 4–5; Feline ideal BCS: 5) on the gut microbial ecosystem of the recipient. Similarly, there are no data available documenting BCS increases in canine FMT recipients from overweight or obese donors. People with a significantly increased body mass index, obesity, or type 2 diabetes are not considered acceptable fecal donors due to their altered gut microbiota compared to individuals with normal body condition [13]. In a clinical trial involving dogs, slight gut microbiota variations were observed between obese and lean individuals [14].

Statement. Donors should not have a history of current (within the last 4 months) or chronic GI signs (eg, vomiting, diarrhea, weight loss, dysorexia, melena, or hematochezia).
Quality of evidence: High.

Comment. Studies indicate that GI disorders in dogs and cats frequently lead to shifts in their gut microbiota, and some causes of GI disease can presumably be transmitted through FMT [15]. Any pathogen that can be transmitted through the fecal–oral route should be assumed to be transmissible via FMT, and some causes of acute GI disease in dogs and cats have fecal–oral transmission potential. In chronic enteropathies, gut microbiota changes can be quite significant and persistent, while in acute gastroenteritis and canine acute hemorrhagic diarrhea syndrome (AHDS), the alterations may be minor and only transient [16–20].

Statement. If acute GI signs (<2 weeks) develop, wait 3 months and then rescreen donor.
Quality of evidence: Low.

Comment. Data obtained from dogs indicate that the gut microbiota undergoes only minor and transient changes during episodes of acute GI disease [21]. After the resolution of clinical signs, the gut microbiota of these dogs characteristically returns to normal within a few weeks [21]. This has been demonstrated in dogs with acute diarrhea and AHDS [15,17,19]. However, there is a lack of comprehensive large-scale studies assessing the duration of infectious agent presence in the GI tract of dogs and cats after an episode with acute GI disease, and it is known that some infectious agents can be shed for weeks. Therefore, the precautionary approach would dictate a restriction period before use as a donor.

Statement. Permanently exclude animals as donors with history of chronic GI signs that have lasted more than 3 weeks, which may suggest possible underlying chronic enteropathy.
Quality of evidence: Low.

Comment. Numerous clinical investigations have demonstrated that the gut microbial ecosystem is altered in a substantial proportion of animals with chronic enteropathies when compared to healthy individuals [16,22]. Given that the objective of FMT is to restore a healthy gut microbial ecosystem in the recipient, it is imperative to exclude dysbiotic animals as donors.

Age, signalment, and environment
Statement. Donors should be a minimum of 12 months and younger than less than 75% of their expected lifespan (eg, <12 years for a breed expected to live 16–17 years).
Quality of evidence: Low.

Comment. The physiologic gut microbiota of dogs younger than 1 year is different compared to that of adult dogs and cats [23,24]. In human medicine, there is evidence that the gut microbial ecosystem changes negatively in older subjects due to various inflammatory processes in the body [25]. In dogs, one study has shown minor alterations in intestinal functional markers in older dogs [26]. The age at which a dog or cat can confidently be assumed to have a stable adult gut microbiota is unknown, but based on expert opinion, 1 year as a cutoff was chosen.

Statement. No exclusion of breeds.
Quality of evidence: Low.

Comment. Studies demonstrating breed-specific changes in the gut microbiota are lacking for both cats and dogs. There is no evidence that specific breeds have an altered gut microbiota compared to other breeds.

Statement. *For donors with farm/wildlife exposure, dog parks, boarding, and so forth:* There is no reason to exclude the donor as long as the animal is healthy with no GI signs.
Quality of evidence: Low.

Comment. The risk of acquiring infectious agents, transmission of enteropathogenic and multidrug-resistant bacteria from other dogs/cats is probably increased in animals that are in close contact with many other individuals (as it is the case in the named circumstances) [27]. However, there are no large-scale studies documenting the degree of risk increase, which is why dogs/cats kept in these circumstances should not be systematically excluded as donors. Testing for certain infectious agents (*see later section*) is, therefore, important.

Statement. Exclude animals that have been hospitalized or boarded for longer than 8 to 10 hours in the previous 4 weeks as this could have increased the risk of acquiring infectious agents.
Quality of evidence: Low.

Comment. To minimize the risk of acquiring infectious agents due to close contact with potentially sick animals, based on expert opinion, it is recommended to temporarily exclude such animals as potential donors.

Statement. Indoor cats from single-cat-households are preferred to minimize risk of infections.
Quality of evidence: Low.

Comment. Cats are prone to harbor parasitic and infectious diseases, regardless of whether they live indoors and/or outdoors. However, hunting of wild animals or scavenging significantly increases their risk of acquiring certain parasites [28]. A comprehensive meta-analysis of parasitic infection risks in indoor and outdoor cats found that limiting outdoor access could help reduce parasitic infections [29]. In geographic regions where the prevalence of free-roaming cats is very high and it is difficult to identify strictly indoor cats, free-roaming cats could be screened as potential donors as described in later discussion.

Statement. Feline fecal donors should ideally be at least 6 weeks in the household prior to undergoing screening.
Quality of evidence: Low.

Comment. As the feline leukemia virus (FeLV) p27 antigen point-of-care test can take up to 6 weeks after infection to become positive [30], a corresponding waiting period should be applied before screening donors. Important to note, no new cats should be introduced within the household during these 6 weeks. If the population of strictly indoor cats is low, the inclusion of free-roaming cats might be a necessity; however, ideally cats would be kept inside for a period of 6 weeks prior to donation.

History of antimicrobials, acid suppressants, and other drugs that induce dysbiosis

The following are the minimum required waiting times (since end of administration) prior to considering fecal donation for each potential dysbiosis-inducing drug.

Statement. *Antimicrobials (oral/parenteral):* At least 6 months and rescreen donor for intestinal dysbiosis.
Quality of evidence: Moderate.

Comment. The aim is to have a fecal donor with a healthy gut microbial ecosystem. Research has demonstrated that antimicrobials have a detrimental impact on the gut microbiota of dogs and cats, resulting in dysbiosis [31]. This is especially true for antimicrobials with anaerobic spectrum, such as metronidazole and tylosin, which can cause severe intestinal dysbiosis [32,33]. Studies indicate that the duration required to recover a normal gut microbiota following cessation of antimicrobial therapy can vary greatly among individuals and may sometimes take several months [24,32,33].

Statement. *Acid suppressants (anything changing gastric pH):* At least 2 weeks.
Quality of evidence: Moderate.

Comment. The reason for acid suppressant administration should be determined to evaluate additional risks. Research suggests that omeprazole and esomeprazole may result in temporary dysbiosis, yet it has been observed that the abundance of the bile acid converting bacterium *Clostridium hiranonis* (newly named *Peptacetobacter hiranonis*) remains within the reference range [34,35]. The gut microbiota typically returns to normal within 1 to 2 weeks after the cessation of treatment [34–36]. These findings have been established in canines and also apply to cats [37]. Studies on the effects of H_2-receptor antagonists on the gut microbiota are lacking.

Diet and other supplements

Statement. Exclude animals that have received raw food diets or raw treats within the last 30 days.
Quality of evidence: Moderate.

Comment. Animals consuming raw food or raw treats are at an increased risk of harboring pathogens and extended spectrum beta-lactamase (ESBL)-producing microorganisms in their feces. Studies suggest that the feces of dogs that were fed a raw diet often contain enteropathogenic bacteria, such as *Campylobacter jejuni*, *Salmonella*, and *Listeria monocytogenes*, at a higher frequency than the feces of dogs that were fed a commercial diet [38,39]. Additionally, the number of these bacteria was higher in dogs that were fed raw diets containing chicken [39]. More than 50% of dogs that were fed a raw diet harbor ESBL-bacteria in their feces [40–42]. Moreover, evidence showed that dogs on a raw diet have an altered gut microbiota [42]. Therefore, it is advised to avoid transferring fecal material containing enteropathogens or multidrug-resistant bacteria, and animals on a raw diet should be excluded as fecal donors. Animals can be switched to processed/cooked diets and then screened after 1 month on the new diet.

No clear recommendation can be given for dietary supplements. Although probiotics can shift the gut microbiota, clinically significant changes are not observed [43]. Currently, there is not enough evidence to provide a statement regarding the administration of probiotics to fecal donors.

Microbiome screening

Statement. Dysbiosis index (DI) should be performed where available to exclude animals with abnormal microbiomes.
Quality of evidence: Moderate.

Comment. The canine and feline fecal DI are validated and standardized tests designed for assessing microbiome shifts [16,22]. A recent meta-analysis of 27 studies revealed that the canine DI, which is calculated based on core bacteria such as *C. hiranonis* (newly named *P. hiranonis*), is a potential useful biomarker of intestinal functionality [44]. Additionally, robust correlation between untargeted metagenomic sequencing and the DI has been demonstrated [45]. The DI is a reliable indicator of shifts in the fecal microbiota in dogs and cats, providing better comparisons across individuals, as well as within the same individual over time, due to its superior reproducibility and analytical sensitivity in comparison to sequencing techniques [45]. The DI for donors should be below 0, and the abundance of all included bacterial taxa should be within their reference ranges. See "Disclosure" section for conflict of interest statement.

Statement. Next-generation sequencing-based technologies for the assessment of the microbiome are not recommended, as they are not validated and there is no standard guidance for interpretation of results for individual animals.
Quality of evidence: Low.

Comment. While recent technologies permit detailed investigation of the microbiota, there is a poor understanding of "normal" at the individual level and its variations [46,47]. There is an inadequate understanding of the gut microbiota to define what constitutes normal/healthy (or acceptable) and abnormal (or unacceptable) results for FMT donors.

Statement. Routine bacterial culture is not an effective tool for assessing the diversity of the entire microbiome, but culture can still be used to test for specific enteropathogens.
Quality of evidence: Moderate.

Comment. Fecal culture is a diagnostic technique used to identify specific or opportunistic enteropathogenic bacteria and fungi in dogs and cats. Many commercial veterinary diagnostic laboratories offer this service to assess the microbial composition of the feces and provide their own interpretation of the balance between normal and abnormal microbial populations. However, this approach has limitations, as aerobic culture-based methods do not adequately represent the mostly anaerobic intestinal microbiota [48]. A study comparing results from 3 commercial laboratories on bacterial culture with the canine DI showed that fecal cultures are not useful for identifying dysbiosis in dogs [49]. In fact, the interpretation of culture results can be misleading.

Infectious disease screening (recommended)

Statement. It is recommended to test for the following infectious diseases in fecal donors:
- *Salmonella* (recommend fecal culture or polymerase chain reaction [PCR])

- *C. jejuni* (recommend PCR or culture by experienced laboratory with the identification on a species level)
- *Giardia* (recommend immunofluorescence assay [IFA], SNAP test, coproantigen, or centrifugal flotation with zinc sulfate, PCR, or a combination of these)
- *Cryptosporidium* (recommend IFA or antigen testing)
- Other intestinal parasites (recommend centrifugal fecal flotation, coproantigen tests, Baermann, and PCR)

  Additional testing in cats includes the following:
- *Tritrichomonas foetus/blagburni* (recommend PCR on fresh fecal sample)
- Enteric coronavirus (recommend PCR; performed once for cats if an indoor cat from a single-cat-household)
- Feline immunodeficiency virus (FIV) and feline leukemia virus (FeLV) (recommend SNAP Triple Test or FeLV antigen enzyme-linked immunosorbent assay [ELISA], FIV antibody testing; Regarding FeLV testing, cat should be indoor and not have contact with known infected cats for at least 6 weeks prior to testing)

Quality of evidence: Moderate.

Comment. The listed organisms have been shown to potentially induce GI disease as well as diseases in other organ systems. Therefore, animals harboring these organisms should be excluded [50].

Optional infectious disease screening
Statement. It is optional to test for the following infectious diseases in fecal donors:
- *Clostridium perfringens* netF-toxin gene (PCR; optional as occurrence is rare in clinically healthy dogs)
  - *Note*: It is not recommended to screen for *C. perfringens* enterotoxin and alpha toxin genes as the clinical significance is unknown in dogs and cats.
- *C. difficile* (PCR; optional as evidence of pathogenicity is weak in dogs and cats and the zoonotic potential is unclear; depending on clinician's preference)

Quality of evidence: Moderate.

Comment. Current evidence suggests that netF, a beta-pore-forming toxin, is likely the major virulence factor in *C. perfringens* strains responsible for canine AHDS [51,52]. Another toxin, *C. perfringens* enterotoxin (CPE) has been found more often in the feces of dogs with AHDS than in the feces of dogs in a control group [53]. Although AHDS is not a transmissible disease, the role

of specific toxins in its development remains unclear, and netF-encoding *C. perfringens* strains are rarely detected in healthy dogs; therefore, it seems prudent to avoid factors/procedures that could increase the risk of exposure to these particular *C. perfringens* strains [51,53,54].

C. difficile is a common pathogen in humans, often leading to pseudomembranous colitis associated with antibiotic use [55]. Companion animals have been shown to carry the same or similar *C. difficile* ribotypes as those found in people, suggesting interspecies transmission [56,57]. However, a recent study demonstrated that interspecies transmission of *C. difficile* occurs infrequently in households with people infected with *C. difficile* [57]. The prevalence of *C. difficile* in dogs is estimated to be as high as 19%, but it rarely produces clinical signs [55]. There appears to be an association between *C. difficile* carriage and intestinal dysbiosis in dogs [58,59].

Frequency of fecal donor screening
Statement. Fecal donors should be screened every 6 months, potentially more frequently based on risk/environment (endemic area).
Quality of evidence: Low.

Comment. There are no clinical trials showing the resilience of the gut microbiota over 6 months or longer, but expert opinion suggests that the gut microbiota remains relatively stable in dogs and cats over the course of several months, provided there are no significant environmental changes or illnesses. Testing should be more frequent in endemic areas at the discretion of the veterinarian.

Part 2: Fecal Microbiota Transplantation Preparation

In this section, general recommendations for fecal collection and FMT preparation are provided. It is important that these recommendations need to be adjusted and optimized according to individual resources and facilities. Considerations include available personnel and equipment (ie, availability of −80°C freezer, lyophilizer, and so forth). Fig. 1 provides an overview of FMT product preparation and processing.

Fecal collection
Statement. Personal protective clothing, gloves, face mask, and eye protection should be worn.
Quality of evidence: Low.

Comment. Fecal samples should be handled in accordance with your local health and safety rules. In

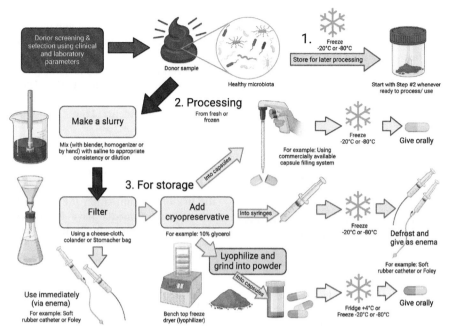

FIG. 1 Overview of FMT product preparation and processing. After a fecal donor screening and selection is complete, naturally voided feces can be used for FMT preparation and processing. Freshly void feces is ideal for FMT administration. If use of fresh feces is not feasible, then feces can be stored until processing and/or use (Step 1). Processing steps for fresh feces and/or frozen feces including making a fecal slurry and filtering the FMT product (Step 2). Once the FMT product is prepared, it can be used immediately or can be stored (Step 3). If the FMT product is to be stored, a cryopreservative can be added. FMT capsules can be administered orally and processed fecal slurries can be administered via rectal enema. (Created with BioRender.com.)

addition, unintentional contamination of individuals handling fecal material may occur, depending on the processing method. Despite the absence of documented cases of people getting diseases following contamination during FMT preparation, feces from small animals can potentially harbor infectious zoonotic pathogens. For this reason, the Companion Animal FMT Consortium advises as part of good laboratory practice to minimize the risk of infection by protecting oneself from contact with fecal material.

Statement. Use naturally voided feces, immediately after defecation.

Quality of evidence: Moderate.

Comment. Although this is usually achievable with dogs, it can be more challenging with cats. One study reported that feline feces did not show significant changes in microbiota composition and diversity over a period of 4 days at room temperature [60]. An additional study obtained the same results for a period of 12 hours at room

temperature [61]. Although neither study investigated bacterial viability, which might affect the clinical efficacy of the final FMT product, these findings suggest that feline feces naturally voided overnight can be processed the following day. As both studies used healthy cats and similar methodology (DNA sequencing), the recommendation is to process cat feces ideally within 24 hours of defecation with the current state of knowledge.

Statement. Collect feces in clean plastic bags, fecal collecting tubes, or glass containers.

Quality of evidence: Low.

Comment. In a clinical setting, it is most practical to use the aforementioned collecting equipment. Adhering to good laboratory practices ensures the preservation of fecal sample quality by reducing the risk of contamination with foreign material. Veterinary studies have demonstrated the clinical efficacy utilizing samples collected in bags and/or leak-proof containers before processing [18,20].

Fecal handling before processing

Statement. Once fresh feces are naturally voided, it should be processed and either administered to the patient or stored as fast as possible and feasible (preferably within 2–6 hours of defecation).

Quality of evidence: Moderate.

Comment. It should be noticed that one study using feces from dogs [62], and other unpublished studies in dogs and cats from the Companion Animal FMT Consortium members have found a significant decrease in the number of viable bacteria after freezing compared to fresh feces.

Statement. If immediate processing is not feasible, freshly voided feces should be stored refrigerated at 4°C and processed as soon as possible.

Quality of evidence: Low.

Comment. Although there is only anecdotal information in dogs, exposure to oxygen might decrease bacterial viability. Therefore, it would be advisable to keep feces in a zip locked bag or sealed container to reduce exposure to oxygen prior to processing.

Statement. *For feline feces if covered in litter:* Manually remove as much litter from the surface of the feces as possible. This can be done using a wooden tongue depressor, spoon, rubber spatula, and/or gloved hand.

Quality of evidence: Low.

Comment. Litter or foreign material adhered to feces may lead to obstruction of the rectal catheter used for enema administration of FMT. If any such material is left after manual removal, it will be eliminated during the filtering of the fecal slurry.

Fecal processing

Statement. Feces can be processed under aerobic conditions and at room temperature.

Quality of evidence: Moderate.

Comment. Studies in human medicine suggest that anaerobic conditions help to preserve bacterial viability of obligate anaerobes while species richness does not seem to be significantly altered under aerobic conditions [63,64]. However, aerobic processing is notably more practical and easier to conduct. Due to the proven clinical efficacy in both human and veterinary medicine in different diseases, the Companion Animal FMT Consortium supports aerobic processing

at room temperature [18,20,65–67]. In veterinary medicine, the potential for the enhancement of FMT efficacy through anaerobic preparation remains uncertain.

Statement. Sterile 0.9% saline (NaCl without additives) or phosphate buffered saline (PBS) can be added to feces to obtain a fecal slurry.

Quality of evidence: Low.

Comment. Although tap water has been described to prepare FMT products, the Companion Animal FMT Consortium prefers using sterile 0.9% saline (routinely available in clinical practice) or PBS to reduce the risk of contamination [68]. In addition, although other dilution media have been reported, such as skimmed milk, most studies have used NaCl or PBS.

Statement. Dilutions of 1:1 to 1:5 (fecal material:-solution) have been used to achieve a desired consistency based on FMT method of administration.

For example, if FMT administered via enema, fecal slurry consistency would be based on catheter size utilized for enema (most commonly 1:1–1:5 dilution). If FMT is administered via endoscopy, a smoothie consistency would be required to easily pass through the endoscopic channel (likely 1:5 dilution used).

Quality of evidence: Low.

Comment. Several FMT dilutions are reported both in human and veterinary medicine. No data are available on the viability and efficacy of the individual mixtures. However, when administered as a rectal enema, the consistency should be as thick as possible to keep the volume low and prevent leakage.

Statement. Various methods can be used to homogenize fecal mixture such as:
- Blending using a dedicated kitchen-style blender/mixer or an immersion blender
- Manual kneading in a clean plastic bag or Stomacher® strainer bag (eg, Stomacher® from Seward Ltd., Bohemia NY, USA)
- Mixing with a spoon in a small container (ideal for small amounts of feces)
Quality of evidence: Low.

Comment. Even though evidence from direct comparisons in FMT preparations is lacking, the possible disadvantage of blending (not kneading/other types of mixing) is that undigested material and foreign substances will also be blenderized and might end up in the filtered FMT slurry.

Statement. In order to remove large particles (such as grass and hair) from the fecal slurry, the fecal slurry can be filtered using the following methods:

- A fine kitchen sieve. A wooden tongue depressor, spoon, or rubber spatula can be used to press thicker fecal slurries through the sieve.
- A cheesecloth (highly absorbent, low-lint cotton fabric). Before use, rinse the cheesecloth to remove lint. Then layer it over a container and fill with fecal slurry. Gather corners and twist the cheesecloth to wring out liquid. With gloved hands, squeeze the middle section of the cheesecloth tightly so the fecal slurry drains out. You can also press down on the strained fecal contents with a wooden tongue depressor, spoon, or rubber spatula to press liquid out.
- An alternative is to use a Stomacher® strainer bag (Stomacher® from Seward Ltd.).
  Quality of evidence: Low.

Comment. The use of a Stomacher® bag has been reported for the preparation of human FMT [69].

Fecal slurry preparation for storage
Statement. If fecal slurry is not intended for immediate use, it should be immediately frozen and stored for future use.
Quality of evidence: Low.

Comment. Immediate freezing of the fecal slurry is recommended for optimal survival of fecal bacteria. See "Fecal product storage after processing" section for additional details.

Statement. The addition of glycerol as a cryoprotectant is recommended in order to improve bacterial viability upon thawing of fecal slurry.

- Recommended: Add glycerol to a final concentration of 10% (1 mL of glycerol to 9 mL of fecal slurry).
  Quality of evidence: Moderate.

Comment. The addition of 10% glycerol improves viability in some bacterial species upon thawing [62]. However, studies have shown clinical improvement without the addition of glycerol [20]. Currently, there is also a lack of clinical studies comparing the FMT effectiveness of adding glycerol or other cryoprotectants.

Statement. Lyophilized FMT products are available commercially. They are prepared by freezing fecal slurries or feces at $-80°C$ and then freeze-dried through sublimation to a powder form. This process uses a commercial lyophilizer and thus is currently only performed in research and commercial facilities.
Quality of evidence: Low.

Comment. In human medicine, lyophilized FMT capsules administered orally are safe and efficacious for recurrent *C. difficile* infection [70]. It appears that spore-forming bacteria are the most important engrafting microbes in lyophilized FMT capsules given orally to people [70]. To date, limited data are available for using lyophilized FMT capsules given orally to dogs and cats [71,72]. Importantly, the shelf-life, based on viability studies, of the commercialized lyophilized FMT products is unknown. Several *in vitro* and *in vivo* engraftment studies are underway in veterinary medicine to investigate the bacterial viability, shelf-life, and clinical efficacy of lyophilized FMT capsules.

Fecal product storage after processing
Statement. After processing, fecal slurries can be stored at $-20°C$ or $-80°C$ for up to 6 months.

- Sealed syringes or conical tubes can be used to store the fecal slurries in aliquots of 50 to 100 mL.
- Fecal slurries can be filled into capsules and then frozen for later administration.
  Quality of evidence: Low.

Comment. Although there is some evidence that storage at $-80°C$ can better preserve bacterial diversity compared to $-20°C$, there is no evidence that this can impact bacterial viability [62]. This recommendation is based on the guidelines used for FMT in humans [9].

Preparation of fecal microbiota transplantation products for administration
Statement. Frozen FMT products should be defrosted in a warm water bath or warming cabinet (up to 37°C/98.6°F) for immediate use, or overnight at fridge temperature before administration to the patient.
Quality of evidence: Low.

Comment. Although defrosting with high temperatures (>40°C) might harm the bacteria, it is unclear if "fast thawing" in a warm water bath or "slow thawing" overnight might influence the viability or efficacy of FMT products. There is clinical evidence for successful FMT after "slow thawing" overnight at fridge temperature in dogs [20].

Statement. Once fecal slurry is thawed, it cannot be refrozen.

Quality of evidence: Moderate.

Comment. Freeze–thaw cycles have been reported to decrease survival of some bacteria [73]. Anecdotal evidence from preliminary results from members of the Companion Animal FMT Consortium supports bacterial degradation caused by thaw and freezing.

Patient preparation based on fecal microbiota transplantation product

Statement. *FMT capsules to be administered orally:* No special patient preparation is recommended. There is no evidence that fasting is required.

Quality of evidence: Low.

Comment. When using commercially available FMT capsules, adhere to manufacturer's instructions. The Companion Animal FMT Consortium declines to make any recommendations regarding patient preparation, as only few studies report on pre-FMT protocols in people [74] and none in veterinary medicine when oral capsules are used. Pretreatment reported include initiation, continuation, or discontinuation of either proton pump inhibitors or antibiotics before oral FMT. The Companion Animal FMT Consortium does not recommend pretreatment with either of those drug categories before any type of FMT.

Statement. *FMT slurries to be administered via enema:*
- Patients should be motivated to defecate before FMT enema administration.
- Cleansing warm water enema is optional.
- Sedation is usually not necessary but depends on patient temperament.
- There is no evidence that fasting is required.

Quality of evidence: Low.

Comment. In patients without diarrhea, the procedure can be scheduled according to the patients' routine of passing feces. It appears logical that engraftment of the FMT might be better if the colon is empty. In a meta-analysis from human medicine, poor bowel preparation was one of the factors associated with failure of FMT [75]; however, there are no data available for dogs and cats to date, and bowel cleansing was not performed in most available studies. Sedation is only recommended for very excited or anxious animals that are unable to tolerate an enema and will not remain quiet for a short period after FMT administration. Cats might require

pregabalin or gabapentin for FMT administration; but if deeper sedation is required, general anesthesia should be preferred to enable protection of the cat's airways. Pretreatment with antimicrobials or proton-pump inhibitors is not recommended.

Statement. *FMT slurries to be administered via endoscopy:*
- No special patient preparation aside from normal endoscopic procedures.

Quality of evidence: Low.

Comment. In people, FMT are frequently delivered via duodenoscopy or colonoscopy [76], whereas this has been rarely reported in dogs [77]. In contrast, most of the veterinary studies have been using rectal enemas [18,20,67]. The Companion Animal FMT Consortium advises that there is limited evidence to make a recommendation on the use of endoscopy to deliver FMT in dogs or cats. However, if endoscopy is clinically indicated, FMT can be administered at the end of the procedure.

Statement. *FMT slurries to be administered via feeding tubes (nasogastric, esophagostomy, percutaneous endoscopic gastrostomy, and gastrostomy tubes):*
- No special patient preparation is recommended. There is no evidence that fasting is required.

Quality of evidence: Low.

Comment. The efficacy of FMT has been reported to be higher with intrarectal (enema) administration compared to other routes for recurrent *C. difficile* infection (rCDI) in people [78]; however, the FMT slurries might be administered orally or intragastrically. Noteworthy, FMT slurries have been given orally with the use of syringes in one canine study [79], but this practice could be associated with a risk of aspiration pneumonia. At this time, the Companion Animal FMT Consortium does not recommend administration of FMT products via feeding tubes.

Part 3: Fecal Microbiota Transplantation Clinical Applications and Dosing

In this section, general recommendations for FMT clinical applications and dosing are provided. Table 1 summarizes the current evidence available for clinical applications and dosing of FMT in companion animals.

Fecal microbiota transplantation indications

Statement. There is a high level of evidence for the use of FMT in acute parvovirus infection and other causes of acute diarrhea in dogs.

Quality of evidence: Moderate.

Comment. Hospitalized puppies with parvoviral diarrhea improved faster and had a shorter hospitalization duration when treated with FMT and standard treatment (eg, intravenous fluids and antimicrobials) as opposed to only standard treatment [67]. The parvovirus-infected puppies received 10 g of feces diluted in a 10 mL saline rectal enema within 6 to 12 hours of being admitted to the hospital. In a study comparing dogs with acute diarrhea treated either with FMT or metronidazole, dogs treated with FMT had a better improvement in fecal scores at day 28 than the metronidazole group [18]. In addition, dogs treated with FMT had an improvement in their DI, whereas dogs treated with metronidazole did not [18].

Statement. There is some evidence for the use of FMT in chronic enteropathy in dogs. The duration of the effect is variable.
Quality of evidence: Moderate.

Comment. In dogs with chronic enteropathies, FMT may be useful as an adjunctive therapy. It has been shown to decrease the Canine IBD Activity Index and Canine Chronic Enteropathy Clinical Activity Index [20,80]. While any dog with chronic enteropathy may respond to FMT, in one study those with a mildly elevated DI were more likely to respond [20]. This finding needs to be further evaluated in a prospective study; therefore, at this time, the Companion Animal FMT Consortium would recommend FMT for any dog with chronic enteropathy regardless of DI result.

Statement. There are anecdotal reports for the use of FMT in cats with acute or chronic enteropathy.
Quality of evidence: Low.

Comment. A cat with ulcerative colitis who failed treatment with conventional therapy responded to 2 rectal enema FMTs within 5 weeks [81]. There was gradual improvement in the stool quality over a 3 month period. The cat had normal feces at an 11 month follow-up.

Fecal microbiota transplantation preparations and technique

Statement. There is a high level of evidence that, despite impact on total and selected bacterial viability, aerobic processing, freezing, lyophilization, and encapsulation of fecal material does not negatively affect safety and clinical efficacy of FMT in people. These

findings are likely to be translated onto small animal medicine.
Quality of evidence: Low.

Comment. The impact of aerobic stool processing on clinical efficacy of FMTs in people and small animals is unknown as almost all cohort and randomized clinical trials (RCTs) available in the literature are based on an aerobic homogenization technique. Recent metanalyses in people with rCDI and Crohn's disease have failed to find any difference in clinical outcomes between FMTs using fresh versus frozen feces [82–84]. Similarly, recent open label single-group or controlled studies demonstrated noninferior safety and short-term clinical efficacy of fresh-frozen, cryopreserved, encapsulated frozen, or lyophilized feces compared to traditional nonoral delivery methods in people with rCDI [70,85]. These findings likely translate onto small animal medicine [86].

Fecal microbiota transplantation route of administration

Statement. There is a high level of evidence in people that the route of administration is not significantly associated with the outcome of FMT for the treatment of GI diseases including CDI, ulcerative colitis, and Crohn's disease. In companion animals, FMT has been administered orally and via rectal enemas, but no study has compared the efficacy of the different routes. Administration via rectal enemas is by far the most common route of administration in humans and companion animals.
Quality of evidence: Low.

Comment. In companion animals, FMT has been administered orally and via rectal enemas, but no study has compared the efficacy of the different routes. The most common route of administration in published studies to date is via rectal enemas in companion animals (see Table 1).

Patient preparation

Statement. There are no studies evaluating the effects of preconditioning the GI tract on patient outcomes including engraftment or improvement of clinical signs of intestinal disease in companion animals. In the absence of such evidence and to maintain good antimicrobial stewardship, the Companion Animal FMT Consortium discourages the use of antimicrobials prior to FMT administration if not otherwise clinically indicated.
Quality of evidence: Low.

TABLE 1
Summary of Studies and Anecdotal Reports Describing Techniques of Fecal Microbiota Transplantation in Dogs and Cats

Author	Species	Study Title	Study Design	Indication	Number of Animals, Frequency of FMT	Route	Technique
Burton et al, [106] 2016	Canine	Evaluation of Fecal Microbiota Transfer as Treatment for Postweaning Diarrhea in Research-Colony Puppies	RCT	Puppies at weaning age, postweaning diarrhea	11 puppies received FMT daily for 5 d, 12 received sham treatment	Oral	10 mL fecal suspension (100 g pooled dam feces mixed with 200 mL 2% fat cow's milk after filtration)
Bottero et al, [80] 2017	Canine	Faecal Microbiota Transplantation in 16 Dogs with Idiopathic Inflammatory Bowel Disease	Case series	IBD refractory to conventional treatment	16 adult dogs with severe, refractory IBD of >1 y duration. Oral treatment group received FMT q48–72h	Endoscopic/oral	Donor feces were mixed with saline at a 1:1 ratio, filtered and mixed with low-fat yoghurt as enrichment solution. 60–80 g feces for dogs <20 kg BW, 100–150 g for dogs >20 kg BW
Pereira et al, [67] 2018	Canine	Fecal Microbiota Transplantation in Puppies with Canine Parvovirus Infection	Non-RCT	Parvovirus infection	33 received standard treatment, 33 received FMT in addition. FMT administered within 6–12 h of admission and q48 h thereafter	Rectal	Donor feces were mixed with saline at a 1:1 ratio. 10 g feces were administered per puppy
Niina et al, [86] 2019	Canine	Fecal Microbiota Transplantation as a New Treatment for Canine Inflammatory Bowel Disease	Case report	IBD refractory to antibiotic and immunosuppressive treatment over time	One 10 y old toy poodle	Rectal	Donor feces were mixed with lactated Ringer at a 1:1 ratio. The dog received approximately 3 g feces/kg BW. Nine treatments within 6 mo
Sugita et al, [107] 2019	Canine	Successful Outcome after a Single Endoscopic Fecal Microbiota	Case report	Intermittent large bowel diarrhea, 4 mo duration, feces positive for C. difficile	One 8 mo old French bulldog	Oral	30 mL fecal suspension (60 g feces diluted in 50 mL tap water after filtration) given orally.

Author	Species	Title	Study type	Condition	Details	Route	Preparation
		Transplantation in a Shiba Dog with Non-responsive Enteropathy during the Treatment with Chlorambucil		(PCR and toxins A and B)		Rectal	Equivalent to approx. 2.5–3 g feces/kg BW
Chaitman et al, [18] 2020	Canine	Fecal Microbial and Metabolic Profiles in Dogs With Acute Diarrhea Receiving Either Fecal Microbiota Transplantation or Oral Metronidazole	Non-RCT	Uncomplicated acute diarrhea of <14 d duration	18 dogs; 11 dogs received a single FMT, 7 dogs received metronidazole 15 mg/kg q12 h for 7 d, 14 healthy control dogs	Rectal	2.5–5 g fresh feces per kg BW recipient, blended with 60 mL 0.9% NaCl until homogenous. For very large dogs a larger volume of saline may be needed to obtain sufficiently liquefied fecal solution
Gal et al, [77] 2021	Canine	One Dog's Waste is Another Dog's Wealth: A Pilot Study of Fecal Microbiota Transplantation in Dogs with Acute Hemorrhagic Diarrhea Syndrome	Case series/uncontrolled clinical trial	Canine AHDS	8 dogs; 4 received a single enteral FMT, 4 received placebo	Rectal via colonoscopy	Donor feces were blended with sterile saline at a ratio of 1:4 and filtered through a sieve. 10–15 mL/kg fecal slurry was administered into the ascending colon during colonoscopy
Sugita et al, [108] 2021	Canine	Successful Outcome after a Single Endoscopic Fecal microbiota Transplantation in a Shiba Dog with Non-responsive Enteropathy during the Treatment with Chlorambucil	Case report	Refractory chronic enteropathy	8 y old male neutered Shiba Dog	Rectal via colonoscopy	100 g donor feces were dissolved in 100 mL saline. The solution was filtered through a gauze pad. 50 mL were administered during colonoscopy into the cecum and colon
Niina et al, [103] 2021	Canine	Fecal Microbiota Transplantation as a New Treatment for	Uncontrolled clinical trial	IBD (FMT as add on treatment)	9 dogs received a single rectal FMT	Rectal	3 g/kg donor feces were dissolved in Ringer's solution and filtered through a gauze pad.

(continued on next page)

TABLE 1 (*continued*)

Author	Species	Study Title	Study Design	Indication	Number of Animals, Frequency of FMT	Route	Technique
							10 mL/kg fecal slurry were administered rectally
Salavati Schmitz, [100], 2022	Canine	Observational Study of Small Animal Practitioners' Awareness, Clinical Practice and Experience With Fecal Microbiota Transplantation in Dogs	NA	Mixed	Summary of FMT practices performed by study participants (155 small animal practitioners)	Variable	Summary of practices: Volume of FMT: 5–50 mL/kg Total volume of FMT: 20–300 mL Weight of FMT: 2-5 g/kg Total weight of FMT in grams (often diluted in water or saline): 1–50 g
Cerquetella et al, [109] 2022	Canine	Case Report: Oral Fecal Microbiota Transplantation in a Dog Suffering From Relapsing Chronic Diarrhea—Clinical Outcome and Follow-Up	Case report	Relapsing chronic diarrhea (FMT as add on treatment)	6 y old male Labrador retriever, 5 capsules/10 kg body weight for 5 consecutive days	Oral	Frozen capsules (size #00) containing 650 µL fecal slurry
Marclay et al, [110] 2022	Canine	Recovery of Fecal Microbiome and Bile Acids in Healthy Dogs after Tylosin Administration with and without Fecal Microbiota Transplantation	RCT	Tylosin-induced intestinal dysbiosis	22 dogs, 10 control dogs (placebo treatment), 6 dogs received a single rectal FMT, 6 dogs received 2 FMT capsules PO q 24 h for 14 consecutive days	Rectal/oral	Rectal FMT: Donor feces were mixed with sterile saline at a ratio of 1:4, filtered, cryopreserved with glycerol at a final concentration of 10% and stored at −80°C for a maximum of 2 mo. Aliquots were thawed at 37°C water bath and 10 mL/kg were administered rectally Oral capsules: Frozen capsules (size #00) containing fecal sediment

Reference	Species	Title	Study design	Condition	Subjects	Route	Protocol
Collier et al, [111] 2022	Canine	Investigating Fecal Microbial Transplant as a Novel Therapy in Dogs with Inflammatory Bowel Disease: A Preliminary Study	RCT	IBD (FMT as add on treatment)	13 dogs, 7 dogs received a single rectal FMT, 6 dogs received placebo	Rectal	Fecal samples from 5 donor dogs were pooled at a total of 50 g. Feces were blended with sterile saline at a ratio of 1:5, filtered using a sieve, stored in 60 mL catheter tip syringes at −20°C for a maximum of 3 mo. Recipients received 10 mL/kg using a rubber catheter
Alves et al, [112] 2023	Canine	Faecal Microbiome Transplantation Improves Clinical Signs of Chronic Idiopathic Large Bowel Diarrhoea in Working Dogs	RCT	Large bowel diarrhea (suspect stress-induced colitis)	30 large breed working dogs, 15 dogs received psyllium husk orally for 30 consecutive days, 15 dogs received a single rectal FMT	Rectal	50–60 g of fresh donor feces was blended with 250 mL of saline and filtered using a gauze. 60 mL of this slurry was rectally administered using a 60 mL catheter tip syringe and a 12 French red rubber catheter
Toresson et al, [20] 2023	Canine	Clinical Effects of Faecal Microbiota Transplantation as Adjunctive Therapy in Dogs with Chronic Enteropathies-A Retrospective Case Series of 41 Dogs	Case series/uncontrolled clinical trial	Dogs with chronic enteropathy that failed prior conventional medical treatment	41 dogs received between 1 and ≥5 FMTs	Rectal	5–7 g/kg of recipient's body weight of fresh frozen feces. Feces was thawed 4–24 h in a fridge. 2–120 mL of sterile saline was added and the mixture was blended. Saline was added until a desirable consistency was reached (a consistency that could be passed through the syringe and rectal catheter with mild-to-moderate pressure)

(continued on next page)

TABLE 1
(continued)

Author	Species	Study Title	Study Design	Indication	Number of Animals, Frequency of FMT	Route	Technique
Sugita et al, [79] 2023	Canine	Pilot Evaluation of a Single Oral Fecal Microbiota Transplantation for Canine Atopic Dermatitis	Clinical trial	Atopic dermatitis	12 dogs with atopic dermatitis, receiving a single oral FMT 20 healthy control dogs	Oral	60 g of feces were dissolved in 50 mL of tap water. Solution was filtered through medical gauze pad. 15–50 mL of this solution were administered orally using a syringe (equivalent to 2–12 g/ kg of donor feces administered)
Lin et al, [113] 2024	Canine	Effects of Fecal Microbial Transplantation on Police Performance and Transportation Stress in Kunming Police Dogs	RCT	Effects of FMT on performance and transportation stress in Kunming police dogs	20 male Wolf Cyan Kunming puppies (45–55 d old) received oral FMTs daily for 14 consecutive days	Oral	Resuspended precipitates of FMTs were used at different dilutions
Rojas et al, [71] 2024	Canine	Microbiome Responses to Oral Fecal Microbiota Transplantation in a Cohort of Domestic Dogs	Uncontrolled clinical trial	Dogs with chronic diarrhea, vomiting, or constipation	54 dogs with chronic diarrhea, vomiting, or constipation	Oral	2 capsules containing lyophilized donor feces for 25 d given with food
Lee et al, [105] 2024	Canine	Safety Profile and Effects on the Peripheral Immune Response of Fecal Microbiota Transplantation in Clinically Healthy Dogs	Case series/ uncontrolled clinical trial	Healthy dogs	10 healthy dogs were treated with a single rectal FMT. AEs and effects on peripheral immune responses were observed	Rectal	Donor feces were mixed in a ziplock bag by kneading with 2.5 mL of nonbacteriostatic sterile saline solution per gram of feces and 30% glycerol to a final glycerol concentration of 10%. The fecal slurry was filtered through mesh sieves, and

(continuation from previous page) stored in 60 mL catheter tip syringes at −80°C for a maximum of 6 mo. FMTs were thawed in a warm water bath at 37°C and administered rectally using a red rubber catheter. Dogs received between 2.5 and 5 g/kg of donor feces (weight before processing/dilution) body weight

Reference	Species	Title	Study type	Population	Route	Protocol	Processing
Vecchiato et al, [114] 2023	Canine	Fecal Microbial Transplantation Effect on Clinical Outcome and Fecal Microbiota and Metabolome in Dogs with Chronic Enteropathy Refractory to Diet	Uncontrolled clinical trial	Dogs with food refractory chronic enteropathy	Rectal	20 dogs with chronic recurrent GI signs that failed a 2 wk dietary trial with hydrolyzed diet or homemade single protein diet—received 1–2 FMTs 2–4 wk apart	2.5–5 g/kg donor feces (fresh: processed within 4 h from collection) mixed by hand in zip bag with 1:1 ratio of nonbacteriostatic sterile saline solution and filtered through fine kitchen sieve
Winston, [99] 2023, Unpublished data	Canine	Scientific and Clinical Assessment of Fecal Microbiota Transplantation to Enhance Weight Loss in Obese Dogs (SLIM Pilot Study)	Randomized, blinded clinical trial	Obese but otherwise clinically healthy dogs	Oral	19 obese dogs received a single induction dose (20 capsules; 5 capsules from each fecal donor), followed by once weekly maintenance dose (12 capsules; 3 capsules per fecal donor) for a total of 12 wk	Feces from 4 lean donors was processed by diluting feces with 1:4 nonbacteriostatic saline. The fecal slurry is filtered in a stomacher bag and double centrifuged. Glycerol is added to a 10% final concentration. Final fecal slurry was pipetted into size 0 delayed released capsules and double

(continued on next page)

TABLE 1
(continued)

Author	Species	Study Title	Study Design	Indication	Number of Animals, Frequency of FMT	Route	Technique
							encapsulated in a size 00) gelatin capsule. Fecal capsules stored at −80°C
Furmanski et al, [81] 2017	Feline	First Case Report of Fecal Microbiota Transplantation in a Cat in Israel	Case report	Ulcerative colitis	10 y old female spayed Abyssinian cat, 2 rectal FMT enemas	Rectal	5 g of donor feces were blended with nonbacteriostatic sterile saline solution at a 1:6 ratio. The suspension as filtered through a strainer yielding a large particle-free fecal slurry. 30 mL of fecal slurry were administered using a 60 mL catheter-tip sterile syringe with an 8 FR 2 way standard sterile balloon silicone-coated latex Foley catheter
Rojas et al, [72] 2023	Feline	Microbiome Responses to Fecal Microbiota Transplantation in Cats with Chronic Digestive Issues	NA	Chronic vomiting, diarrhea and/or constipation (FMT as add on treatment to standard care)	46 cats received daily oral FMTs	Oral	1–2 capsules containing lyophilized feces q24 h for until a minimum of 50 capsules were administered
Procoli, unpublished data, 2024	Feline	Cats with Food and Steroid Refractory Chronic GI Signs and Dysbiosis (Based on Fecal DI)	NA	Diarrhea, weight loss	5 cats	Rectal	2.5 g/kg fresh frozen donor feces mixed by hand in zip bag with sterile nonbacteriostatic saline solution at 1:2 ratio then filtered on a

Marsilio, unpublished data, 2024	Feline	NA	NA	Therapy-resistant diarrhea in kittens	5 kittens	Rectal	Donor feces are processed by removing litter, mixing feces with 2.5 mL/g of nonbacteriostatic saline and 30% glycerol to a final glycerol concentration of 10%. The fecal slurry is filtered through mesh sieves and stored in 60 mL catheter tip syringes at −80°C for a maximum of 6 mo	fine kitchen sieve and frozen with 10% glycerol at −20°C for max 3 mo. Max volume enema 25 mL. Administered after thawing at 37°C on day of procedure

Abbreviations: BW, body weight; DI, dysbiosis index; FMT, fecal microbiota transplantation; IBD, inflammatory bowel disease; NA, not applicable; RCT, randomized clinical trial.

Comment. Preconditioning of the bowel refers to procedures or treatments to prepare the bowel for the administration of an FMT with the goal to improve engraftment and, by extension, the outcome of a patient. Preconditioning can entail fasting, bowel lavage, and treatment with antimicrobials. The European Consensus Conference on FMT in humans recommends preconditioning with oral antimicrobials before FMT administration for patients with rCDI only and with the goal to reduce the abundance of *C. difficile* [9]. However, preconditioning with antimicrobials has shown to negatively affect engraftment in patients with irritable bowel syndrome [87]. The most common indication for FMT in companion animals is currently chronic enteropathy, which is a distinctively different disorder than rCDI. Therefore, the Companion Animal FMT Consortium advises against preconditioning of the GI tract with antimicrobials, and their use should be strictly limited to situations where clinically indicated for other reasons. The effect of bowel lavages and cleansing enemas on FMT engraftment and patient outcome is unknown; therefore, the Companion Animal FMT Consortium does not recommend such procedures unless required for patient procedure preparation. To reduce residual fecal matter in the recipient prior to FMT and possibly prolong FMT retention, the Companion Animal FMT Consortium recommends fasting patients prior to FMT administration.

Fecal microbiota transplantation dosing

Statement. No evidence-based dosing regimen for administration of FMTs in any form (fresh, frozen, or lyophilized) or through any route (oral or rectal) can be provided at this point.

Quality of evidence: Low.

Comment. The techniques for FMT administration in the literature and among members of the Companion Animal FMT Consortium vary widely. For FMTs administered via rectal enemas, some FMT Consortium members prefer smaller volumes of concentrated fecal slurries to increase the retention time, while others prefer larger volumes to increase mucosal surface contact. There are currently no studies supporting either technique. To provide guidance, the Companion Animal FMT Consortium summarized doses and techniques that have previously been published and/or used by members of the FMT Consortium (see Table 1). It is important to note that the administration of rectal enemas may cause vomiting and subsequently aspiration, especially in cats. The effect is mostly volume

dependent. Companion Animal FMT Consortium members routinely administer the following fecal slurry volumes via rectal enema to dogs and cats:

- Medium-to-large-sized dogs: 10 to 20 mL/kg body weight of the recipient
- Small dogs and cats: 5 to 10 mL/kg body weight of the recipient

Statement. While some preliminary data exist that FMT may be of value for some extra-GI diseases (eg, diabetes mellitus and obesity), the level of evidence or even anecdotal reports are scarce. The routine use of FMT for the treatment of extra-GI diseases cannot be recommended at this point.

Quality of evidence: Low.

Comment. It has recently been suggested that in complex extra-GI diseases, precise manipulation of microbes and microbial metabolism may be more tractable than modulating host physiology, in part, due to the plasticity of the microbial ecosystems [88]. The gut microbiota influences the pathogenesis of metabolic diseases like diabetes mellitus, metabolic syndrome, and obesity through mechanisms such as the production of bacterial metabolites (eg, short-chain fatty acids, secondary bile acids, and indole metabolites) that can compromise intestinal barrier integrity, promote chronic inflammation, and affect glucose homeostasis; however, these sequelae may be potentially reversible by FMT [89,90].

FMT studies in humans with type 2 diabetes mellitus have shown minimal clinical effects but significant shifts in gut microbial communities, indicating a complex relationship between the microbiota and metabolic health [91]. In type 1 diabetes mellitus (T1DM), FMT has been observed to prolong beta cell function, with microbial composition and certain biomarkers predicting the preservation of this function, highlighting the potential of microbiome modulation in the management of T1DM [92]. A meta-analysis and various clinical trials on metabolic syndrome and obesity have shown mixed short-term benefits of FMT, including improved hemoglobin A1c (HbA1C) levels and lipid profiles in some cases, but no consistent effects on obesity, illustrating the nuanced impact of FMT on metabolic parameters [93]. A small pilot, prospective, randomized, double-blinded, controlled veterinary clinical trial on diabetic dogs showed that FMT decreased water consumption and had a modest effect on host metabolism but did not change key diabetic indicators, expanding the interest in microbiome intervention in dogs [94].

For obesity, there are multiple human placebo controlled RCTs that highlight the important role that the gut microbiota play in obesity and metabolic disease and demonstrate that engraftment of lean microbes into an obesogenic gut ecosystem is possible [95,96]. Dysbiosis is noted in obese companion animals [97,98], indicating that microbial targeted intervention, such as FMT, may be beneficial. Currently in veterinary medicine, there are 2 ongoing clinical trials (SLIM studies) evaluating the scientific and clinical utility of FMT to enhance weight loss in obese dogs and cats. The SLIM studies are the first to evaluate the efficacy of FMT as an adjunctive therapy for canine and feline obesity management and will shed light on the role(s) that the gut ecosystem plays during treatment and recovery from an obesogenic disease state [99].

Fecal microbiota transplantation frequency

Statement. Repeated FMT treatments can be beneficial in dogs with chronic enteropathy, but the specific number of FMTs and the administration frequency are dependent upon individual patient factors.
Quality of evidence: Low.

Comment. In a survey for veterinarians assessing FMT practices in small animal patients, approximately two-thirds of participants reported that FMTs were routinely administered to patients more than once, yet the frequency of repeated administrations ranged from daily to every 2 weeks [100]. Repeated FMTs may improve engraftment and clinical response after the initial treatment in some dogs, particularly in patients with more severe dysbiosis. In a retrospective study examining the clinical effects of adjunctive FMT therapy in 41 dogs with chronic enteropathy, a median of 3 FMTs was administered to each dog via rectal enema, with most dogs receiving treatments at 10 to 20 day intervals [20]. Additionally in 74% of FMT responders, further clinical improvement was observed after receiving a second FMT, as compared to the first [20]. Factors such as clinical response to FMT, adverse effects, patient tolerance of the procedure, and client factors should be considered when determining the number and administration intervals of FMTs in individual patients.

Statement. Fewer total FMTs may be required for acute diarrhea in dogs, with one study in dogs with parvovirus infection requiring an average of 1.8 (range 1–3) transplants until improvement of diarrhea.
Quality of evidence: Moderate.

Comment. As in dogs with chronic enteropathy, the specific number of FMTs for dogs with acute diarrhea is dependent on the individual patient and is typically based on clinical response, adverse effects, patient tolerance of the procedure, and client-related factors. In a study of dogs with canine parvovirus infection, a mean of 1.8 FMTs were administered [67], as compared to a median of 3 FMTs reported in dogs with chronic enteropathy [20]. A single FMT dose has also produced positive clinical outcomes in dogs with acute uncomplicated diarrhea [18]. Thus, fewer total FMTs might be sufficient in dogs with acute diarrhea as compared to dogs with chronic enteropathy.

Statement. There are currently no data or reports available on the frequency of administration of FMTs for cats with acute or chronic enteropathy.
Quality of evidence: Low.

Comment. Data regarding the frequency of administration of FMTs in cats are not available. As in dogs, the number of FMTs and the frequency of administration should be determined on a case-by-case basis and based on the clinical response to initial FMT, adverse effects, tolerance of the procedure, and client-related factors.

Fecal microbiota transplantation retention times

Statement. No studies on the effect of retention time on the outcome of patients have been conducted in humans or companion animals. Members of the Companion Animal FMT Consortium are generally aiming for a minimum retention time of 30 to 45 minutes.
Quality of evidence: Low.

Comment. Improved engraftment of donated microbes is a theoretic benefit of prolonged retention of transplanted material, though a consensus recommendation for ideal retention time has not been established. For Companion Animal FMT Consortium members, a retention time of at least 30 to 45 minutes is targeted in dogs and cats receiving FMT via rectal enema, but defecation of the transplanted material prior to that time should not be considered a treatment failure. In one study of 41 dogs receiving an FMT via rectal enema, only one dog defecated within 30 minutes of the procedure [20]. The remaining dogs had an owner-reported minimum retention time ranging from 1 to 15 hours [20].

Patient sedation

Statement. Sedation should be considered on a case-by-case basis, with particular consideration given to patients that are anxious, aggressive, intolerant of the procedure, or unable to retain the transplant.

Quality of evidence: Low.

Comment. The decision to use sedation is made on a case-by-case basis and determined by patient temperament. No prospective, controlled studies have neither evaluated whether sedation prolongs retention time in dogs and cats nor evaluated how the use of sedation impacts overall efficacy of the procedure. The majority of the Companion Animal FMT Consortium members (67%) report never or rarely using sedation in dogs receiving FMT, whereas 40% report never or rarely using sedation in cats. For patients with severe colitis-associated rectal pain, local analgesia (eg, rectal suppositories containing a local anesthetic) could be considered if available and applicable to the patient.

Endpoints for fecal microbiota transplantation

Statement. Different endpoints for measuring the success of an FMT need to be considered including quality of life, clinical signs, and/or reduction or discontinuation of concurrent medication such as immunosuppressants or antimicrobials. Further studies are needed to assess biomarker-based endpoints such as the DI or other measures of the intestinal microbiota as tools to assess treatment success.

Quality of evidence: Low.

Comment. While the canine and feline DI might be helpful as biomarker to guide FMT-based therapy in individual cases, the DI does not normalize in every patient and/or long term despite improvement or resolution of clinical signs.

Statement. While FMT is generally considered a safe treatment and often helpful in a variety of primary GI diseases, it should be considered as part of a multimodal treatment approach rather than a sole treatment option.

Quality of evidence: Low.

Comment. While anecdotal reports of FMT as the sole successful treatment of acute or chronic GI disorders exist, most trials in humans and small animals have used FMT as an adjunct treatment in conjunction with other treatment modalities.

Adverse events for fecal microbiota transplantation

Statement. While there is a scarcity of data on adverse events (AEs) in dogs and cats, data in human medicine and reports in veterinary medicine show that FMTs are generally considered safe with few serious side effects reported even in immunocompromised patients (eg, dogs with parvovirus infection) and patients on immunotherapy (eg, corticosteroids).

Quality of evidence: Moderate.

Comment. In a 2021 metanalysis evaluating 9 high-quality studies from which data were collected for 756 FMTs performed in 388 patients for the treatment of *C. difficile* infection, the total pooled rate of AE was 39.3% with most AEs being mild (eg, self-limiting signs such as flatulence, abdominal pain, vomiting, bloating, nausea, constipation, headaches, dizziness, or fever) [101]. In a 2018 Cochrane review evaluating 4 studies with a total of 277 participants with ulcerative colitis, the authors noted that it was challenging to differentiate serious AEs (eg, aspiration pneumonia, bowel perforation, sepsis, or death) related to the FMT itself, the procedure involved with the delivery, or the underlying disease [102]. A total of 7% (10 out of 140) of FMT participants had serious AEs compared to 5% (7 out of 137) of control participants (RR 1.40, 95% CI 0.55–3.58; 4 studies; IO = 0%; low certainty evidence). A total of 78% (50 out of 64) FMT participants had mild AEs compared to 75% (49 out of 65) in the control group (RR 1.03, 95% CI 0.81–1.31; IO = 31%; moderate certainty evidence). As with the predisposition of chronic enteropathy, several factors likely play a role in the development of FMT-related AEs including the method of FMT administration, presence of comorbidities and immunocompetence, concurrent medications, the integrity of the gut mucosal barrier of the recipient, and the rigor of the fecal donor screening process.

Statement. The most commonly reported adverse effects (AEs) associated with FMT in both humans and companion animals include worsening of diarrhea, bloating, flatulence, abdominal pain, nausea, vomiting, and dysorexia. Rarely fever and dehydration have been reported in companion animals.

Quality of evidence: Moderate.

Comment. As described in the statement earlier, the majority of AEs associated with FMT administration to humans is mild. In studies where FMT has been performed in dogs and cats [18,20,72,86,103], very few have reported AEs although it is unclear if a monitoring protocol was in place to detect AEs in all studies. In an unpublished, uncontrolled study, mild AEs (eg, fever, diarrhea, vomiting, inappetence, and abdominal pain) were described in a group of colony cats and cats with chronic enteropathy [104]. These signs were not observed in a study of client owned, healthy dogs where a monitoring system was in place to detect AEs [105]. Systematic controlled studies are needed to determine the prevalence of AEs in dogs and cats receiving FMT. Additionally, a unified standard for screening of donors for FMT administration to dogs and cats as well as a central repository for reporting FMT-related AEs are strongly recommended to help minimize FMT-related AEs and to better describe their occurrence in veterinary medicine. Until then, clients should be made aware of the possibility, albeit low, of FMT-related AEs.

SUMMARY

The gut microbiota is an intricate and complex ecosystem that has substantial impacts on the host during health and disease [115]. As demonstrated herein, dysbiosis has been noted in a variety of disease states in veterinary medicine and FMT should be considered as microbial-directed therapeutic. To increase accessibility of FMT to dogs and cats, establishment of a fecal donor program should be considered in any practice setting where FMT would be utilized on a regular basis. The Companion Animal FMT Consortium developed these clinical guidelines specifically to provide veterinarians with guidance for fecal donor selection and screening, standardized FMT preparations, and current recommended FMT clinical applications. These clinical guidelines are the first available to provide veterinarians with evidence-based statements to increase the accessibility of FMT as a microbial-directed therapeutic in veterinary medicine.

As we continue to acquire knowledge about the therapeutic potential of FMT in companion animals, rational decisions about how to manipulate gut microbial ecosystems given a specific dysbiotic state will become available. Aligned with the Companion Animal FMT Consortium's mission, to promote accessibility of FMT to veterinarians in diverse practice settings, the FMT Consortium plans to provide updated clinical FMT guidelines for dogs and cats every 5 years as new evidence for FMT emerges in small animal medicine.

CLINICS CARE POINTS

- A fecal donor program can readily be established in any practice type; thus, increasing the accessibility of FMT to dogs and cats.
- FMT processing and preparation can be modified based on the availability of equipment and resources. Ideally, fresh feces should be utilized for FMT whenever possible.
- Substantial evidence for use of FMT in patients suffering from canine parvovirus enteritis, canine acute diarrhea, and chronic enteropathy is currently available. FMT should be considered as an adjunctive therapeutic in these diseases. Active research into other clinical applications for FMT in veterinary medicine are actively underway.
- Although no specific FMT dosing can be recommended at this time, Table 1 provides an overview of FMT formulation, dosing, and frequency of administration based on the available veterinary evidence.

CONTRIBUTORS

The Companion Animal FMT Consortium chair (J.A Winston) planned all the virtual meetings and organized members of the consortium. All consortium members established the main topics. Working groups leads (J.S. Suchodolski, F. Gaschen, K. Busch, and S. Marsilio) orchestrated the development of topic statements. Once statements were finalized, each working group provided supporting evidence and drafted the text of commentary relevant to their statements. J.A. Winston wrote the initial draft of the article. All consortium members read and revised the article for important intellectual content and approved the final article.

DISCLOSURE

J.S. Suchodolski and M. Katherine Tolbert are employees of the Gastrointestinal Laboratory at Texas A&M University, which offers microbiome testing including the DI on a fee-for-service basis. Both authors refrained from contributing to the microbiome screening section of these clinical guidelines.

SUPPLEMENTARY DATA

Supplementary data to this article can be found online at https://doi.org/10.1016/j.yasa.2024.06.006.

REFERENCES

[1] Libertucci J, Young VB. The role of the microbiota in infectious diseases. Nat Microbiol 2019;4(1):35–45.

[2] Tan P, Li X, Shen J, et al. Fecal Microbiota Transplantation for the Treatment of Inflammatory Bowel Disease: An Update. Front Pharmacol 2020;11:574533.

[3] Napolitano M, Covasa M. Microbiota Transplant in the Treatment of Obesity and Diabetes: Current and Future Perspectives. Front Microbiol 2020;11:590370.

[4] Vendrik KEW, Ooijevaar RE, de Jong PRC, et al. Fecal Microbiota Transplantation in Neurological Disorders. Front Cell Infect Microbiol 2020;10:98.

[5] Chen D, Wu J, Jin D, et al. Fecal microbiota transplantation in cancer management: Current status and perspectives. Int J Cancer 2019;145(8):2021–31.

[6] McDonald LC, Gerding DN, Johnson S, et al. Clinical Practice Guidelines for *Clostridium difficile* Infection in Adults and Children: 2017 Update by the Infectious Diseases Society of America (IDSA) and Society for Healthcare Epidemiology of America (SHEA). Clin Infect Dis 2018;66(7):987–94.

[7] Chaitman J, Jergens AE, Gaschen F, et al. Commentary on key aspects of fecal microbiota transplantation in small animal practice. Vet Med Auckl NZ 2016;7:71–4.

[8] Chaitman J, Gaschen F. Fecal Microbiota Transplantation in Dogs. Vet Clin North Am Small Anim Pract 2021;51(1):219–33.

[9] Cammarota G, Ianiro G, Tilg H, et al. European consensus conference on faecal microbiota transplantation in clinical practice. Gut 2017;66(4):569–80.

[10] Hsu CC, Sandford BA. The Delphi Technique: Making Sense of Consensus. doi:10.7275/PDZ9-TH90.

[11] Guyatt GH, Oxman AD, Vist GE, et al. GRADE: an emerging consensus on rating quality of evidence and strength of recommendations. BMJ 2008;336(7650):924–6, AD.

[12] Atkins D, Best D, Briss PA, et al. Grading quality of evidence and strength of recommendations. BMJ 2004; 328(7454):1490.

[13] Woodworth MH, Carpentieri C, Sitchenko KL, et al. Challenges in fecal donor selection and screening for fecal microbiota transplantation: a review. Gut Microb 2017;8(3):225–37.

[14] Vecchiato CG, Golinelli S, Pinna C, et al. Fecal microbiota and inflammatory and antioxidant status of obese and lean dogs, and the effect of caloric restriction. Front Microbiol 2022;13:1050474.

[15] Suchodolski JS, Markel ME, Garcia-Mazcorro JF, et al. The fecal microbiome in dogs with acute diarrhea and idiopathic inflammatory bowel disease. PLoS One 2012;7(12):e51907.

[16] Sung CH, Marsilio S, Chow B, et al. Dysbiosis index to evaluate the fecal microbiota in healthy cats and cats with chronic enteropathies. J Feline Med Surg 2022; 24(6):e1–12.

[17] Ziese AL, Suchodolski JS, Hartmann K, et al. Effect of probiotic treatment on the clinical course, intestinal microbiome, and toxigenic *Clostridium perfringens* in dogs with acute hemorrhagic diarrhea. PLoS One 2018;13(9):e0204691.

[18] Chaitman J, Ziese AL, Pilla R, et al. Fecal Microbial and Metabolic Profiles in Dogs With Acute Diarrhea Receiving Either Fecal Microbiota Transplantation or Oral Metronidazole. Front Vet Sci 2020;7:192.

[19] Werner M, Suchodolski JS, Straubinger RK, et al. Effect of amoxicillin-clavulanic acid on clinical scores, intestinal microbiome, and amoxicillin-resistant *Escherichia coli* in dogs with uncomplicated acute diarrhea. J Vet Intern Med 2020;34(3):1166–76.

[20] Toresson L, Spillmann T, Pilla R, et al. Clinical Effects of Faecal Microbiota Transplantation as Adjunctive Therapy in Dogs with Chronic Enteropathies-A Retrospective Case Series of 41 Dogs. Vet Sci 2023;10(4):271.

[21] Stübing H, Suchodolski JS, Reisinger A, et al. The Effect of Metronidazole versus a Synbiotic on Clinical Course and Core Intestinal Microbiota in Dogs with Acute Diarrhea. Vet Sci 2024;11(5):197.

[22] AlShawaqfeh MK, Wajid B, Minamoto Y, et al. A dysbiosis index to assess microbial changes in fecal samples of dogs with chronic inflammatory enteropathy. FEMS Microbiol Ecol 2017;93(11).

[23] Blake AB, Cigarroa A, Klein HL, et al. Developmental stages in microbiota, bile acids, and clostridial species in healthy puppies. J Vet Intern Med 2020;34(6): 2345–56.

[24] Stavroulaki EM, Suchodolski JS, Pilla R, et al. Short- and long-term effects of amoxicillin/clavulanic acid or doxycycline on the gastrointestinal microbiome of growing cats. PLoS One 2021;16(12):e0253031.

[25] Leite G, Pimentel M, Barlow GM, et al. Age and the aging process significantly alter the small bowel microbiome. Cell Rep 2021;36(13):109765.

[26] Fernández-Pinteño A, Pilla R, Manteca X, et al. Age-associated changes in intestinal health biomarkers in dogs. Front Vet Sci 2023;10:1213287.

[27] Lefebvre SL, Reid-Smith RJ, Waltner-Toews D, et al. Incidence of acquisition of methicillin-resistant *Staphylococcus aureus*, *Clostridium difficile*, and other health-care-associated pathogens by dogs that participate in animal-assisted interventions. J Am Vet Med Assoc 2009;234(11):1404–17.

[28] Mendoza Roldan JA, Otranto D. Zoonotic parasites associated with predation by dogs and cats. Parasit Vectors 2023;16(1):55.

[29] Chalkowski K, Wilson AE, Lepczyk CA, et al. Who let the cats out? A global meta-analysis on risk of parasitic infection in indoor versus outdoor domestic cats (*Felis catus*). Biol Lett 2019;15(4):20180840.

[30] Hofmann-Lehmann R, Hartmann K. Feline leukaemia virus infection: A practical approach to diagnosis. J Feline Med Surg 2020;22(9):831–46.

[31] Stavroulaki EM, Suchodolski JS, Xenoulis PG. Effects of antimicrobials on the gastrointestinal microbiota

of dogs and cats. Vet J Lond Engl 1997 2023;291: 105929.

[32] Pilla R, Gaschen FP, Barr JW, et al. Effects of metronidazole on the fecal microbiome and metabolome in healthy dogs. J Vet Intern Med 2020;34(5):1853–66.

[33] Manchester AC, Webb CB, Blake AB, et al. Long-term impact of tylosin on fecal microbiota and fecal bile acids of healthy dogs. J Vet Intern Med 2019;33(6): 2605–17.

[34] Jones SM, Gaier A, Enomoto H, et al. The effect of combined carprofen and omeprazole administration on gastrointestinal permeability and inflammation in dogs. J Vet Intern Med 2020;34(5):1886–93.

[35] McAtee R, Schmid SM, Tolbert MK, et al. Effect of esomeprazole with and without a probiotic on fecal dysbiosis, intestinal inflammation, and fecal short-chain fatty acid concentrations in healthy dogs. J Vet Intern Med 2023;37(6):2109–18.

[36] Garcia-Mazcorro JF, Suchodolski JS, Jones KR, et al. Effect of the proton pump inhibitor omeprazole on the gastrointestinal bacterial microbiota of healthy dogs. FEMS Microbiol Ecol 2012;80(3):624–36.

[37] Schmid SM, Suchodolski JS, Price JM, et al. Omeprazole Minimally Alters the Fecal Microbial Community in Six Cats: A Pilot Study. Front Vet Sci 2018;5:79.

[38] Mounsey O, Wareham K, Hammond A, et al. Evidence that faecal carriage of resistant *Escherichia coli* by 16-week-old dogs in the United Kingdom is associated with raw feeding. One Health Amst Neth 2022;14: 100370.

[39] Finley R, Ribble C, Aramini J, et al. The risk of salmonellae shedding by dogs fed *Salmonella*-contaminated commercial raw food diets. Can Vet J 2007;48(1): 69–75.

[40] Solís D, Toro M, Navarrete P, et al. Microbiological Quality and Presence of Foodborne Pathogens in Raw and Extruded Canine Diets and Canine Fecal Samples. Front Vet Sci 2022;9:799710.

[41] Runesvärd E, Wikström C, Fernström LL, et al. Presence of pathogenic bacteria in faeces from dogs fed raw meat-based diets or dry kibble. Vet Rec 2020;187(9): e71.

[42] Schmidt M, Unterer S, Suchodolski JS, et al. The fecal microbiome and metabolome differs between dogs fed Bones and Raw Food (BARF) diets and dogs fed commercial diets. PLoS One 2018;13(8):e0201279.

[43] Garcia-Mazcorro JF, Lanerie DJ, Dowd SE, et al. Effect of a multi-species synbiotic formulation on fecal bacterial microbiota of healthy cats and dogs as evaluated by pyrosequencing. FEMS Microbiol Ecol 2011;78(3): 542–54.

[44] Félix AP, Souza CMM, de Oliveira SG. Biomarkers of gastrointestinal functionality in dogs: A systematic review and meta-analysis. Anim Feed Sci Technol 2022; 283:115183.

[45] Sung CH, Pilla R, Chen CC, et al. Correlation between Targeted qPCR Assays and Untargeted DNA Shotgun Metagenomic Sequencing for Assessing the Fecal Microbiota in Dogs. Anim Open Access J MDPI 2023;13(16): 2597.

[46] Roume H, Mondot S, Saliou A, et al. Multicenter evaluation of gut microbiome profiling by next-generation sequencing reveals major biases in partial-length metabarcoding approach. Sci Rep 2023;13(1):22593.

[47] Forry SP, Servetas SL, Kralj JG, et al. Variability and bias in microbiome metagenomic sequencing: an interlaboratory study comparing experimental protocols. Sci Rep 2024;14(1):9785.

[48] Hitch TCA, Afrizal A, Riedel T, et al. Recent advances in culture-based gut microbiome research. Int J Med Microbiol IJMM 2021;311(3):151485.

[49] Werner M, Suchodolski JS, Lidbury JA, et al. Diagnostic value of fecal cultures in dogs with chronic diarrhea. J Vet Intern Med 2021;35(1):199–208.

[50] Companion Animal Parasite Council Parasite Guidelines. Companion Animal Parasite Council. Available at: https://capcvet.org/guidelines/.

[51] Leipig-Rudolph M, Busch K, Prescott JF, et al. Intestinal lesions in dogs with acute hemorrhagic diarrhea syndrome associated with netF-positive *Clostridium perfringens* type A. J Vet Diagn Investig Off Publ Am Assoc Vet Lab Diagn Inc 2018;30(4):495–503.

[52] Mehdizadeh Gohari I, Parreira VR, Nowell VJ, et al. A novel pore-forming toxin in type A *Clostridium perfringens* is associated with both fatal canine hemorrhagic gastroenteritis and fatal foal necrotizing enterocolitis. PLoS One 2015;10(4):e0122684.

[53] Sindern N, Suchodolski JS, Leutenegger CM, et al. Prevalence of *Clostridium perfringens* netE and netF toxin genes in the feces of dogs with acute hemorrhagic diarrhea syndrome. J Vet Intern Med 2019;33(1):100–5.

[54] Busch K, Suchodolski JS, Kuhner KA, et al. *Clostridium perfringens* enterotoxin and *Clostridium difficile* toxin A/B do not play a role in acute haemorrhagic diarrhoea syndrome in dogs. Vet Rec 2015;176(10):253.

[55] Weese JS. *Clostridium* (*Clostridioides*) *difficile* in animals. J Vet Diagn Investig Off Publ Am Assoc Vet Lab Diagn Inc 2020;32(2):213–21.

[56] Loo VG, Brassard P, Miller MA. Household Transmission of *Clostridium difficile* to Family Members and Domestic Pets. Infect Control Hosp Epidemiol 2016; 37(11):1342–8.

[57] Redding LE, Habing GG, Tu V, et al. Infrequent intrahousehold transmission of *Clostridioides difficile* between pet owners and their pets. Zoonoses Public Health 2023;70(4):341–51.

[58] Werner M, Ishii PE, Pilla R, et al. Prevalence of *Clostridioides difficile* in Canine Feces and Its Association with Intestinal Dysbiosis. Anim Open Access J MDPI 2023;13(15):2441.

[59] Thanissery R, McLaren MR, Rivera A, et al. *Clostridioides difficile* carriage in animals and the associated changes in the host fecal microbiota. Anaerobe 2020;66: 102279.

[60] Tal M, Verbrugghe A, Gomez DE, et al. The effect of storage at ambient temperature on the feline fecal microbiota. BMC Vet Res 2017;13(1):256.

[61] Langon X. Validation of method for faecal sampling in cats and dogs for faecal microbiome analysis. BMC Vet Res 2023;19(1):274.

[62] Barko P, Nguyen-Edquilang J, Williams DA, et al. Fecal microbiome composition and diversity of cryopreserved canine stool at different duration and storage conditions. PLoS One 2024;19(2):e0294730.

[63] Bénard MV, Arretxe I, Wortelboer K, et al. Anaerobic Feces Processing for Fecal Microbiota Transplantation Improves Viability of Obligate Anaerobes. Microorganisms 2023;11(9):2238.

[64] Shimizu H, Arai K, Asahara T, et al. Stool preparation under anaerobic conditions contributes to retention of obligate anaerobes: potential improvement for fecal microbiota transplantation. BMC Microbiol 2021;21(1):275.

[65] Allegretti JR, Elliott RJ, Ladha A, et al. Stool processing speed and storage duration do not impact the clinical effectiveness of fecal microbiota transplantation. Gut Microb 2020;11(6):1806–8.

[66] Lee CH, Steiner T, Petrof EO, et al. Frozen vs Fresh Fecal Microbiota Transplantation and Clinical Resolution of Diarrhea in Patients With Recurrent Clostridium difficile Infection: A Randomized Clinical Trial. JAMA 2016;315(2):142–9.

[67] Pereira GQ, Gomes LA, Santos IS, et al. Fecal microbiota transplantation in puppies with canine parvovirus infection. J Vet Intern Med 2018;32(2):707–11.

[68] Abkar L, Moghaddam HS, Fowler SJ. Microbial ecology of drinking water from source to tap. Sci Total Environ 2024;908:168077.

[69] Kao D, Roach B, Silva M, et al. Effect of Oral Capsule- vs Colonoscopy-Delivered Fecal Microbiota Transplantation on Recurrent Clostridium difficile Infection: A Randomized Clinical Trial. JAMA 2017;318(20):1985–93.

[70] Jiang ZD, Jenq RR, Ajami NJ, et al. Safety and preliminary efficacy of orally administered lyophilized fecal microbiota product compared with frozen product given by enema for recurrent Clostridium difficile infection: A randomized clinical trial. PLoS One 2018;13(11):e0205064.

[71] Rojas CA, Entrolezo Z, Jarett JK, et al. Microbiome Responses to Oral Fecal Microbiota Transplantation in a Cohort of Domestic Dogs. Vet Sci 2024;11(1):42.

[72] Rojas CA, Entrolezo Z, Jarett JK, et al. Microbiome Responses to Fecal Microbiota Transplantation in Cats with Chronic Digestive Issues. Vet Sci 2023;10(9):561.

[73] Saliba R, Zahar JR, El Allaoui F, et al. Impact of freeze/thaw cycles and single freezing at -80 °C on the viability of aerobic bacteria from rectal swabs performed with the ESwabTM system. Diagn Microbiol Infect Dis 2020;96(3):114895.

[74] Du C, Luo Y, Walsh S, et al. Oral Fecal Microbiota Transplant Capsules Are Safe and Effective for Recurrent Clostridioides difficile Infection: A Systematic Review and Meta-Analysis. J Clin Gastroenterol 2021;55(4):300–8.

[75] Tariq R, Hayat M, Pardi D, et al. Predictors of failure after fecal microbiota transplantation for recurrent Clostridioides difficile infection: a systematic review and meta-analysis. Eur J Clin Microbiol Infect Dis 2021;40(7):1383–92.

[76] Lee EH, Lee SK, Cheon JH, et al. Comparing the efficacy of different methods of faecal microbiota transplantation via oral capsule, oesophagogastroduodenoscopy, colonoscopy, or gastric tube. J Hosp Infect 2023;131:234–43.

[77] Gal A, Barko PC, Biggs PJ, et al. One dog's waste is another dog's wealth: A pilot study of fecal microbiota transplantation in dogs with acute hemorrhagic diarrhea syndrome. PLoS One 2021;16(4):e0250344.

[78] Gough E, Shaikh H, Manges AR. Systematic review of intestinal microbiota transplantation (fecal bacteriotherapy) for recurrent Clostridium difficile infection. Clin Infect Dis 2011;53(10):994–1002.

[79] Sugita K, Shima A, Takahashi K, et al. Pilot evaluation of a single oral fecal microbiota transplantation for canine atopic dermatitis. Sci Rep 2023;13(1):8824.

[80] Bottero E, Benvenuti E, Ruggiero P. Fecal microbiota transplantation (FMT) in 16 dogs with idiopatic IBD. Published online 2017.

[81] Furmanski S, Mor T. First case report of fecal microbiota transplantation in a cat in Israel. Isr J Vet Med 2017;72(3):35–41.

[82] Tang G, Yin W, Liu W. Is frozen fecal microbiota transplantation as effective as fresh fecal microbiota transplantation in patients with recurrent or refractory Clostridium difficile infection: A meta-analysis? Diagn Microbiol Infect Dis 2017;88(4):322–9.

[83] Hui W, Li T, Liu W, et al. Fecal microbiota transplantation for treatment of recurrent C. difficile infection: An updated randomized controlled trial meta-analysis. PLoS One 2019;14(1):e0210016.

[84] Fehily SR, Basnayake C, Wright EK, et al. Fecal microbiota transplantation therapy in Crohn's disease: Systematic review. J Gastroenterol Hepatol 2021;36(10):2672–86.

[85] Youngster I, Mahabamunuge J, Systrom HK, et al. Oral, frozen fecal microbiota transplant (FMT) capsules for recurrent Clostridium difficile infection. BMC Med 2016;14(1):134.

[86] Niina A, Kibe R, Suzuki R, et al. Improvement in Clinical Symptoms and Fecal Microbiome After Fecal Microbiota Transplantation in a Dog with Inflammatory Bowel Disease. Vet Med Auckl NZ 2019;10:197–201.

[87] Singh P, Alm EJ, Kelley JM, et al. Effect of antibiotic pretreatment on bacterial engraftment after Fecal Microbiota Transplant (FMT) in IBS-D. Gut Microb 2022;14(1):2020067.

[88] Maruvada P, Leone V, Kaplan LM, et al. The Human Microbiome and Obesity: Moving beyond Associations. Cell Host Microbe 2017;22(5):589–99.

[89] Fuhri Snethlage CM, Nieuwdorp M, Hanssen NMJ. Faecal microbiota transplantation in endocrine diseases and obesity. Best Pract Res Clin Endocrinol Metab 2021;35(3):101483.

[90] Okubo H, Nakatsu Y, Kushiyama A, et al. Gut Microbiota as a Therapeutic Target for Metabolic Disorders. Curr Med Chem 2018;25(9):984–1001.

[91] Su L, Hong Z, Zhou T, et al. Health improvements of type 2 diabetic patients through diet and diet plus fecal microbiota transplantation. Sci Rep 2022;12(1):1152.

[92] de Groot P, Nikolic T, Pellegrini S, et al. Faecal microbiota transplantation halts progression of human new-onset type 1 diabetes in a randomised controlled trial. Gut 2021;70(1):92–105.

[93] Leong KSW, Jayasinghe TN, Wilson BC, et al. Effects of Fecal Microbiome Transfer in Adolescents With Obesity: The Gut Bugs Randomized Controlled Trial. JAMA Netw Open 2020;3(12):e2030415.

[94] A. Gal, Interim analysis of a prospective clinical trial of fecal microbial transplantation in diabetic dogs, Presented at ACVIM Forum (2022).

[95] Allegretti JR, Kassam Z, Mullish BH, et al. Effects of Fecal Microbiota Transplantation With Oral Capsules in Obese Patients. Clin Gastroenterol Hepatol 2020;18(4):855–63.e2.

[96] Yu EW, Gao L, Stastka P, et al. Fecal microbiota transplantation for the improvement of metabolism in obesity: The FMT-TRIM double-blind placebo-controlled pilot trial. PLoS Med 2020;17(3):e1003051.

[97] Thomson P, Santibáñez R, Rodríguez-Salas C, et al. Differences in the composition and predicted functions of the intestinal microbiome of obese and normal weight adult dogs. PeerJ 2022;10:e12695.

[98] Ma X, Brinker E, Graff EC, et al. Whole-Genome Shotgun Metagenomic Sequencing Reveals Distinct Gut Microbiome Signatures of Obese Cats. Microbiol Spectr 2022;10(3):e0083722.

[99] Winston JA. Harnessing the Power of Microbes to Fight Obesity. Presented at ACVIM Forum; 2023.

[100] Salavati Schmitz S. Observational Study of Small Animal Practitioners' Awareness, Clinical Practice and Experience With Fecal Microbiota Transplantation in Dogs. Top Companion Anim Med 2022;47:100630.

[101] Michailidis L, Currier AC, Le M, et al. Adverse events of fecal microbiota transplantation: a meta-analysis of high-quality studies. Ann Gastroenterol 2021;34(6):802–14.

[102] Imdad A, Pandit NG, Zaman M, et al. Fecal transplantation for treatment of inflammatory bowel disease. Cochrane Database Syst Rev 2023;4(4):CD012774.

[103] Niina A, Kibe R, Suzuki R, et al. Fecal microbiota transplantation as a new treatment for canine inflammatory bowel disease. Biosci Microbiota Food Health 2021;40(2):98–104.

[104] M.A. Lee, T. Slead, M.K. Tolbert, et al., Adverse Events Following Repeat Fecal Microbiota Transplantation in Cats: A Case Series, Presented at ACVIM Forum (2023).

[105] Lee MA, Questa M, Wanakumjorn P, et al. Safety profile and effects on the peripheral immune response of fecal microbiota transplantation in clinically healthy dogs. J Vet Intern Med 2024;38(3):1425–36.

[106] Burton EN, O'Connor E, Ericsson AC, et al. Evaluation of Fecal Microbiota Transfer as Treatment for Post-weaning Diarrhea in Research-Colony Puppies. J Am Assoc Lab Anim Sci JAALAS 2016;55(5):582–7. Available at: https://www.ncbi.nlm.nih.gov/pmc/articles/PMC5029830/. [Accessed 31 May 2024].

[107] Sugita K, Yanuma N, Ohno H, et al. Oral faecal microbiota transplantation for the treatment of *Clostridium difficile*-associated diarrhoea in a dog: a case report. BMC Vet Res 2019;15(1):11.

[108] Sugita K, Shima A, Takahashi K, et al. Successful outcome after a single endoscopic fecal microbiota transplantation in a Shiba dog with non-responsive enteropathy during the treatment with chlorambucil. J Vet Med Sci 2021;83(6):984–9. Available at: https://www.jstage.jst.go.jp/article/jvms/83/6/83_21-0063/_article/-char/ja/. [Accessed 31 May 2024].

[109] Cerquetella M, Marchegiani A, Rossi G, et al. Case Report: Oral Fecal Microbiota Transplantation in a Dog Suffering From Relapsing Chronic Diarrhea—Clinical Outcome and Follow-Up. Front Vet Sci 2022;9.

[110] Marclay M, Dwyer E, Suchodolski JS, et al. Recovery of Fecal Microbiome and Bile Acids in Healthy Dogs after Tylosin Administration with and without Fecal Microbiota Transplantation. Vet Sci 2022;9(7):324.

[111] Collier AJ, Gomez DE, Monteith G, et al. Investigating fecal microbial transplant as a novel therapy in dogs with inflammatory bowel disease: A preliminary study. PLoS One 2022;17(10):e0276295.

[112] Alves JC, Santos A, Jorge P, et al. Faecal microbiome transplantation improves clinical signs of chronic idiopathic large bowel diarrhoea in working dogs. Vet Rec 2023;193(10):e3052.

[113] Lin QY, Du JJ, Xu H, et al. Effects of fecal microbial transplantation on police performance and transportation stress in Kunming police dogs. Appl Microbiol Biotechnol 2024;108(1):46.

[114] C.G. Vecchiato, F. Sportelli, C. Delsante, et al., Fecal microbial transplantation effect on clinical outcome and fecal microbiota and metabolome in dogs with chronic enteropathy refractory to diet. Congress Proceedings 33rd ECVIM-CA Annual Congress. 2023.

[115] Pilla R, Suchodolski JS. The Role of the Canine Gut Microbiome and Metabolome in Health and Gastrointestinal Disease. Front Vet Sci 2019;6:498.

Advances in Small Animal Care 5 (2024) 109–119

ADVANCES IN SMALL ANIMAL CARE

MicroRNA as Biomarkers in Small Animal Gastrointestinal Inflammation and Cancer

Janne Graarup-Hansen Lyngby, DVM, PhD, DACVIM (SAIM)*, Lise Nikolic Nielsen, DVM, PhD, CertSAM

Department of Veterinary Clinical Science, University of Copenhagen, Dyrlaegevej 16, Frederiksberg C 1870, Denmark

---

KEYWORDS

• Dogs • Cats • miRNAs • Chronic inflammatory enteropathy • IBD • Biomarker • Gastrointestinal neoplasia

KEY POINTS

- It remains a clinical challenge to discriminate between inflammatory gastrointestinal (GI) diseases and cancer of the GI tract in dogs and cats.
- MicroRNAs are small noncoding RNAs involved with posttranscriptional gene regulation in health and disease. Their potential as diagnostic biomarkers is gaining increased interest in the veterinary community.
- Differential expression of microRNAs in tissue, serum, and feces from dogs and to a small extent in cats with GI disease has been investigated with varying results.
- Further studies are needed to validate the putative microRNA biomarkers in GI disease in dogs and cats in a larger clinical setting.

INTRODUCTION

Chronic gastrointestinal (GI) diseases are common in dogs and cats [1–3]. The underlying etiology includes a wide range of conditions, from endoparasites to chronic inflammatory enteropathy (CIE) and gastrointestinal cancer (GIC) [4–10]. The clinical presentation may vary but will often manifest as vomiting, diarrhea, weight loss, anorexia, and abdominal discomfort [8,11–13]. Unfortunately, the clinical signs do not necessarily direct the veterinarian to the underlying etiology, and this proposes a clinical challenge, requiring a thorough diagnostic work-up including elaborate blood work, fecal examination, imaging studies, and ultimately biopsies from the GI tract [7,8,14]. Such a work-up can be costly, potentially invasive, and extend over several weeks to months. This can prolong the time to reach a final diagnosis and potentially lead to disease progression, increased morbidity, and even mortality.

There is an ongoing search for new biomarkers in human and veterinary medicine. MicroRNAs have proven to be promising diagnostic and prognostic biomarkers in human colorectal cancer as well as other inflammatory and neoplastic diseases [15–21]. MicroRNAs are small 20 to 23 nucleotide single-stranded, endogenous RNAs involved with epigenetic gene regulation as microRNAs impair translation of messenger RNA (mRNA) by binding to it, thereby inhibiting its function [22–24]. MicroRNAs are currently gaining much attention in the veterinary community and this review aims to introduce microRNA in general and specifically the applicability of microRNA as biomarkers in GI inflammatory diseases and GIC. A secondary aim is to describe current challenges and future perspectives of using microRNA as a biomarker in GI diseases in dogs and cats.

---

*Corresponding author, E-mail address: janne.lyngby@sund.ku.dk

https://doi.org/10.1016/j.yasa.2024.06.007

2666-450X/24/

CHRONIC INFLAMMATORY ENTEROPATHY

CIE is a diagnosis of exclusion and is defined as persistent or recurrent GI signs for 3 weeks or more, the presence of mucosal inflammation on histopathology of GI biopsies, and the exclusion of other underlying diseases [4,7,8,12,25].

In dogs, CIE is retrospectively subclassified based on response to therapy, into (1) food-responsive enteropathy (FRE), (2) antibiotic-responsive enteropathy (ARE), (3) steroid-responsive enteropathy (SRE), which is also known as idiopathic inflammatory bowel disease (IBD), and (4) nonresponsive enteropathy—a subgroup of dogs that do not respond sufficiently to medical management [5,7]. The justification of the subgroup of ARE is currently being debated, and it has been suggested to rename this subgroup "idiopathic intestinal dysbiosis" [7]. Despite the lack of consistent subclassification of CIE in cats, the terminology of (1) FRE, (2) SRE, and (3) nonresponsive enteropathy can likewise be applied; however, the ARE subtype has not been convincingly documented in cats [4,8]. In dogs with CIE, the FRE subgroup accounts for approximately 60% to 65%, the ARE approximately 16%, and SRE approximately 19% [26,27]. In a study in cats, the prevalence of FRE is approximately 40% to 50% and SRE around 30% [28,29].

Protein-losing enteropathy, a syndrome characterized by intestinal intraluminal protein loss, is considered a special type of chronic enteropathy parallel to the subgroups mentioned earlier and often with a guarded prognosis [5,7,30]. As there are currently no publications investigating microRNA in protein-losing enteropathy, this will not be further discussed in this review.

GASTROINTESTINAL NEOPLASIA

Overall, GIC accounts for 1.5% to 8% of tumors in dogs [31,32] and 4% to 13.5% in cats [33–35]. The etiology for development of GIC remains unknown in dogs and cats, and no organism or chemical has been consistently proven to contribute to the development of GIC in companion animals, except for the influence of feline retroviral infections on lymphoma [36]. Even so, genetic susceptibility is observed in several cat and dog breeds [35,37]. For cases of gastric carcinoma, the Belgian Tervuren, Bouvier des Flandres, Chow Chow, Collie, Groenendael, Norwegian Elkhound, Norwegian Lundehund, and Standard Poodle are predisposed [37–42], and both German Shepherds and Boxer dogs are predisposed to colorectal carcinoma[43,44]. In cats, a significantly increased risk of lymphoma is seen in "mixed breed cats" and Siamese cats [35].

As with other diseases affecting the GI tract, the clinical signs are more commonly related to the anatomic location than to the actual tumor type. However, paraneoplastic syndromes for specific tumors, cancer cachexia, as well as side effects of therapy can contribute to the clinical picture [44–46]. The onset of disease can be insidious in nature in several cancer types and clinical signs can be present for several months prior to diagnosis [47].

The most prevalent GIC in dogs is carcinoma, followed by lymphoma and leiomyosarcoma or gastrointestinal stromal tumors (GISTs) [48]. In cats, lymphoma represents the most prevalent cancer type of the GI tract, followed by carcinoma and mast cell tumors [35,36,48–51]. Of cats with GI lymphoma, the majority present with small cell lymphoma (SCL) [14,49]. SCL of the GI tract is regarded as an indolent disease, but it remains challenging to differentiate from inflammatory lymphocytic infiltrates as often seen in CIE [14,52]. The majority (60%–75%) of GI lymphomas in cats are SCL of T-cell immunophenotype [14,27,49,52,53]. Gastrointestinal SCL is considered uncommon in dogs but has been described [54,55]. The diagnostic challenges of SCL in dogs are comparable to that of cats, and the challenge might be greater due to the decreased prevalence of this disease in dogs and hence a decreased awareness from the clinician.

While some solid tumors may be more easily differentiated from nonneoplastic enteropathies with the use of diagnostic imaging, more diffusely spread neoplasia such as SCL and specific types of disseminated carcinoma(s) displays similar clinical, laboratory, and imaging characteristics as nonneoplastic enteropathies and will require additional testing. Tissue biopsy with histopathology remains the gold standard technique, even though additional diagnostic tests such as immunohistochemistry are often indicated [7,52].

THE USE OF BIOMARKERS IN GASTROINTESTINAL INFLAMMATORY DISEASE AND IN GASTROINTESTINAL CANCER

As CIE and GIC may display similar clinical signs and laboratory findings, blood-derived or fecal biomarkers could play a vital part in order to differentiate these conditions in not just a timely manner but ultimately also with a focus on advancing the use of noninvasive testing modalities [13,56]. Currently, no ideal biomarkers exist. Generally, valuable diagnostic biomarkers may be indicative of specific natural biologic or pathologic processes or a response to an exposure or intervention

[57]. An ideal biomarker can diagnose a condition but should also be able to differentiate it from other conditions with a high degree of reliability and precision, that is, excellent diagnostic performance [57–59]. Conceptually, biomarkers can be histopathologic, imaging, or physiologic characteristics, but they are commonly molecules present in biological fluids or tissue. In addition, biomarkers for commercial use need to have a strong consistent diagnostic sensitivity and specificity, a methodology suited for commercial use including robustness for transport to specialized laboratories and a rapid analysis turnover rate [57–59].

MicroRNA

One group of biomarkers gaining increased attention these years are microRNAs [16,21,60]. MicroRNAs are small, 21 to 23 nucleotide long, noncoding, single-stranded RNAs that target mRNA [22,23]. They regulate gene expression and play a pivotal role in development and normal physiology [61]. Their role as diagnostic and prognostic biomarkers in health and disease is being broadly investigated in both human and veterinary medicine [17,62–65].

The Historical Perspective

In 1993, 2 independent research groups discovered the first microRNA [66,67]. The gene, lin-4, involved in the larval development of *Caenorhabditis elegans* from the first to the second larval stage, did not encode for a protein but for small RNAs. In addition, they discovered 22 distinct nucleotides and 61 nucleotide fragments of RNA, with the longer pieces suggested to be a stem loop and a precursor for the shorter one [66,67]. Seven years later, Let-7 was discovered, likewise in *C elegans*, and, shortly thereafter, in drosophila flies, followed by mammals including humans. In 2001, these molecules were named microRNAs [60,68,69]. Hundreds of microRNAs have since been found in humans, and the majority of them are conserved in closely related species. Likewise, many microRNAs are conserved more broadly among species, that is, 1 out of 3 of microRNAs in *C elegans* has been found in humans [21,22,70]. When searching miRBase, a database for published microRNA sequences and annotations, a total of 38,589 entries for all species are listed, with 962 belonging to dogs (*Canis lupus familiaris*)[a] [1]. miRbase is dependent on volunteer researchers submitting novel

microRNA sequences; currently no microRNAs from cats have been annotated in the database.

The Canonical Pathway of Biogenesis

The majority of microRNAs are processed through the canonical pathway of microRNA biogenesis [22,71,72]. They get their unique structure from processing of a stem-loop region of longer RNA transcripts [73] as illustrated and described in Fig. 1. Noncanonical biogenesis and alternative modification of microRNA have been described but will not be further discussed in this review.

A microRNA gene is transcribed from the DNA in the nucleus by RNA polymerase II or III [74] into the primary-microRNA (pri-miRNA) and is hundreds to a few thousands of nucleotides long [71,72]. The pri-miRNA is then cleaved in the nucleus by the microprocessor complex consisting of Drosha RNase III endonucleases and its cofactor DiGeorge syndrome chromosomal region 8. The microprocessor complex cleaves both of the pri-miRNA strands near the primary stem loop, liberating an approximately 60 to 70 nucleotide stem-loop intermediate—the hairpin microRNA precursor (pre-miRNA) [74].The pre-miRNA is actively transported from the nucleus into the cytoplasm via the export receptor Exportin-5 [75]. In the cytoplasm, the RNase III endonuclease, Dicer, recognizes the double-stranded RNA of the pre-miRNA and cuts both strands of the duplex, separating the terminal base pair with the stem loop and leaving a microRNA duplex [22]. The "guide strand" of the microRNA duplex is bound to an Argonaute protein (Ago), the microRNA duplex is separated, and, in general, the "passenger strand" is degraded. However, in some cases, the "passenger strand" is functionally active [76]. The mature microRNA is now ready to bind to mRNA [22].

The mature microRNA bound to Ago is the main component of the RNA-induced silencing complex [22]. This complex represses translation of mRNA by causing translational inhibition or cleavage of the mRNA transcript [71,72,77]. Whether the microRNA causes translational inhibition or target cleavage depends on the potential catalytic activity of the Ago protein and the degree of complementarity of the seed sequence [71,78]. However, target cleavage appears uncommonly in mammals compared to plants, and, hence, translational repression is the most common posttranscriptional regulation by microRNAs [77].

The Role of MicroRNA

MicroRNAs play an important role in all biological pathways in multicellular organisms as referred to

---

[a]Release 22.1, mirBase, www.miRBase.org accessed on 03.01. 2024.

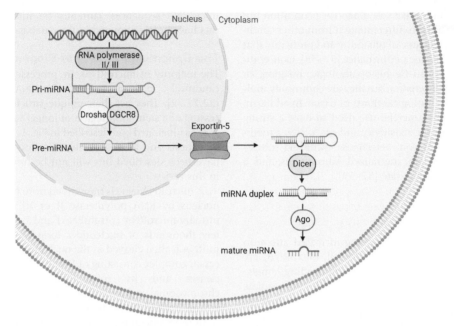

FIG. 1 miRNA biogenesis: MicroRNA is transcripted from DNA and undergoes specific modification in the cell. The mature miRNA can now bind to messenger RNA and inhibit its translation. Ago, Argonaute protein; DGCR8, DiGeorge syndrome chromosomal region 8; miRNA, microRNA; pre-miRNA, precursor microRNA; pri-miRNA, primary-miRNA. (Created with BioRender.com.)

above with the example of the first described micro-RNA, lin-4 [66,67,72]. The roles and functions of micro-RNA are continuously gaining attention, as more microRNAs and their functions are being discovered [22].

A single microRNA has the ability to target numerous mRNAs, whereas, conversely, a single mRNA can be targeted by many microRNAs [71,77,79,80]. Target regions for microRNAs on the mRNA are often clustered, adding to their effect [79,81].

Most of the microRNAs will remain within the cells; however, microRNAs may circulate in the bloodstream within extracellular vesicles or be secreted into either urine or feces [82–84]. MicroRNAs have been implicated as both cause and relation in human colorectal cancer[15,65,85] as well as in chronic enteropathies in people including ulcerative colitis and Crohn's disease [19,86,87].

MicroRNAs in Dogs and Cats
In dogs, microRNAs have been detected in tissue and different body fluids including serum, plasma, cerebrospinal fluid, and feces [88–91]. The diagnostic and prognostic potentials of microRNAs in dogs have been investigated in a number of diseases including liver disease, GI disease, and multiple neoplasms [64,92–96].

In cats, microRNA investigation is still in its infancy, but microRNAs have been detected in tissue and body fluids including serum, urine, and feces in this species [97–100]. MicroRNAs have been investigated in cardiac disease, CIE, GI SCL and other GIC, liver disease, and a number of infectious diseases including pyelonephritis in cats [97,100–102].

MicroRNA IN GASTROINTESTINAL INFLAMMATION AND CANCER IN DOGS AND CATS
Dogs
A summary of studies from the available literature on microRNA in dogs can be found in Table 1. In large bowel IBD in dogs, an increased differential expression in both serum and tissue of several microRNAs was found [105]. Several studies investigated microRNA expression in tissue from the GI tract including formalin-fixed paraffin-embedded (FFPE) tissue from

TABLE 1
microRNA expression in gastrointestinal inflammation and cancer in dogs and cats

Dogs:

	Groups	Feces	Serum	Tissue
Ishii et al, [103] 2019 (oral abstract ACVIM 2019)	• 22 CIE, (7 FRE, 15 SRE) • 23 healthy controls	*Increase:* miR 29a in all CIE and SRE dogs compared to healthy control	NA	NA
Joos et al, [104] 2020	• 8 T-cell lymphoma, • 8 LPE, • 8 healthy controls	NA	NA	*Increase:* miR-18b, miR-20b, miR-363 *Decrease:* miR-141, miR-192, miR-194, and miR-203
Konstantinidis et al, [105] 2020	• 26 colonic IBD, • 16 healthy controls	NA	*Increase:* miR-16, miR-21, miR-122, miR-146a, and miR-147 *Decrease:* miR-185, miR-192 and miR-223	*Increase:* miR-16, miR-21, miR-122 and miR-147 *Decrease:* miR-185, miR-192 and miR-223
Lyngby et al, [94] 2022	• 24 GIC, • 10 CIE, • 10 healthy controls	*Increase:* miR-451, miR-223, and miR 27a in GIC compared to CIE	*Increase:* miR-20b, miR-148a-3p, and miR-652, in GIC compared to CIE	NA
Kehl et al, [106] 2023	• 17 healthy controls • 18 GI inflammation • 27 intestinal lymphoma • 27 intestinal carcinoma	NA	NA	*Decrease:* miR-126 and miR-214 (T-cell and B-cell lymphoma, as well as in carcinomas and LPE)

(continued on next page)

TABLE 1
(continued)

	Groups	Feces	Serum	Tissue
Irving et al, [107] 2023	• 12 minimal inflammation • 10 severe inflammation • 9 T-cell lymphoma	NA	NA	*Increase:* miR-200c in mild inflammation compared to the other groups. miR-363 in severe inflammation, and miR-146b expression in both severe inflammation and T-cell lymphoma. *Decrease:* miR-200c in severe inflammation and lymphoma
Cats:				
Kehl et al, [108] 2022	• 11 lymphoma • 5 carcinoma • 5 controls			*Increase:* miR-20b in all cancers, miR-192 in carcinomas and B-cell lymphomas only.
Brogaard et al, [102] 2023	• 10 GIC (4 SCL, 4 intermediate or large cell lymphoma, 2 carcinoma) • 9 CIE • 10 healthy controls	*Decrease:* miR-148-3p in SCL compared to CIE	*Increase:* miR-223 in GIC and SCL compared to CIE and healthy controls	NA

Abbreviations: CIE, chronic inflammatory enteropathy; FRE, food-responsive enteropathy; GIC, gastrointestinal cancer; LPE, lymphoplasmacytic enteritis; miR, microRNA; NA, not assessed; SRE, steroid-responsive enteropathy.

dogs. When assessing microRNA expression in FFPE tissue from dogs with intestinal T-cell lymphoma, lymphoplasmacytic enteritis (LPE), and healthy dogs using quantitative PCR (qPCR), a downregulation of tumor-suppressor microRNAs and an upregulation of microRNAs involved in oncogenesis were documented [104]. Irving and colleagues [107] demonstrated that microRNA from archived FFPE duodenal tissue from dogs can be extracted and utilized for next-generation sequencing and qPCR. They found that tissue microRNA expression profiles varied between minimal inflammation (mild IBD) compared to severe inflammation (severe IBD) and T-cell lymphoma. In this study, microRNAs expression separated mild IBD from severe IBD and T-cell lymphoma, respectively, but could not be used to distinguish between severe IBD and T-cell lymphoma from each other.

Digital droplet polymerase chain reaction (PCR) has been successfully used to detect and quantify aberrant microRNA profiles in FFPE intestinal tissue from dogs with GI lymphoma or carcinoma compared to dogs with enteritis and healthy controls [106].

In another study, microRNA abundance in serum and feces from dogs with GI neoplasia, including carcinoma, lymphoma, and leiomyosarcomas/GISTs, was compared to dogs with CIE using small RNA sequencing and reverse transcription quantitative real-time PCR (RT-qPCR) [94]. In this study, several microRNAs were able to differentiate CIE from GIC in both serum and feces with excellent diagnostic performance that further improved when combining several microRNAs [94]. When investigating microRNA expression in fecal samples from dogs using RT-qPCR, an overall increase in all cases of CIE (SRE + FRE), particularly dogs with SRE compared to healthy dogs, was found [103].

Overall, though several microRNAs have been assessed from different biological materials, using different techniques, no perfect diagnostic assay using microRNA that is consistently superior to others has been identified.

Cats
A summary of studies regarding microRNA in cats can be found in Table 1. When investigating microRNA expression in FFPE tissue from GI masses in cats, lymphoma and carcinoma samples showed upregulated microRNA-20b values, but only carcinomas and B-cell lymphomas showed increased expression of microRNA-192 [108].

Cats with CIE showed differential expression of miR-223-3p in serum compared to cats with GIC (lymphoma and carcinoma), but not in feces [102]. When cats with SCL within the GIC group were compared to cats with CIE, miR-223-3p was found to be significantly increased [102]. Fecal miR-148-3p was decreased in SCL when comparing with cats with CIE. As the sample size was small in this study [102], and the differentiation between CIE and SCL is especially challenging in cats, further studies investigating the potential of microRNAs as diagnostic biomarkers are warranted.

A number of different microRNAs have hence been suggested to diagnose or differentiate GI inflammation and cancer in dogs and cats, but very few microRNA expression profiles overlap between the studies. Further investigations in using specific panels of microRNAs or even combining microRNAs with other biomarkers in a composite score could be attempted in relevant clinical populations to increase diagnostic accuracy and usefulness.

CHALLENGES OF USING microRNA AS DIAGNOSTIC BIOMARKERS
Although these initial positive findings of microRNAs being able to differentiate CIE from GIC in dogs and cats, several steps remain before a commercialized test is available for clinical practice.

Shipment of samples from practice to specialized laboratories for microRNA analysis appears possible, as studies have shown that microRNAs can be preserved both in serum and plasma samples from dogs [90] and fecal microRNAs show relative robustness in dogs [88] and in cats [99]. However, at this time, no studies assessing the stability of serum from cats have been performed. Several studies have been able to prove that microRNA expression from FFPE tissue can be assessed; however, at the stage in the diagnostic approach, where biopsies have already been obtained, other and better validated assessment methods are currently available. Though the idea of microRNA as a diagnostic or prognostic tissue biomarker in GI disease in cats and dogs should not be discarded, the true potential and biggest need lie in (minimally invasive) biomarkers, that is, from serum or feces, that can be performed earlier in the diagnostic work-up.

When profiling microRNAs by small RNA sequencing or qPCR, data normalization is required in order to remove as much technical variation as possible [109,110]. Unfortunately, different studies employ various normalization strategies to report microRNA levels, challenging the comparison of results between studies and potentially leading to erroneous conclusions [110]. Currently, no consensus has been reached on the most appropriate normalization technique or use of normalizers for qPCR on microRNAs analysis, and this lack of standardization is a significant challenge in microRNA research and its applicability [21,110]. As good normalizers may not always be found simply in the literature, it should be emphasized that proper selection of multiple endogenous normalizers for the specific study is key to reliable results.

FUTURE IMPLEMENTATION OF microRNAs FOR GASTROINTESTINAL DISEASE IN SMALL ANIMAL CARE

The study of microRNAs as diagnostic biomarkers of specific disease categories continues to be a heavily explored area within research and a small panel of microRNAs are already commercially available for the diagnosis of thyroid cancer in people [111,112]. Although the recent studies of microRNAs in GI disease in dogs and cats show promise, well-standardized validation and verification protocols for the microRNA assays to ensure trustworthy results will still need to be implemented and examined in larger patient groups in order for these panels of microRNAs to become commercially available.

Diagnostic microRNAs for CIE or GIC may even transform from being diagnostic biomarkers into therapeutic targets. In humans, it is speculated that upregulated microRNAs in cancer should be inhibited with specific antagonists, while patients with downregulated essential microRNAs should be supplied with synthetic nucleotides [113–115].

In addition, combining multiple microRNAs in a panel or combining microRNAs with other biomarkers in a composite score could increase the diagnostic utility.

SUMMARY

Despite the increasing number of publications and investigations of microRNA in dogs and cats, there are currently no commercially available biomarkers for diagnosis or prognosis of GI inflammation and GIC. Composite scores including microRNA as well as other biomarkers could be an alternative to sole microRNA panels. However, further assessment of the suggested biomarkers' performance in larger patient populations in a clinical setting is needed before strong diagnostic recommendation and routine use can be recommended.

DISCLOSURE

The authors have nothing to disclose.

REFERENCES

[1] O'Neill DG, Church DB, McGreevy PD, et al. Prevalence of disorders recorded in dogs attending primary-care veterinary practices in England. PLoS One 2014;9(3). https://doi.org/10.1371/JOURNAL.PONE.0090501.

[2] Robinson NJ, Dean RS, Cobb M, et al. Investigating common clinical presentations in first opinion small animal consultations using direct observation. Vet Rec 2015;176(18):463.

[3] Wolf S, Selinger J, Ward MP, et al. Incidence of presenting complaints and diagnoses in insured Australian dogs. Aust Vet J 2020;98(7):326–32.

[4] Bandara Y, Priestnall SL, Chang YM, et al. Outcome of chronic inflammatory enteropathy in cats: 65 cases (2011-2021). J Small Anim Pract 2023;64(3):121–9 [Article].

[5] Dandrieux JRS. Inflammatory bowel disease versus chronic enteropathy in dogs: are they one and the same? J Small Anim Pract 2016;57(11):589–99, Blackwell Publishing Ltd.

[6] Gualtieri M, Monzeglio MG, Scanziani E. Gastric neoplasia. Vet Clin Small Anim Pract 1999;29(2):415–40.

[7] Jergens AE, Heilmann RM. Canine chronic enteropathy-Current state-of-the-art and emerging concepts. Front Vet Sci 2022;9. https://doi.org/10.3389/FVETS.2022.923013.

[8] Marsilio S. Feline chronic enteropathy. J Small Anim Pract 2021b;62(6):409–19.

[9] Turk MAM, Gallina AM, Russell TS. Nonhematopoietic gastrointestinal neoplasia in cats: A retrospective study of 44 cases. Veterinary Pathology 1981;18(5):614–20.

[10] Willard MD. Alimentary neoplasia in geriatric dogs and cats. Vet Clin Small Anim Pract 2012;42(4):693–706.

[11] Allenspach K, Wieland B, Gröne A, et al. Chronic enteropathies in dogs: Evaluation of risk factors for negative outcome [Article]. J Vet Intern Med 2007;21(4):700–8.

[12] Allenspach K, Mochel JP. Current diagnostics for chronic enteropathies in dogs. Vet Clin Pathol 2022;50(S1):18–28, American Society for Veterinary Clinical Pathology.

[13] Jergens AE, Crandell JM, Evans R, et al. A clinical index for disease activity in cats with chronic enteropathy. J Vet Intern Med 2010;24(5):1027–33.

[14] Marsilio S. Differentiating Inflammatory Bowel Disease from Alimentary Lymphoma in Cats: Does It Matter? [Article]. Vet Clin Small Anim Pract 2021a;51(1):93–109.

[15] Akao Y, Nakagawa Y, Naoe T. MicroRNA-143 and -145 in colon cancer [Article]. DNA Cell Biol 2007;26(5):311–20.

[16] Dalmay T, Edwards DR. MicroRNAs and the hallmarks of cancer. Oncogene 2006;25(46):6170–5.

[17] Li C, Yan G, Yin L, et al. Prognostic roles of microRNA 143 and microRNA 145 in colorectal cancer: A meta-analysis [Article]. Int J Biol Markers 2019;34(1):6–14.

[18] Liu T, Tang H, Lang Y, et al. MicroRNA-27a functions as an oncogene in gastric adenocarcinoma by targeting prohibitin. Cancer Lett 2009;273(2):233–42 [Article].

[19] Schönauen K, Le N, von Arnim U, et al. Circulating and Fecal microRNAs as Biomarkers for Inflammatory Bowel Diseases. Inflamm Bowel Dis 2018;24(7):1547–57 [Article].

[20] Song Y-X, Yue Z-Y, Wang Z-N, et al. MicroRNA-148b is frequently down-regulated in gastric cancer and acts as a tumor suppressor by inhibiting cell proliferation. Mol Cancer 2011;10(1):1 [Article].

[21] Zuo Z, Jiang Y, Zeng S, et al. The value of microRNAs as the novel biomarkers for colorectal cancer diagnosis: A meta-analysis. Pathol Res Pract 2020;216(10):153130 [Article].

[22] Bartel DP. MicroRNAs: Genomics, Biogenesis, Mechanism, and Function. Cell 2004;116(2):281–97 [Article].

[23] Bartel DP. MicroRNAs: Target Recognition and Regulatory Functions. Cell 2009;136(2):215–33 [Article].

[24] Winter J, Jung S, Keller S, et al. Many roads to maturity: MicroRNA biogenesis pathways and their regulation. Nat Cell Biol 2009;11(3):228–34.

[25] Allenspach K, Culverwell C, Chan D. Long-term outcome in dogs with chronic enteropathies: 203 cases. Vet Rec 2016;178(15):368 [Article].

[26] Kathrani A. Dietary and Nutritional Approaches to the Management of Chronic Enteropathy in Dogs and Cats. Vet Clin Small Anim Pract 2021;51(1):123–36.

[27] Freiche V, Fages J, Paulin MV, et al. Clinical, laboratory and ultrasonographic findings differentiating low-grade intestinal T-cell lymphoma from lymphoplasmacytic enteritis in cats. J Vet Intern Med 2021;35(6):2685–96.

[28] Dzięcioł M, Nizański W, Jezierski T, et al. Evaluation of clinicopathological features in cats with chronic gastrointestinal signs. Pol J Vet Sci 2017;20(2):429–37.

[29] Grant Guilford W, Jones BR, Markwell PJ, et al. Food Sensitivity in Cats with Chronic Idiopathic Gastrointestinal Problems. J Vet Intern Med 2001;15(1):7–13.

[30] Allenspach K, Iennarella-Servantez C. Canine Protein Losing Enteropathies and Systemic Complications. Vet Clin Small Anim Pract 2021;51(1):111–22.

[31] Dobson JM, Samuel S, Milstein H, et al. Canine neoplasia in the UK: Estimates of incidence rates from a population of insured dogs. J Small Anim Pract 2002;43(6):240–6.

[32] Grüntzig K, Graf R, Hässig M, et al. The Swiss canine cancer registry: A retrospective study on the occurrence of tumours in dogs in Switzerland from 1955 to 2008. J Comp Pathol 2015;152(2–3):161–71.

[33] Bastianello SS. A survey of neoplasia in domestic species over a 40-year period from 1935 to 1974 in the Republic of South Africa. V. Tumours occurring in the cat. Onderstepoort J Vet Res 1983;50(2):105–10.

[34] Manuali E, Forte C, Vichi G, et al. Tumours in European Shorthair cats: a retrospective study of 680 cases. J Feline Med Surg 2020;22(12):1095–102.

[35] Rissetto K, Villamil JA, Selting KA, et al. Recent trends in feline intestinal neoplasia: an epidemiologic study of 1,129 cases in the veterinary medical database from 1964 to 2004. J Am Anim Hosp Assoc 2011;47(1):28–36.

[36] Louwerens M, London CA, Pedersen NC, et al. Feline Lymphoma in the Post-Feline Leukemia Virus Era. J Vet Intern Med 2005;19(3):329–35.

[37] Hugen S, Thomas RE, German AJ, et al. Gastric carcinoma in canines and humans, a review. Vet Comp Oncol 2017;15(3):692–705.

[38] Candido MV, Syrjä P, Kilpinen S, et al. Canine breeds associated with gastric carcinoma, metaplasia and dysplasia diagnosed by histopathology of endoscopic biopsy samples. Acta Vet Scand 2018;60(1). https://doi.org/10.1186/S13028-018-0392-6.

[39] Kolbjørnsen Ø, Press MC, Landsverk T. Gastropathies in the Lundehund: I. Gastritis and gastric neoplasia associated with intestinal lymphangiectasia. APMIS 1994;102(7–12):647–61.

[40] Koterbay AM, Muthupalani S, Fox JG, et al. Risk and characteristics of gastric carcinoma in the chow chow dog. Can Vet J 2020;61(4):396–400 [Article].

[41] Qvigstad G, Skancke E, Waldum HL. Gastric Neuroendocrine Carcinoma Associated with Atrophic Gastritis in the Norwegian Lundehund. J Comp Pathol 2008;139(4):194–201.

[42] Seim-Wikse T, Jörundsson E, Nødtvedt A, et al. Breed predisposition to canine gastric carcinoma–a study based on the Norwegian canine cancer register. Acta Vet Scand 2013;55:25.

[43] Patnaik AK, Hurvitz AI, Johnson GF. Canine gastrointestinal neoplasms. Veterinary Pathology 1977;14(6):547–55.

[44] Spuzak J, Ciaputa R, Kubiak K, et al. Adenocarcinoma of the posterior segment of the gastrointestinal tract in dogs-clinical, endoscopic, histopathological and immunohistochemical findings. Pol J Vet Sci 2017;20(3):539–49.

[45] Baez JL, Michel KE, Sorenmo K, et al. A prospective investigation of the prevalence and prognostic significance of weight loss and changes in body condition in feline cancer patients. J Feline Med Surg 2007;9(5):411–7.

[46] Cribb AE. Feline Gastrointestinal Adenocarcinoma: A Review and Retrospective Study. Can Vet J 1988;29(9):709–12.

[47] Sogame N, Risbon R, Burgess KE. Intestinal lymphoma in dogs: 84 cases (1997-2012). J Am Vet Med Assoc 2018;252(4):440–7.

[48] Vail DM, Thamm DH, Liptak JM. Cancer of the Gastrointestinal Tract [Book]. In: Withrow and MacEwen's small animal clinical oncology. 6th edition. Elsevier - Health Sciences Division; 2019.

[49] Gieger T. Alimentary Lymphoma in Cats and Dogs. Vet Clin Small Anim Pract 2011;41(2):419–32.

[50] Richter KP. Feline gastrointestinal lymphoma. Vet Clin Small Anim Pract 2003;33(5):1083–98.

[51] Sabattini S, Bottero E, Turba ME, et al. Differentiating feline inflammatory bowel disease from alimentary lymphoma in duodenal endoscopic biopsies. J Small Anim Pract 2016;57(8):396–401.

[52] Marsilio S, Freiche V, Johnson E, et al. ACVIM consensus statement guidelines on diagnosing and distinguishing low-grade neoplastic from inflammatory

lymphocytic chronic enteropathies in cats [Article]. J Vet Intern Med 2023;37(3):794–816.

[53] Paulin MV, Couronné L, Beguin J, et al. Feline low-grade alimentary lymphoma: an emerging entity and a potential animal model for human disease. BMC Vet Res 2018;14(1). https://doi.org/10.1186/S12917-018-1635-5.

[54] Couto KM, Moore PF, Zwingenberger AL, et al. Clinical characteristics and outcome in dogs with small cell T-cell intestinal lymphoma [Article]. Vet Comp Oncol 2018;16(3):337–43.

[55] Lane J, Price J, Moore A, et al. Low-grade gastrointestinal lymphoma in dogs: 20 cases (2010 to 2016). J Small Anim Pract 2018;59(3):147–53 [Article].

[56] Heilmann RM, Steiner JM. Clinical utility of currently available biomarkers in inflammatory enteropathies of dogs. J Vet Intern Med 2018;32(5):1495–508.

[57] Califf RM. Biomarker definitions and their applications. Exp Biol Med 2018;243(3):213–21.

[58] Atkinson AJ, Colburn WA, DeGruttola VG, et al. Biomarkers and surrogate endpoints: preferred definitions and conceptual framework. Clin Pharmacol Therapeut 2001;69(3):89–95.

[59] Bennett MR, Devarajan P. Characteristics of an Ideal Biomarker of Kidney Diseases [Bookitem]. In: Biomarkers of kidney disease. Second edition; 2017. 2017. p. 1–20. https://doi.org/10.1016/B978-0-12-803014-1.00001-7.

[60] Bartel DP, Chen C-Z. Micromanagers of gene expression: the potentially widespread influence of metazoan microRNAs [Article]. Nat Rev Genet 2004;5(5):396–400.

[61] He L, Hannon GJ. MicroRNAs: Small RNAs with a big role in gene regulation. Nat Rev Genet 2004;5(7):522–31.

[62] Calin GA, Ferracin M, Cimmino A, et al. A MicroRNA Signature Associated with Prognosis and Progression in Chronic Lymphocytic Leukemia. N Engl J Med 2005;353(17):1793–801 [Article].

[63] Chang P-Y, Chen C-C, Chang Y-S, et al. MicroRNA-223 and microRNA-92a in stool and plasma samples act as complementary biomarkers to increase colorectal cancer detection [Article]. Oncotarget 2016;7(9):10663–75.

[64] Fish EJ, Martinez-Romero EG, DeInnocentes P, et al. Circulating microRNA as biomarkers of canine mammary carcinoma in dogs. J Vet Intern Med 2020;34(3):1282–90.

[65] Link A, Balaguer F, Shen Y, et al. Fecal microRNAs as novel biomarkers for colon cancer screening. Cancer Epidemiol Biomarkers Prev 2010;19(7):1766–74.

[66] Lee RC, Feinbaum RL, Ambros V. The C. elegans heterochronic gene lin-4 encodes small RNAs with antisense complementarity to lin-14. Cell 1993;75(5):843–54.

[67] Wightman B, Ha I, Ruvkun G. Posttranscriptional regulation of the heterochronic gene lin-14 by lin-4 mediates temporal pattern formation in C. elegans. Cell 1993;75(5):855–62.

[68] Lagos-Quintana M, Rauhut R, Lendeckel W, et al. Identification of novel genes coding for small expressed RNAs. Science (New York, N.Y.) 2001;294(5543):853–8.

[69] Lau NC, Lim LP, Weinstein EG, et al. An abundant class of tiny RNAs with probable regulatory roles in Caenorhabditis elegans. Science 2001;294(5543):858–62.

[70] Friedman RC, Farh KKH, Burge CB, et al. Most mammalian mRNAs are conserved targets of microRNAs. Genome Res 2009;19(1):92–105.

[71] Pal AS, Kasinski AL. Animal Models to Study MicroRNA Function [Article]. Adv Cancer Res 2017;135:53–118.

[72] Sahabi K, Selvarajah GT, Abdullah R, et al. Comparative aspects of microRNA expression in canine and human cancers. J Vet Sci 2018;19(2):162–71.

[73] Bartel DP. Metazoan MicroRNAs. Cell 2018;173(1):20–51, Cell Press.

[74] Lee Y, Kim M, Han J, et al. MicroRNA genes are transcribed by RNA polymerase II. EMBO J 2004;23(20):4051–60.

[75] Yi R, Qin Y, Macara IG, et al. Exportin-5 mediates the nuclear export of pre-microRNAs and short hairpin RNAs. Gene Dev 2003;17(24):3011–6.

[76] Guo L, Lu Z. The fate of miRNA* strand through evolutionary analysis: implication for degradation as merely carrier strand or potential regulatory molecule? PLoS One 2010;5(6). https://doi.org/10.1371/JOURNAL.PONE.0011387.

[77] Selbach M, Schwanhäusser B, Thierfelder N, et al. Widespread changes in protein synthesis induced by microRNAs. Nature 2008;455(7209):58–63.

[78] Moore MJ, Scheel TKH, Luna JM, et al. miRNA-target chimeras reveal miRNA 3′-end pairing as a major determinant of Argonaute target specificity. Nat Commun 2015;6. https://doi.org/10.1038/NCOMMS9864.

[79] Plotnikova O, Baranova A, Skoblov M. Comprehensive Analysis of Human microRNA-mRNA Interactome. Front Genet 2019;10:933.

[80] Uhlmann S, Mannsperger H, Zhang JD, et al. Global microRNA level regulation of EGFR-driven cell-cycle protein network in breast cancer. Mol Syst Biol 2012;8. https://doi.org/10.1038/MSB.2011.100.

[81] Grimson A, Farh KKH, Johnston WK, et al. MicroRNA targeting specificity in mammals: determinants beyond seed pairing. Mol Cell 2007;27(1):91–105.

[82] Aguilera-Rojas M, Sharbati S, Stein T, et al. Systematic analysis of different degrees of haemolysis on miRNA levels in serum and serum-derived extracellular vesicles from dogs. BMC Vet Res 2022;18(1). https://doi.org/10.1186/s12917-022-03445-8.

[83] Mori MA, Ludwig RG, Garcia-Martin R, et al. Extracellular miRNAs: From Biomarkers to Mediators of Physiology and Disease. Cell Metabol 2019;30(4):656–73 [Article].

[84] Turchinovich A, Cho WC. The origin, function and diagnostic potential of extracellular microRNA in human body fluids. Front Genet 2014;5:30 [Article].

[85] Yau TO, Tang CM, Harriss EK, et al. Faecal microRNAs as a non-invasive tool in the diagnosis of colonic adenomas and

colorectal cancer: A meta-analysis. Sci Rep 2019;9(1). https://doi.org/10.1038/s41598-019-45570-9.

[86] Feng Y, Zhang Y, Zhou D, et al. MicroRNAs, intestinal inflammatory and tumor. Bioorg Med Chem Lett 2019;29(16):2051–8 [Article].

[87] James JP, Riis LB, Malham M, et al. MicroRNA biomarkers in IBD-differential diagnosis and prediction of colitis-associated cancer [Unknown]. Int J Mol Sci 2020;21(Issue 21).

[88] Cirera S, Willumsen LM, Johansen TT, et al. Evaluation of microRNA stability in feces from healthy dogs. Vet Clin Pathol 2018;47(1):115–21 [Article].

[89] Mármol-Sánchez E, Heidemann PL, Gredal H, et al. MicroRNA profiling of cerebrospinal fluid from dogs with steroid responsive meningitis-arteritis and meningoencephalitis of unknown origin [Unknown]. Front Vet Sci 2023;5(10). https://doi.org/10.3389/fvets.2023.1144084.

[90] Enelund L, Nielsen LN, Cirera S. Evaluation of microRNA Stability in Plasma and Serum from Healthy Dogs. MicroRNA 2017;6(1):42–52 [Article].

[91] Koenig EM, Fisher C, Bernard H, et al. The beagle dog MicroRNA tissue atlas: Identifying translatable biomarkers of organ toxicity. BMC Genom 2016;17(1): 649 [Article].

[92] Armstrong SK, Hunter RW, Oosthyuzen W, et al. Candidate circulating microRNA biomarkers in dogs with chronic pancreatitis. J Vet Intern Med 2024. https://doi.org/10.1111/jvim.17009.

[93] Cherry AD, Chu CP, Cianciolo RE, et al. MicroRNA-126 in dogs with immune complex-mediated glomerulonephritis. J Vet Intern Med 2023. https://doi.org/10.1111/jvim.16932.

[94] Lyngby JG, Gòdia M, Brogaard L, et al. Association of fecal and serum microRNA profiles with gastrointestinal cancer and chronic inflammatory enteropathy in dogs. J Vet Intern Med 2022;36(6):1989–2001.

[95] Oosthuyzen W, Ten Berg PWL, Francis B, et al. Sensitivity and specificity of microRNA-122 for liver disease in dogs. J Vet Intern Med 2018;32(5):1637–44.

[96] Zheng W-B, Cai L, Zou Y, et al. Altered miRNA Expression Profiles in the Serum of Beagle Dogs Experimentally Infected with Toxocara canis. Animals : An Open Access Journal from MDPI 2023;13(2). https://doi.org/10.3390/ani13020299.

[97] Godia M, Brogaard L, Marmol-Sanchez E, et al. Urinary microRNAome in healthy cats and cats with pyelonephritis or other urological conditions. PLoS One 2022;17(7). https://doi.org/10.1371/JOURNAL.PONE.0270067.

[98] Laganà A, Dirksen WP, Supsavhad W, et al. Discovery and characterization of the feline miRNAome. Sci Rep 2017; 7(1). https://doi.org/10.1038/S41598-017-10164-W.

[99] Lyngby JG, Kristensen AT, Fredholm M, et al. Evaluation of fecal microRNA stability in healthy cats. Vet Clin Pathol 2019;48(3):455–60.

[100] Weber K, Rostert N, Bauersachs S, et al. Serum microRNA profiles in cats with hypertrophic cardiomyopathy. Mol Cell Biochem 2015;402(1–2):171–80.

[101] Armstrong SK, Oosthuyzen W, Gow AG, et al. Investigation of a relationship between serum concentrations of microRNA-122 and alanine aminotransferase activity in hospitalised cats. J Feline Med Surg 2022;24(8): e289–94.

[102] Brogaard L, Lyngby JG, Kristensen AT, et al. Association of serum and fecal microRNA profiles in cats with gastrointestinal cancer and chronic inflammatory enteropathy. J Vet Intern Med 2023;37(5):1738–49.

[103] Ishii PE, Pilla R, Blake AB, et al. Fecal MicroRNA 29a is Increased in Dogs with Chronic Enteropathy (2019 ACVIM Forum, Abstract GI10). J Vet Intern Med 2019; 33(5):2469–70.

[104] Joos D, Leipig-Rudolph M, Weber K. Tumour-specific microRNA expression pattern in canine intestinal T-cell-lymphomas. Vet Comp Oncol 2020;18(4):502–8.

[105] Konstantinidis AO, Pardali D, Adamama-Moraitou KK, et al. Colonic mucosal and serum expression of microRNAs in canine large intestinal inflammatory bowel disease. BMC Vet Res 2020;16(1):69 [Article].

[106] Kehl A, Valkai M, Van de Weyer A-L, et al. miRNA Profiles of Canine Intestinal Carcinomas, Lymphomas and Enteritis Analysed by Digital Droplet PCR from FFPE Material. Veterinary Sciences 2023;10(2). https://doi.org/10.3390/vetsci10020125.

[107] Irving JR, Hiron TK, Davison LJ, et al. Characterization of canine intestinal microRNA expression in inflammatory bowel disease and T-cell lymphoma. J Comp Pathol 2023;204:23–9.

[108] Kehl A, Törner K, Jordan A, et al. Pathological Findings in Gastrointestinal Neoplasms and Polyps in 860 Cats and a Pilot Study on miRNA Analyses. Veterinary Sciences 2022;9(9). https://doi.org/10.3390/vetsci9090477.

[109] Mohammadian A, Mowla SJ, Elahi E, et al. Normalization of miRNA qPCR high-throughput data: a comparison of methods. Biotechnol Lett 2013;35(6):843–51.

[110] Schwarzenbach H, Da Silva AM, Calin G, et al. Data normalization strategies for microRNA quantification [Article]. Clin Chem 2015;61(11):1333–42.

[111] Ho PTB, Clark IM, Le LTT. MicroRNA-Based Diagnosis and Therapy. Int J Mol Sci 2022;23(13). https://doi.org/10.3390/ijms23137167:MDPI.

[112] Interpace Biosciences. 2023. Available at: https://thygenext-thyramir.com/combination-testing/.

[113] Khalilian S, Abedinlou H, Hussen BM, et al. The emerging role of miR-20b in human cancer and other disorders: Pathophysiology and therapeutic implications. Front Oncol 2022;12:985457 [Article].

[114] Khordadmehr M, Jigari-Asl F, Ezzati H, et al. A comprehensive review on miR-451: A promising cancer biomarker with therapeutic potential. J Cell Physiol 2019;234(12):21716–31, Wiley-Liss Inc.

[115] Li X, Xu M, Ding L, et al. MiR-27a: A novel biomarker and potential therapeutic target in tumors. J Cancer 2019;10(12):2836–48 [Article].

Advances in Small Animal Care 5 (2024) 121–132

ADVANCES IN SMALL ANIMAL CARE

Vitamin D Metabolism in Canine Protein-Losing Enteropathy

Glynn Woods, BVMS, MSc, SFHEA, DipECVIM-CA, MRCVS[a,b,*],
Julien R.S. Dandrieux, BSc, Dr med vet, PhD, GCUT, DACVIM(SAIM) MRCVS[a,b]

[a]University of Edinburgh, Roslin, Scotland, UK; [b]Hospital for Small Animals, The Royal (Dick) School of Veterinary Studies, Easter Bush Campus, Midlothian EH25 9RG, UK

KEYWORDS
- Albumin • Supplementation • Calcitriol • Prognosis • Dog • PLE • Vitamin D

KEY POINTS
- Decreased vitamin D concentration is a common finding in canine protein-losing enteropathy (PLE). Whether hypovitaminosis D contributes to the pathogenesis or is secondary to PLE is currently undetermined.
- Canine PLE can be a cause of ionized hypocalcemia, which, if severe or with rapid onset, can cause clinical signs such as seizures. Vitamin D supplementation should be considered for dogs with PLE that develop clinical signs secondary associated with ionized hypocalcemia.
- Although low serum vitamin D concentration has been reported to be a negative prognostic factor in canine PLE, it remains unknown whether there are benefits to supplementing vitamin D in dogs that do not show clinical signs of hypocalcemia.
- Dogs with PLE who are supplemented with vitamin D need to have their ionized calcium monitored regularly to avoid iatrogenic hypercalcemia.
- Prospective, longitudinal studies of dogs diagnosed with PLE are required to ascertain whether (1) treatment response is associated with normalization of serum vitamin D concentration without supplementation and (2) supplementation in depleted dogs improves their outcome.

 Video content accompanies this article at https://www.advancesinsmallanimalcare.com.

VITAMIN D METABOLISM

Vitamin D metabolism is complex, perpetuated by interchangeable nomenclature and multiple vitamin D metabolites (Table 1). The 2 main forms of naturally occurring vitamin D are vitamin D2 (ergocalciferol or D2) and vitamin D3 (cholecalciferol or D3) that only differ by the presence of a carbon 22 to 23 double bond and a methyl group on the D2 side chain. D2 is found in plant material arising from a photosynthetic conversion of ergosterol present in the plant cell wall, whereas D3 is formed in the dermis of many mammals by ultraviolet B light-mediated conversion of 7-dehydrocholesterol (a cholesterol hormone intermediate) [1].

In contrast to humans, dogs cannot synthesize meaningful amounts of D3 in their skin and therefore depend on nutritional sources, typically a combination of D2 and D3 to meet their vitamin D requirement [2,3]. As it stands currently, the National Research Council (NRC, Ad Hoc Committee on Dog and Cat Nutrition), the Association of American Feed Control Officials (AAFCO, https://www.aafco.org/wp-content/uploads/2023/01/FINAL_Committee_Report_Book_w_Cover.pdf), and the European Pet and Food Industry

*Corresponding author, *E-mail address:* glynnawoods@gmail.com

https://doi.org/10.1016/j.yasa.2024.06.012
2666-450X/24/

TABLE 1
List of Vitamin D Metabolites, Their Synonyms, and Conversion to the International System of Units (Abbreviated SI from the French "système international d'unités")

Vitamin D Metabolite	Synonym	Abbreviation	Chemical Formula	Molar Mass (g/mol)	Metric Units[a]	SI Units[a]	Conversion Metric to SI[a]
Vitamin D_2	Ergocalciferol	D2	$C_{28}H_{44}O$	396.659	ng/mL	nmol/L	2.496
Vitamin D_3	Cholecalciferol	D3	$C_{27}H_{44}O$	384.648	ng/mL	nmol/L	2.496
1-hydroxycholecalciferol	Alfacalcidol	1(OH)D3					
25-hydroxyvitamin D	Calcidiol, calcifediol	25(OH)D	$C_{27}H_{44}O_2$	400.64	ng/mL	nmol/L	2.496
1,25-dihydroxyvitamin D_3	Calcitriol	1,25(OH)2D3	$C_{27}H_{44}O_3$	416.646	pg/mL	pmol/L	2.6

[a] Multiply by the factor to convert from metric to SI units and divide to convert from SI to metric. NOTE: One international unit (IU) of D2 or D3 = 0.025 mcg = 25 ng = 0.65 pmol.

(FEDIAF, https://europeanpetfood.org/wp-content/uploads/2022/03/Updated-Nutritional-Guidelines.pdf) deem vitamin D essential in canine diets [4]. Although the need for oral vitamin D supplementation is widely accepted, puppies can grow adequately when fed a vitamin D-depleted diet [5]. These findings suggest that oral vitamin D intake is not always essential for dogs, but rather depends on the calcium and phosphorus balance within diet. Further research into the extent of vitamin D production in canine skin, the characterization of enzyme expression, and the relationship among dietary calcium, phosphorus, and vitamin D is warranted to establish these physiologic relationships.

It is important to note, especially in the context of protein-losing enteropathy, that vitamin D is a fat-soluble steroid-like hormone. As such it passively diffuses the phospholipid bilayer of cells. Once D2 and D3 reach portal circulation, both are bound, for the most part, to vitamin D-binding protein (VDBP). Albumin also transports a small proportion of D2 and D3, while 1% of vitamin D remains unbound in circulation and is available for cellular processes. The VDBP provides a large reservoir of vitamin D that when released can diffuse through cell membranes into cell nuclei and activate gene transcription. While it is the unbound vitamin D that promotes nuclear transcription, recent research has also suggested a biological role of the VDBP–vitamin D complex in maximizing vitamin D reabsorption, as receptors for this compound have been located within the kidneys and parathyroid glands [6,7].

After binding to either VDBP or albumin, D2 and D3 are transported to the liver. Within the endoplasmic reticulum of hepatocytes, the cytochrome P450 enzyme family (CYP), namely CYP2R1 (25 hydroxylases), catalyzes the hydroxylation of D2 and D3 into 25-hydroxyergocalciferol and 25-hydroxycholecalciferol, respectively. Collectively, these 2 hydroxylated prohormones are 25-hydroxyvitamin-D2/3 (25(OH)D2/3 or 25(OH)D), also named calcidiol or calcifediol [8]. Both prohormones are routinely measured together and define the individual's total "vitamin D" status. Subsequently, 25(OH)D is transported to the kidney bound to VDBP. Within the renal proximal tubules, 25(OH)D is converted by alpha 1 hydroxylase (CYP27B1) to 1,25 dihydroxyvitamin D2/3 (1,25(OH)2D2/3 or 1,25(OH)2D), also named calcitriol [9].

The main role of 1,25(OH)2D is to maintain calcium and phosphorus homeostasis. This tightly controlled balance depends on the constant interplay among calcitriol, parathyroid hormone (PTH), calcitonin, and fibroblast growth factor 23(FGF23), which is summarized in Fig. 1.

1,25(OH)2D is the metabolically active form of vitamin D and exerts its actions on almost all canine tissues through the vitamin D receptor (VDR). The VDR is found inside cells and within all cell membranes. Once bound by 1,25(OH)2D, membranous VDR receptors give rise to rapid transmembrane movement of calcium. Two physiologic examples of this non-genomic effect of 1,25(OH)2D include the absorption of calcium across the gut brush border and the docking of calcium channels in the distal convoluted tube of the nephron. The VDR is also a ligand-activated transcription factor. Once activated by 1,25(OH)2D, and much like a steroid hormone, the cytoplasmic VDR translocates to the nucleus where it acts as a transcription factor with genomic activity and influences various physiologic functions [10,11].

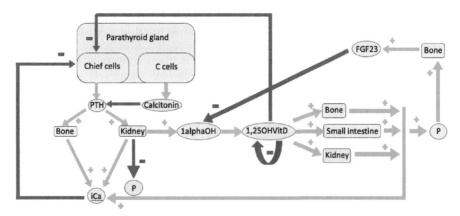

FIG. 1 Summary of the hormones involved in the control of ionized calcium concentration. Ionized hypocalcemia, through decreased occupation of the calcium-sensing receptor within chief cells of the parathyroid gland, promotes increased exocytosis of PTH. PTH acts directly on bone and kidney, and indirectly via calcitriol (1,25OHVitD) to increase blood ionized calcium (iCa) concentration by osteoclast resorption, as well as renal and intestinal calcium reabsorption. Calcitonin released by C cells of the parathyroid glands inhibits the action of PTH on the bone, acting to limit further calcium resorption. The increase in ionized calcium leads to increase binding of calcium-sensing receptor within Chief cells, which reduces PTH release. In addition, 1,25OHVitD directly exerts negative feedback on itself and mediates increased intestinal absorption of phosphorus(P), which in turns leads to fibroblast growth factor 23 (FGF23) release from bone. FGF23 promotes phosphaturesis and simultaneously inhibits 1-alphahydroxylase (1alphaOH) within the kidney, which reduces 1,25OHVitD activation.

LIMITATIONS OF THE CURRENT LITERATURE

Despite recent advances in our understanding of vitamin D and an exponential increase in the number of publications in both human and animal medicine over the past 10 years, the studies have several limitations, especially in canine protein-losing enteropathy (PLE), which the clinician needs to be aware of [12].

Proof of Causation

First, and perhaps most importantly, is that although hypovitaminosis D is well reported in canine gastroenterology literature, there is still no definitive evidence for the underlying mechanism. Although it is possible that the main driver for hypovitaminosis D is loss from the gut, as supported by the fact that dogs with PLE had lower vitamin D concentration than dogs with chronic enteropathy (CE), it is likely that it is a multifactorial process and further studies are required to refine our understanding [13]. For this reason, treatment of the underlying gut disease might be sufficient to restore adequate vitamin D concentration.

Prospective Studies Are Required

To date, there has been no prospective literature investigating vitamin D in canine PLE. In addition, 2 publications, which highlighted a possible prognostic role of hypovitaminosis D in canine PLE and CE, lacked control groups [14,15]. As such, their conclusions are weakened and these publications have additional limitations, which are common among vitamin D literature such as small cohort size, no dietary conformity, lack of treatment protocol, and use of less accurate measurement techniques.

Is Vitamin D a Glorified Acute Phase Protein?

It is also important for clinicians to understand that alongside its implication in PLE, hypovitaminosis D occurs in a wide variety of non- "protein-losing" diseases both in animals and humans given its role as a negative acute phase reactant [16]. Vitamin D is also well known to modulate the immune response and a depleted vitamin D state can impact a range of local gastrointestinal (GI) immune surveillance strategies perhaps contributing to PLE pathogenesis [17,18]. There have been few attempts to eliminate this as a confounding factor in canine GI disease and many studies site this as a concern. Future studies comparing serum vitamin D concentration across a range of dogs with accurate phenotype such as noninflammatory (ie, primary lymphangiectasia) and inflammatory (ie, lymphocytic plasmocytic enteritis) PLE would help conclude etiology of hypovitaminosis D in canine PLE.

Are We Measuring the Most Appropriate Metabolite?

Recently, the accuracy of 25(OH)D has been brought into question as it fails to consider differences in VDBP, which can account for a wide range in vitamin D concentration. To address this concern, the vitamin D metabolite ratio has grown in popularity [19]. This ratio accounts for the degradation of 25(OH)D to $24,25(OH)_2D$ but requires measurement of 24, 25-dihydroxyvitamin D [$24,25(OH)_2D$], a test not available to most veterinary laboratories. Until canine metabolites are being measured collectively, inaccuracies in the management of PLE cases might persist.

Can We Draw Conclusions from a Single Value?

As it stands, there are currently no longitudinal data following vitamin D concentrations in canine PLE. Allenspach and colleagues [15] found that severity of hypovitaminosis D was associated with poorer outcomes. However, this study does not answer whether specific vitamin D supplementation is required to improve outcome. One case report published by one of the authors would dispute the need to supplement vitamin D in canine PLE as improvement was achieved by controlling the PLE rather than supplementing vitamin D with normalization of vitamin D concentration [20]. Hence, further work is required to determine when vitamin D supplementation is indicated and the best protocol to achieve resolution of the hypovitaminosis D.

VITAMIN D IN PROTEIN-LOSING ENTEROPATHY

The impact of vitamin D on serum calcium concentration in canine PLE is most significant. Calcium has historically been associated with bone health, but in the last 20 years, attention has turned to its plethora of nonskeletal roles. Calcium is one of the most tightly regulated electrolytes of the body and circulates either protein-bound, ionized ("free"), or complexed (Fig. 2). Hence, serum calcium concentration is dependent on protein concentration, particularly albumin, which is the most abundant serum protein. For this reason, it is not unexpected for dogs with PLE to present with total hypocalcemia.

Although a decrease in total calcium is expected due to the reduction in protein-bound calcium, there is evidence that concurrent ionized hypocalcemia is also frequently present in dogs with PLE [13,21]. Ionized

calcium is the metabolically active component, capable of binding to calcium-sensing receptors and therefore also more clinically relevant. The cause for the hypocalcemia in PLE is likely multifactorial [14]. Despite documentation of vitamin D depletion and concurrent hypocalcemia, there is no evidence for a reduction in VDBP or intestinal VDR in dogs with CE [22,23].

Mechanisms that have been reported as a cause for the ionized hypocalcemia include

1. Hypovitaminosis D [13–15,23]. It is unclear whether the reduction in vitamin D is due to GI loss, malnutrition, or malabsorption of vitamin D. The rarity of bleeding disorders in dogs with PLE suggests that malabsorption is less likely as there is no evidence for vitamin K deficiency.
2. Hypomagnesaemia has also been reported in dogs with PLE and concurrent hypomagnesaemia and hypocalcemia have been noted to be more frequent in dogs with GI disease [24–26]. Magnesium is involved in several steps of vitamin D metabolism and it is possible that hypomagnesemia contributes to hypovitaminosis D [27].
3. PTH response might also be blunted in dogs with PLE as it is also dependent on magnesium [28]. This functional deficiency in PTH may deplete 1,25(OH)2D. There is currently no strong evidence that dogs with severe PLE lose vitamin D bound to VDBP, although this could in theory contribute to the overall hypovitaminosis D.

It is important to recognize that the hypocalcemia from PLE can be so severe that clinical signs can develop that might require prompt supplementation [20,24,29]. The most common clinical signs reported in dogs with hypocalcemia are listed in Table 2.

Overall, ionized calcium concentration has not been reported to be a significant prognostic factor in dogs with PLE [15]. On the contrary, hypovitaminosis D is a negative prognostic factor in dogs with CE both with normal and decreased albumin concentrations (ie, PLE) [14,15].

When ionized hypocalcemia is identified in a dog diagnosed with PLE, it needs to be determined whether this finding is clinically relevant and whether supplementation with vitamin D and/or calcium is (immediately or chronically) indicated, which is further discussed later.

HOW TO MEASURE VITAMIN D?

Several methodologies have been developed to measure vitamin D metabolites and include methods with complete removal of protein and lipids prior to analysis

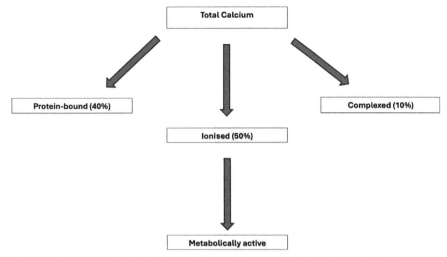

FIG. 2 Forms of calcium in the body. Total calcium in blood is divided into ionized, protein-bound, and complexed to low molecular weight ligands, such as bicarbonate, phosphate, and citrate. Ionized calcium is the metabolically active component and the metabolite of clinical interest; although the exact proportion varies, on average it is about 50% of the total calcium in dogs and cats.

(such as liquid chromatography-tandem mass spectrometric [LC–MS/MS]) or without removal (such as immunoassays) [30]. Overall, LC-MS/MS methods are deemed superior to detect all vitamin D metabolites

TABLE 2
Common Clinical Signs Reported Due to Clinically Significant Hypocalcemia

Clinical Sign	Note
Muscle tremors or twitching	Focal or diffuse
Facial rubbing	
Biting or licking of paws	
Generalised seizures	
Rear leg muscle cramping/stiff gait (Video 1)	More common in rear than front legs
Behavior changes	**Restless, aggressive, hypersensitive,** reduced activity
Decreased appetite	
Weight loss	

The signs in bold should increase the clinical suspicion for significant hypocalcemia in dogs with PLE. A thorough history is required as these signs can be only episodic.

(free or protein bound) and yield typically higher concentration of vitamin D metabolites than immunoassays. The reader is referred to a recent review for additional information on the subject of dogs [1].

In view of the plethora of methodologies, a certification program has been developed for human samples, the Vitamin D External Quality Assessment Scheme (DEQAS), to ensure that results between different protocols are comparable to a validated reference method. Of note, this scheme is currently not available specifically for canine samples but veterinarians should strive, when possible, to use a DEQAS laboratory for quality assurance. Commercial laboratories should ideally have a species-specific reference interval to enable interpretation of the result. In the United Kingdom, the general data protection regulation prevents the releasing of a list of DEQAS participating laboratories. For this reason, the clinician should request this information, from their testing laboratory.

In view of the challenges to quantify vitamin D metabolites, it is expected that measurements from one laboratory to the other will yield different results, especially if different methodologies are used (eg, LC-MS/MS vs immunoassay). For this reason, the ideal scenario is to identify a DEQAS-accredited laboratory with a well-defined reference interval for dogs to analyze samples. Alternatively, if this is not possible, the samples, especially if serially monitored, should be sent to the same, ideally DEQAS accredited, laboratory.

Historically, 25(OH)D has been measured to assess overall body stores of vitamin D. This is the most abundant metabolite in circulation, and it has a longer half-life (3 weeks) than the active metabolite 1,25(OH)2D (4-6 hours). For these reasons, 25(OH)D is deemed more reflective of total vitamin D stores than 1,25(OH)2D, as the latter is produced to demand. Supporting this concept is the fact that 25(OH)D was significantly lower in patients with Crohn's disease (CD) than healthy controls, whereas 1,25(OH)2D was not significantly different [31]. In accordance, 25(OH)D is also the metabolite that has been measured in the majority of large studies on vitamin D in canine PLE [13–15,25]. The indication for measuring both 25(OH)D versus 1-25(OH)$_2$D is currently under debate, but this might be useful in instances (ie, Rickets type 1 in humans) where there is inadequate conversion from 25(OH)D to 1 to 25(OH)$_2$D [32]. The utility of measuring 1 to 25(OH)$_2$D in veterinary medicine is currently unknown.

WHEN AND HOW TO SUPPLEMENT VITAMIN D?

In clinical practice, it is unclear, when or if there is a benefit of measuring 25(OH)D and a lack of evidence on when and how to supplement, especially in canine PLE. To the authors' knowledge, other than nutritional studies performed in puppies, there is a paucity of literature determining vitamin D reference intervals and requirements in different life stages of dogs. Furthermore, there are no data regarding specific breed requirements or disease states [5,33,34].

Vitamin D Supplementation in People

In people, a sufficient concentration of vitamin D is based on the concentration required to suppress PTH secretion [35,36]. This definition of physiologic "sufficiency" is widely accepted; however, different guidelines advise different cut-offs and supplementary recommendations (such as the Endocrine Society 2011, https://www.nogg.org.uk/full-guideline) [37,38]. Most of these studies suggest that a serum value of approximately 50 nmol/L (20 ng/mL) of D3 is adequate in an adult, but some suggest a value in excess of 75 nmol/L (30 ng/mL). This equates to an oral intake of 38 to 50 mcg (1500-2000 IU) of vitamin D3 per day [37].

25(OH)D Blood Concentration in Healthy Dogs

A canine study that used PTH suppression as a marker for sufficiency of vitamin D supplementation reported that a 25(OH)D blood concentration of 250 to 300 nmol/L (100–120 ng/mL) was required to reach this target using a competitive chemiluminescence immunoassay (LIASION 25[OH]D assay) [39]. This value is similar to the reference interval for dogs used by 2 regularly cited DEQAS-approved, canine reference laboratories. The Veterinary Diagnostic Laboratory of the Michigan State University reports a 25(OH)D blood concentration reference interval of 112 to 366 nmol/L, slightly higher than the reference interval established by the Vitamin D Animal Laboratory of the University of Edinburgh (39.5–172.7 nmol/L), which offer the test commercially [40]. These differences are not unexpected, because while LC-MS/MS is used by both laboratories, the exact methodologies differ, and they have each obtained assay-specific reference intervals for their test. Despite variation in reference intervals, dogs with hypercalcemia due to excessive dietary supplementation of vitamin D consistently have markedly higher 25(OH)D concentration of over 400 nmol/L, supporting the specificity of this finding across laboratories [41].

Vitamin D Supplementation in Dogs

There is no widely accepted recommendation on vitamin D supplementation in dogs. When recommendations are made, the advice is further complicated by the presence of both the minimum adequate intake and the minimum recommended allowance that differs with different guidelines (National Research Council 2006, AAFCO 2014 [https://www.aafco.org/wp-content/uploads/2023/01/FINAL_Committee_Report_Book_w_Cover.pdf], and FEDIAF 2014 [https://europeanpetfood.org/wp-content/uploads/2022/03/Updated-Nutritional-Guidelines.pdf]) [4]. Current nutritional recommendations from the AAFCO, the NRC, and the FEDIAF suggest a concentration of 500 to 640 IU/100 g Dry Matter (DM) of vitamin D in canine diet with lower concentration (320 IU/100 g DM) for giant breed puppies [34].

Hypovitaminosis D in People with Gastrointestinal Disease

Within the context of human GI disease, complications of hypovitaminosis D are well recognized [42–44]. Patients with CD are particularly at risk, with up to 80% of newly diagnosed patients being vitamin D deficient [45]. Similar to dogs, hypoproteinemia is one of the main risk factors for the development of hypovitaminosis D in CD [42]. A seminal gastroenterology study on hypovitaminosis D documented that a D2 dose of 900 IU per day was sufficient to correct the hypovitaminosis in patients with a range of GI diseases [46]. The authors of this study also reported that D2 was absorbed despite the presence of severe steatorrhea.

This study highlighted that even in the face of malabsorptive disease, vitamin D deficiency can be prevented by relatively small oral doses of D2. Recent publications have since proven that oral doses of 25 mcg (1,000 IU) per day can maintain serum concentration within the recommended reference range in different disease states [47,48]. However, it is important to note that other vitamin D metabolites have different oral potency. One study reported that a much higher daily dose (5,000 IU) of D3 was required in patients with CD [49].

Hypovitaminosis D in Dogs with Gastrointestinal Disease

Hypovitaminosis D is regularly identified in CE and as with human disease, dogs with PLE are more likely to be deficient [13,15,24,25,50,51]. Unfortunately, no studies have serially monitored vitamin D concentration in canine PLE. For this reason, many questions remain unanswered, such as

1. Is or when is supplementation required and which vitamin D metabolite to use?
2. Is vitamin D status correlated with response to treatment?
3. Is control of the underlying GI disease without vitamin D supplementation sufficient to normalize vitamin D concentration?
4. Does vitamin D treatment in PLE dogs with hypovitaminosis lead to a better outcome?

The main vitamin D metabolites used for supplementation in dogs include D2 (ergocalciferol), D3 (cholecalciferol), 25(OH)D (calcidiol), and 1-25(OH)2D3 (calcitriol). The main disadvantage of D2 and D3 supplementation is that relatively high doses are required, and the biological half-life and time-to-peak effect are long (5–21 days). In other words, if the dog is overdosed, there will be a long period between reduction of the supplement and resolution of the toxicity (typically 1–4 weeks). 25(OH)D is an alternative, which is more potent than D2 and with a shorter time to peak effect (1–4 days). Finally, 1-25(OH)2D3 is the most potent metabolite with a similar biological time than 25(OH)D. Hence, the risk of overdosing is higher with 1-25(OH)2D3, but the time for resolution of toxicity is shorter than for D2 or D3.

Clinical Decision-Making Using Available Evidence
Scenario 1: dog diagnosed with protein-losing enteropathy and ionized hypocalcemia ± hypovitaminosis D with clinical signs of hypocalcemia

If clinical signs, as listed in Table 2, are present and suspected to be secondary to ionized hypocalcemia, then supplementation is justified, especially with a concurrent demonstration of hypovitaminosis D. The animal should be initially stabilized with calcium supplementation. Oral and intravenous forms of calcium supplementation are available. Oral supplementation is sufficient for most patients and intravenous supplementation is reserved for dogs unable to tolerate oral medication (ie, seizuring). Due to differing amount of elemental calcium (Table 3), the authors advise care when prescribing oral supplementation at the regular dose of 1 to 4 g of calcium per day in divided doses or 25 to 50 mg/kg/day of elemental calcium divided in 2 to 3 daily doses. Similarly, an electrocardiogram is advised during intravenous administration.

Once the dog is clinically stable, and the ionized calcium is above 0.8 mmol/L, then vitamin D supplementation can be considered. In this setting, 1,25(OH)2D3 (calcitriol) is often preferred due to its fast onset of action and short biological half-life as mentioned earlier.

Current recommendations for dogs include dosages of 20 to 30 ng/kg per os q24 h of 1,25(OH)2D3, ideally with food for 3 to 4 days followed by half the dose per os q24 h thereafter. Monitoring includes ionized calcium and serum phosphorus twice a week for the first week and then a week later. Ongoing monitoring (see further discussion) is dependent on the progress of the dog and resolution of the hypocalcemia with the aim of discontinuing the drug once the dog's calcium has normalized and the albumin concentration has improved.

Scenario 2: dog diagnosed with protein-losing enteropathy and hypovitaminosis D ± ionized hypocalcemia without clinical signs suggestive of hypocalcemia

There is currently no evidence to suggest that supplementation of vitamin D in this scenario will improve the outcome of the dogs. The authors do not routinely supplement but rather monitor for clinical signs

TABLE 3
Commonly Used Calcium Preparations and Their Respective Elemental Calcium Content

Calcium Formulation	Elemental Calcium (%)	Elemental Calcium per 1 g (mg)
Calcium carbonate	40	400
Calcium gluconate	9	90
Calcium lactate	13	130

suggestive of hypocalcemia or absence of clinical response to standard treatment.

Some clinicians might elect to supplement PLE dogs with vitamin D and justify their decision with the evidence that lower vitamin D concentrations at the time of diagnosis are associated with a poorer outcome [15]. However, causation between hypovitaminosis D and poor outcome has not been proven, nor has a positive impact of vitamin D supplementation on outcome been demonstrated.

With no agreed dose range for vitamin D supplementation in canine PLE, clinicians draw on human guidelines as well as employing veterinary literature pertaining to primary hypoparathyroidism and secondary renal hyperparathyroidism [52]. This approach is not risk free: First, it presumes that doses used to treat one pathophysiological mechanism of hypovitaminosis D are appropriate for all patients with PLE. Second, it is assumed that human doses are transferable to canine patients. This is unlikely to be the case as a recent study showed higher than normal (2.3 ug/kg $BW^{0.75}$) oral doses of D3 supplementation failed to improve 25(OH)D concentrations in deficient dogs [53]. Furthermore, in contrast to human studies that typically use D2 as a supplement, a recent canine study using oral 25(OH)D documented a rapid rise in plasma concentrations in dogs with naturally occurring hypovitaminosis D [54,55]. As more evidence comes to light, it is likely that stark differences arise between canine and human supplementation strategies.

Although evidence is lacking, if treatment of hypovitaminosis D in PLE is considered, calcitriol should be avoided in view of the risk of over-supplementation versus any benefit from supplementation. Instead the authors recommend D3 (cholecalciferol) as there is a randomized, blinded placebo-controlled study reporting the use of D3 in dogs with atopic dermatitis [56]. The starting dose was 300 IU/kg orally per day with dose doubling every 2 weeks based on blood-ionized calcium concentrations. Most dogs responded to a final dose of 1,000 to 1,400 IU/kg orally per day with a significant increase in serum 25(OH)D within a period of 8 weeks compared to a decrease in the placebo group. This protocol can be considered in PLE dogs without clinical signs of hypocalcemia (see Table 2) and concurrent hypovitaminosis D. If the clinician opts to supplement 25OHVitD, this approach is preferred and considered safe, because an increase in VitD metabolites will likely be observed and adverse effects have not been reported.

Although serum 25(OH)D concentrations can be measured in dogs, the lack of consensus on an appropriate reference interval and a lack of data to suggest that supplementation improves outcome in canine PLE make it difficult to justify measuring 25-(OH)D concentration routinely in canine PLE.

MONITORING VITAMIN D SUPPLEMENTATION IN PROTEIN-LOSING ENTEROPATHY

Human patients started on D3 (cholecalciferol) supplementation are monitored closely [57]. Particular attention is paid to patients with GI pathology as vitamin D supplementation is often inadequate because of variable uptake of oral supplementation requiring dosage tailoring [58].

The use of low-fat diets to treat canine PLE also provides another reason to monitor serum 25(OH)D. Vitamin D is a fat-soluble vitamin, and therefore, despite the clinical effectiveness of low and ultra-low-fat diets in treating PLE, the low-fat content may hinder the dogs' ability to replenish their vitamin D store [59–62]. Supporting this argument, low-fat diets result in suboptimal concentrations of serum 25(OH)D (calcidiol) in people, necessitating higher doses of vitamin D supplementation [63,64].

Murine, cell line, and human GI studies have shown that glucocorticoids, which are often used to treat canine PLE, can increase 24-hydroxylase activity, resulting in decreased 25(OH)D serum concentrations by enhancing active metabolite degradation [65–67]. It is not known whether the same principle is applicable to dogs generally or in PLE, but it was not suggested by a study in atopic dogs, where treatment with prednisolone for 30 days did not result in a change in serum vitamin D concentrations [68].

It remains uncertain if serum 25(OH)D concentration normalizes without supplementation with resolution of GI clinical signs and normalization of biochemical parameters, in particular albumin, in canine PLE. One case report suggests that even severe hypovitaminosis D and severe clinical ionized hypocalcemia can normalize in PLE dogs without supplementation of vitamin D [20].

As D3 absorption in dogs is highly variable and PLE may impact GI vitamin D absorption [53,56], monitoring is indicated and can include

1. Clinical signs (if present due to the hypocalcemia).
2. Ionized calcium, phosphate, and albumin (normalization suggests control of the underlying disease and further supplementation might not be required).

3. 25(OH)D concentration to ensure that 25(OH)D concentration is, ideally, within a reference interval from a laboratory with dog-specific data.

IATROGENIC VITAMIN D TOXICITY

In human, medicine evidence of hypervitaminosis D is not based on serum vitamin D concentration alone, but rather on a combination of hypervitaminosis D and hypercalcemia. In the absence of hypercalcemia, hypervitaminosis D in human patients is not deemed an emergency [69].

In hypervitaminosis D, both calcium and phosphorus rise in serum. The use of calcium–phosphorus ratio can help identify patients at risk of the nephrotoxic effects [70]. Dogs receiving vitamin D supplementation should have regular measurement of their calcium concentration (ideally ionized calcium) and be monitored for clinical signs of hypercalcemia including weakness, lethargy, anorexia, polyuria, polydipsia, and depression [71]. In rare cases, tissue calcification leading to acute kidney injury has been reported [72].

Healthy laboratory dogs fed diets with increasing concentrations of vitamin D3 (cholecalciferol) did not show adverse effects up to the maximum concentration of 9,992 IU/kg of D3 of dry matter fed for 6 months [73]. Therefore, the risk of hypercalcemia by supplementing dogs with D3 at a starting dose of 300 IU/kg, as outlined earlier, in addition to the recommended dietary allowance for vitamin D of 500 IU/kg DM is likely negligible. Whether a dose of 300 IU/kg of D3 leads to an increase in serum 25(OH)VitD in canine PLE has yet to be determined and individual dose adjustments are likely to be required.

Overall, in keeping with human recommendations, authors recommend monitoring serum calcium and associated signs as a surrogate for vitamin D toxicity.

SUMMARY

Hypovitaminosis D is common in canine PLE and can lead to clinically significant ionized hypocalcemia. Considering the available literature, vitamin D loss from diseased intestines likely contributes most to hypovitaminosis D. Hypovitaminosis D at diagnosis is associated with poorer outcome and as such many clinicians elect to supplement accordingly. There is currently a lack of prospective and longitudinal data with a sufficiently large number of dogs to investigate changes in vitamin D concentration in canine PLE and the benefits from supplementation. Current dose recommendations

vary greatly, are extrapolated from other disease processes, and fail to consider the specifics of canine PLE pathology or confounding factors from other treatments. The authors believe that currently supplementation should be mostly considered in dogs with clinical signs of ionized hypocalcemia and documented inappropriate vitamin D concentrations until there is evidence-based literature to support supplementation in other scenarios. In addition, close monitoring of ionized calcium in dogs receiving vitamin D supplementation is recommended to avoid over-supplementation in lieu of repeated vitamin D measurements.

CLINICS CARE POINTS

- There is no evidence to support vitamin D supplementation in dogs that do not have clinical signs suggestive of hypocalcaemia.
- Calcium should be tested promptly and ideally under anaerobic conditions to limit spurious results.
- Take care when prescribing calcium and vitamin D supplementation to limit the chance of dose miscalculation.
- If hypocalcaemia is documented concurrently with clinical signs suggestive of hypocalcaemia, then calcitriol supplementation should be considered given its rapid onset of action and short half-life.
- Given the current evidence, resolution of clinical signs and serum ionised calcium is an appropriate way of assessing vitamin D status, especially when finances or testing availability is limited.

DISCLOSURE

The authors have nothing to disclose.

SUPPLEMENTARY DATA

Supplementary data to this article can be found online at https://doi.org/10.1016/j.yasa.2024.06.012.

REFERENCES

[1] Hurst EA, Homer NZ, Mellanby RJ. Vitamin D Metabolism and Profiling in Veterinary Species. Metabolites 2020;10(9):371.

[2] How KL, Hazewinkel HA, Mol JA. Dietary vitamin D dependence of cat and dog due to inadequate cutaneous

synthesis of vitamin D. Gen Comp Endocrinol 1994; 96(1):12–8.

[3] Wheatley VR, Sher DW. Studies of the lipids of dog skin. I. The chemical composition of dog skin lipids. J Invest Dermatol 1961;36:169–70.

[4] Nutrient requirements of dogs and cats. National Academies Press; 2006.

[5] Kealy RD, Lawler DF, Monti KL. Some observations on the dietary vitamin D requirement of weanling pups. J Nutr 1991;121(11 Suppl):S66–9.

[6] Schwartz JB, Gallagher JC, Jorde R, et al. Determination of Free 25(OH)D Concentrations and Their Relationships to Total 25(OH)D in Multiple Clinical Populations. J Clin Endocrinol Metab 2018;103(9): 3278–88.

[7] Bikle DD. Vitamin D: Production, Metabolism and Mechanisms of Action. In: Feingold KR, Anawalt B, Blackman MR, et al, editors. Endotext. MDText.com, Inc.; 2000. Available at: http://www.ncbi.nlm.nih.gov/books/NBK278935/. [Accessed 20 February 2024].

[8] Jones G, Prosser DE, Kaufmann M. Cytochrome P450-mediated metabolism of vitamin D. J Lipid Res 2014; 55(1):13–31.

[9] Zehnder D, Bland R, Walker EA, et al. Expression of 25-hydroxyvitamin D3-1alpha-hydroxylase in the human kidney. J Am Soc Nephrol JASN 1999;10(12):2465–73.

[10] Bikle DD. Vitamin D Metabolism, Mechanism of Action, and Clinical Applications. Chem Biol 2014;21(3): 319–29.

[11] Haussler MR, Jurutka PW, Mizwicki M, et al. Vitamin D receptor (VDR)-mediated actions of 1α,25(OH)2vitamin D3: Genomic and non-genomic mechanisms. Best Pract Res Clin Endocrinol Metab 2011;25(4):543–59.

[12] Crowe FL, Jolly K, MacArthur C, et al. Trends in the incidence of testing for vitamin D deficiency in primary care in the UK: a retrospective analysis of The Health Improvement Network (THIN), 2005-2015. BMJ Open 2019;9(6):e028355.

[13] Gow AG, Else R, Evans H, et al. Hypovitaminosis D in dogs with inflammatory bowel disease and hypoalbuminaemia. J Small Anim Pr 2011;52:411–8.

[14] Titmarsh H, Gow AG, Kilpatrick S, et al. Association of Vitamin D Status and Clinical Outcome in Dogs with a Chronic Enteropathy. J Vet Intern Med 2015;29:1473–8.

[15] Allenspach K, Rizzo J, Jergens AE, et al. Hypovitaminosis D is associated with negative outcome in dogs with protein losing enteropathy: a retrospective study of 43 cases. BMC Vet Res 2017;13(1).

[16] Amer M, Qayyum R. Relation between serum 25-hydroxyvitamin D and C-reactive protein in asymptomatic adults (from the continuous National Health and Nutrition Examination Survey 2001 to 2006). Am J Cardiol 2012;109(2):226–30.

[17] Fakhoury HMA, Kvietys PR, AlKattan W, et al. Vitamin D and intestinal homeostasis: Barrier, microbiota, and immune modulation. J Steroid Biochem Mol Biol 2020; 200:105663.

[18] Schwalfenberg GK. A review of the critical role of vitamin D in the functioning of the immune system and the clinical implications of vitamin D deficiency. Mol Nutr Food Res 2011;55(1):96–108.

[19] Ginsberg C, Hoofnagle AN, Katz R, et al. The Vitamin D Metabolite Ratio Is Independent of Vitamin D Binding Protein Concentration. Clin Chem 2021;67(2):385–93.

[20] Woods GA, Willems A, Hurst E, et al. Epileptic seizure in a cocker spaniel associated with hypocalcaemia, hypovitaminosis D and a protein-losing enteropathy. Vet Rec Case Rep 2019;7(2):e000813.

[21] Kull PA, Hess RS, Craig LE, et al. Clinical, clinicopathologic, radiographic, and ultrasonographic characteristics of intestinal lymphangiectasia in dogs: 17 cases (1996?1998). J Am Vet Med Assoc 2001;219(2):197–202.

[22] Cartwright JA, Gow AG, Milne E, et al. Vitamin D Receptor Expression in Dogs. J Vet Intern Med 2018;32(2): 764–74.

[23] Jablonski Wennogle SA, Priestnall SL, Suárez-Bonnet A, et al. Comparison of clinical, clinicopathologic, and histologic variables in dogs with chronic inflammatory enteropathy and low or normal serum 25-hydroxycholecalciferol concentrations. J Vet Intern Med 2019;33(5): 1995–2004.

[24] Kimmel SE, Waddell LS, Michel KE. Hypomagnesemia and hypocalcemia associated with protein-losing enteropathy in Yorkshire terriers: five cases (1992-1998). J Am Vet Med Assoc 2000;217:703–6.

[25] Jones C, Jablonski SA, Petroff BK, et al. Relationship between serum magnesium, calcium, and parathyroid concentrations in dogs with abnormally low serum 25-hydroxyvitamin D concentration and chronic or protein-losing enteropathy. J Vet Intern Med 2023; 37(1):101–9.

[26] Woods GA, Oikonomidis IL, Gow AG, et al. Investigation of hypomagnesaemia prevalence and underlying aetiology in a hospitalised cohort of dogs with ionised hypocalcaemia. Vet Rec 2021;189(9).

[27] Matias P, Ávila G, Ferreira AC, et al. Hypomagnesemia: a potential underlooked cause of persistent vitamin D deficiency in chronic kidney disease. Clin Kidney J 2023; 16(11):1776–85.

[28] Vetter T, Lohse MJ. Magnesium and the parathyroid. Curr Opin Nephrol Hypertens 2002;11(4):403–10.

[29] Whitehead J, Quimby J, Bayliss D. Seizures Associated With Hypocalcemia in a Yorkshire Terrier With Protein-Losing Enteropathy. J Am Anim Hosp Assoc 2015; 51(6):380–4.

[30] Alonso N, Zelzer S, Eibinger G, et al. Vitamin D Metabolites: Analytical Challenges and Clinical Relevance. Calcif Tissue Int 2023;112(2):158–77.

[31] Sadeghian M, Saneei P, Siassi F, et al. Vitamin D status in relation to Crohn's disease: Meta-analysis of observational studies. Nutr Burbank Los Angel Cty Calif 2016; 32(5):505–14.

[32] Kim CJ, Kaplan LE, Perwad F, et al. Vitamin D 1α-Hydroxylase Gene Mutations in Patients with 1α-

Hydroxylase Deficiency. J Clin Endocrinol Metab 2007; 92(8):3177–82.

[33] Goedegebuure SA, Hazewinkel HAW. Morphological Findings in Young Dogs Chronically Fed a Diet Containing Excess Calcium. Vet Pathol 1986;23(5):594–605.

[34] Tryfonidou MA, Stevenhagen JJ, van den Bemd GJCM, et al. Moderate cholecalciferol supplementation depresses intestinal calcium absorption in growing dogs. J Nutr 2002;132(9):2644–50.

[35] Institute of Medicine (US) Committee to Review Dietary Reference Intakes for Vitamin D and Calcium. In: Ross AC, Taylor CL, Yaktine AL, editors. Dietary reference intakes for calcium and vitamin D. National Academies Press (US); 2011. Available at: http://www.ncbi.nlm.nih.gov/books/NBK56070/. [Accessed 20 February 2024].

[36] Hollis BW. Circulating 25-hydroxyvitamin D levels indicative of vitamin D sufficiency: implications for establishing a new effective dietary intake recommendation for vitamin D. J Nutr 2005;135(2):317–22.

[37] Holick MF, Binkley NC, Bischoff-Ferrari HA, et al. Evaluation, Treatment, and Prevention of Vitamin D Deficiency: an Endocrine Society Clinical Practice Guideline. J Clin Endocrinol Metab 2011;96(7):1911–30.

[38] Godel JC, Canadian Paediatric Society, First Nations I and MHC. Vitamin D supplementation: Recommendations for Canadian mothers and infants. Paediatr Child Health 2007;12(7):583–9.

[39] Selting KA, Sharp CR, Ringold R, et al. Serum 25-hydroxyvitamin D concentrations in dogs – correlation with health and cancer risk. Vet Comp Oncol 2016;14(3):295–305.

[40] Hurst EA, Homer NZ, Denham SG, et al. Development and application of a LC–MS/MS assay for simultaneous analysis of 25-hydroxyvitamin-D and 3-epi-25-hydroxyvitamin-D metabolites in canine serum. J Steroid Biochem Mol Biol 2020;199:105598.

[41] Mellanby RJ, Mee AP, Berry JL, et al. Hypercalcaemia in two dogs caused by excessive dietary supplementation of vitamin D. J Small Anim Pr 2005;46:334–8.

[42] Siffledeen JS, Siminoski K, Steinhart H, et al. The Frequency of Vitamin D Deficiency in Adults with Crohn's Disease. Can J Gastroenterol Hepatol 2003;17:473–8.

[43] Tajika M, Matsuura A, Nakamura T, et al. Risk factors for vitamin D deficiency in patients with Crohn's disease. J Gastroenterol 2004;39(6):527–33.

[44] Ulitsky A, Ananthakrishnan AN, Naik A, et al. Vitamin D deficiency in patients with inflammatory bowel disease: association with disease activity and quality of life. JPEN J Parenter Enteral Nutr 2011;35(3):308–16.

[45] Leslie WD, Miller N, Rogala L, et al. Vitamin D status and bone density in recently diagnosed inflammatory bowel disease: the Manitoba IBD Cohort Study. Am J Gastroenterol 2008;103(6):1451–9.

[46] Davies M, Mawer EB, Krawitt EL. Comparative absorption of vitamin D3 and 25-hydroxyvitamin D3 in intestinal disease. Gut 1980;21(4):287–92.

[47] Heaney RP. Vitamin D in Health and Disease. Clin J Am Soc Nephrol 2008;3(5):1535.

[48] Grant WB, Holick MF. Benefits and requirements of vitamin D for optimal health: a review. Altern Med Rev J Clin Ther 2005;10(2):94–111.

[49] Yang L, Weaver V, Smith JP, et al. Therapeutic Effect of Vitamin D Supplementation in a Pilot Study of Crohn's Patients. Clin Transl Gastroenterol 2013;4(4):e33.

[50] Allenspach K, Wieland B, Grone A, et al. Chronic enteropathies in dogs: evaluation of risk factors for negative outcome. J Vet Intern Med 2007;21:700–8.

[51] Bush WW, Kimmel SE, Wosar MA, et al. Secondary hypoparathyroidism attributed to hypomagnesemia in a dog with protein-losing enteropathy. J Am Vet Med Assoc 2001;219(12):1732–4.

[52] Miller M, Quimby J, Langston C, et al. Effect of calcifediol supplementation on renin-angiotensin-aldosterone system mediators in dogs with chronic kidney disease. J Vet Intern Med 2022;36(5):1693–9.

[53] Young LR, Backus RC. Oral vitamin D supplementation at five times the recommended allowance marginally affects serum 25-hydroxyvitamin D concentrations in dogs. J Nutr Sci 2016;5:e31.

[54] Kurzbard RA, Backus RC, Yu S. Rapid improvement in vitamin D status with dietary 25-hydroxycholecalciferol in vitamin D insufficient dogs. J Nutr Sci 2021;10:e12.

[55] Young LR, Backus RC. Serum 25-hydroxyvitamin D3 and 24R,25-dihydroxyvitamin D3 concentrations in adult dogs are more substantially increased by oral supplementation of 25-hydroxyvitamin D3 than by vitamin D3. J Nutr Sci 2017;6:e30.

[56] Klinger CJ, Hobi S, Johansen C, et al. Vitamin D shows in vivo efficacy in a placebo-controlled, double-blinded, randomised clinical trial on canine atopic dermatitis. Vet Rec 2018;182(14):406.

[57] Hanley DA, Cranney A, Jones G, et al. Vitamin D in adult health and disease: a review and guideline statement from Osteoporosis Canada (summary). CMAJ (Can Med Assoc J) 2010;182(12):1315–9.

[58] Raftery T, O'Sullivan M. Optimal vitamin D levels in Crohn's disease: a review. Proc Nutr Soc 2015;74(1):56–66.

[59] Okanishi H, Yoshioka R, Kagawa Y, et al. The clinical efficacy of dietary fat restriction in treatment of dogs with intestinal lymphangiectasia. J Vet Intern Med 2014;28:809–17.

[60] Nagata N, Ohta H, Yokoyama N, et al. Clinical characteristics of dogs with food-responsive protein-losing enteropathy. J Vet Intern Med 2020;34(2):659–68.

[61] Myers M, Martinez SA, Shiroma JT, et al. Prospective Evaluation of Low-Fat Diet Monotherapy in Dogs with Presumptive Protein-Losing Enteropathy. J Am Anim Hosp Assoc 2023;59(2):74–84.

[62] Wennogle SA, Stockman J, Webb CB. Prospective evaluation of a change in dietary therapy in dogs with steroid-resistant protein-losing enteropathy. J Small Anim Pract 2021;62(9):756–64.

[63] Raimundo FV, Faulhaber GAM, Menegatti PK, et al. Effect of High- versus Low-Fat Meal on Serum 25-Hydroxyvitamin D Levels after a Single Oral Dose of Vitamin D: A Single-Blind, Parallel, Randomized Trial. Int J Endocrinol 2011;2011:809069.

[64] Dawson-Hughes B, Harris SS, Lichtenstein AH, et al. Dietary fat increases vitamin D-3 absorption. J Acad Nutr Diet 2015;115(2):225–30.

[65] Akeno N, Matsunuma A, Maeda T, et al. Regulation of vitamin D-1alpha-hydroxylase and -24-hydroxylase expression by dexamethasone in mouse kidney. J Endocrinol 2000;164(3):339–48.

[66] Kurahashi I, Matsunuma A, Kawane T, et al. Dexamethasone enhances vitamin D-24-hydroxylase expression in osteoblastic (UMR-106) and renal (LLC-PK1) cells treated with 1alpha,25-dihydroxyvitamin D3. Endocrine 2002;17(2):109–18.

[67] Skversky AL, Kumar J, Abramowitz MK, et al. Association of glucocorticoid use and low 25-hydroxyvitamin D levels: results from the National Health and Nutrition Examination Survey (NHANES): 2001-2006. J Clin Endocrinol Metab 2011;96(12):3838–45.

[68] Kovalik M, Thoday KL, Berry J, et al. Prednisolone therapy for atopic dermatitis is less effective in dogs with lower pretreatment serum 25-hydroxyvitamin D concentrations. Vet Dermatol 2012;23(2):125–30, e27-e28.

[69] Kennel KA, Drake MT, Hurley DL. Vitamin D deficiency in adults: when to test and how to treat. Mayo Clin Proc 2010;85(8):752–7, quiz 757-758.

[70] Lippi I, Guidi G, Marchetti V, et al. Prognostic role of the product of serum calcium and phosphorus concentrations in dogs with chronic kidney disease: 31 cases (2008–2010). J Am Vet Med Assoc 2014;245(10):1135–40.

[71] de Brito Galvão JF, Schenck PA, Chew DJ. A Quick Reference on Hypocalcemia. Vet Clin North Am Small Anim Pract 2017;47(2):249–56.

[72] Hilbe M, Sydler T, Fischer L, et al. Metastatic calcification in a dog attributable to ingestion of a tacalcitol ointment. Vet Pathol 2000;37(5):490–2.

[73] Jewell DE, Panickar KS. Increased dietary vitamin D was associated with increased circulating vitamin D with no observable adverse effects in adult dogs. Front Vet Sci 2023;10:1242851.

Advances in Small Animal Care 5 (2024) 133–149

ADVANCES IN SMALL ANIMAL CARE

Comparative Cytology and Histology in Canine and Feline Gastrointestinal Neoplasia

Advantages and Challenges

Paola Cazzini, DVM, MS, DiplACVP (Clin Path), MRCVS*,
Alexandra Malbon, BVSc, BSc(hons), Dr med vet, PhD, DiplECVP, MRCVS,
Linda Morrison, BVMS, FRCPath, DiplECVP MRCVS

Easter Bush Pathology, Royal (Dick) School of Veterinary Studies and the Roslin Institute, University of Edinburgh, Roslin 0131 6517458, UK

KEYWORDS
- Cytology • Histology • Biopsy • Sampling • Neoplasia • Gastrointestinal • Stomach • Intestine

KEY POINTS
- Understanding the advantages and disadvantages of the various techniques is key to deciding the most appropriate sampling method in cases of gastrointestinal neoplasia.
- Cytologic evaluation of samples is a less invasive and expensive technique than histology and has a faster turnaround time; however, additional diagnostics are needed in some cases.
- Histologic evaluation of samples is more invasive and expensive, but in some cases it is essential, as evaluation of tissue architecture can give key diagnostic information.

INTRODUCTION

Gastrointestinal (GI) neoplasms in dogs and cats are reported to represent less than 1% to 11.9% of all tumors [1–9]. This location poses unique challenges during the diagnostic process. However, reaching a final diagnosis is essential for prognostication and to allow the selection of therapeutic options. Choosing the right sampling technique depends both on the lesion location, and on the suspected type of neoplasia. Cytology is less invasive, fast, and relatively cheap. However, it is more useful for certain tumors than others, depending on cellular exfoliation and other factors; for example, it has high diagnostic utility for most round cell tumors, but its usefulness can be limited for mesenchymal neoplasia. More invasive techniques and expensive procedures are

required when acquiring samples for histologic investigation, and selection of the appropriate sampling method is key to obtaining a diagnostic sample. In some cases, histology is essential to reach an accurate diagnosis, for example, assessment of invasion, and tumor grading. For this reason, understanding advantages and challenges of these diagnostic techniques empowers clinicians to make better choices.

SAMPLING

When deciding on how to sample a lesion for cytologic or histologic evaluation there are many factors to consider, such as clinical status of the patient, costs, and potential complications. Regardless of the sampling

---

*Corresponding author, E-mail address: paola.cazzini@ed.ac.uk

https://doi.org/10.1016/j.yasa.2024.06.008
2666-450X/24/

method selected, it is important to provide the signalment and clinical history, which should include any prior test results, lesion location and description (including images), and method of sampling [10,11].

Cytology

Although histology remains the reference standard for the diagnosis of many GI tumors, cytology has several advantages: it is generally a less invasive and expensive technique and has a faster turnaround time [12,13]. Different techniques can be used to collect cytologic samples, each with their own advantages and limitations.

Fine needle aspiration

With the use of imaging techniques such as ultrasound and computed tomography, masses and pathologic areas can be identified and sampled through fine needle aspiration (FNA). The center of large or fast-growing masses is often necrotic and therefore of limited diagnostic utility; aspirating multiple areas within the lesion increases the probability of a diagnostic sample [12]. In a study where histology was compared with FNA cytology of GI tumors, cytology demonstrated sensitivity and specificity of 71% and 100% for the diagnosis of lymphoma, 63% and 98% for epithelial tumors, and 44% and 100% for mesenchymal neoplasia, respectively [14]. In this study, FNAs of intestinal lesions were more rewarding than gastric ones, which were more often inconclusive or in which the main process was masked by inflammation or necrosis [14]. The needle rinse technique, where an FNA is taken and the needle rinsed through with saline rather than a smear prepared, allows a cell block to be obtained [15]. This can then be used to prepare histologic sections, allowing recuts and the use of immunohistochemistry (IHC) [15].The advantages of this technique were highlighted in the diagnosis of GI lymphoma in a cat and a dog, and a case of gastrointestinal stromal tumor (GIST) in a dog in a recent case series [15].

Brush, touch imprint, or squash cytology from gastrointestinal endoscopy

A cytology brush can be passed through the working channel of a flexible endoscope and rubbed vigorously onto the mucosa, before being rolled on a glass slide; or a mucosal endoscopic biopsy can be used to make impression smears or squash preparations [16–18]. Advantages include limited invasiveness and rapid diagnosis; however, only mucosal and occasionally submucosal layers are sampled using this technique. In a study comparing cytology and histology obtained through

endoscopy, brush cytology from intestinal lesions had adequate numbers of epithelial cells, although some iatrogenic haemorrhage and cell lysis was observed [16]. Gastric brush cytologies were contaminated by oropharyngeal bacteria and leukocytes which made interpretation more difficult. Although both techniques (especially brush cytology) demonstrated good diagnostic accuracy, in this study most lesions were inflammatory rather than neoplastic, with only a few cases of lymphoma included. In a study in which squash endoscopic biopsies were compared with histology, when differentiating between intestinal lymphoma and enteritis in dogs, there was 81.4% agreement; cytology had sensitivity and specificity of 98.6% and 73.5%, respectively [18]. A significant proportion of lymphocytic enteritis cases were misdiagnosed in cytology as small cell lymphoma. This is not surprising as differentiation is challenging also in histology. In this study 99% of squash preparations were of diagnostic quality, and they performed better than imprints and brush cytology samples used in other studies [18]. Samples of good diagnostic quality were also obtained in a study on gastric adenocarcinomas which compared endoscopic squash cytology and histology [19].

Impression smears from surgical biopsies

When biopsies are taken during laparotomy, impression smears can be prepared before tissue fixation. It is important to dab the sample on gauze or tissue paper until sticky, before making imprints on glass slides, to avoid excessive blood contamination. For imprints it is also useful to note the anatomic orientation [12]. In a study comparing cytology of GI neoplasia with histology, impression smears had a higher concordance with surgical biopsies than did FNAs [14]. In cases of lymphoma and smooth muscle tumors, sensitivity and specificity were both 100%, whilst for epithelial neoplasias they were 90% and 100%, respectively. In these cases, cytology can be useful not only for a faster diagnosis, but also to detect malignant cells at margins intraoperatively. When simultaneously sampling cytology and biopsy samples, it is imperative to avoid exposure of cytologic smears to formalin or formalin fumes as this alters staining, rendering slides poorly or nondiagnostic [12].

Rectal scrapings

Scraping is a relatively non-invasive and easy technique which can aid in the diagnosis of masses and lesions located in the distal part of the large intestine. An ear curette or conjunctival scraper can be introduced with a gloved finger. Care must be taken when scraping the lesion to avoid perforation. During extraction the material on the scraper can be protected by the glove. Squash preparations can be made from the material obtained [13]. The use of lubricant gel should be avoided or minimised, as gel on the slide will stain, masking cytologic features.

Histology

There are several publications describing how to get the optimum result from histology samples, both in general and from GI biopsies [10,11,20,21]. Overall, taking endoscopic biopsies is a less invasive procedure than taking full-thickness biopsies, with a shorter surgical time, lower risk of complications and allows the mucosal surface to be visualised at the time of sampling, facilitating targeted sampling of mucosal lesions (Table 1) [10,11,20,22]. In addition, endoscopy allows sampling of multiple areas of mucosa, which is useful for lesions with a patchy distribution (eg, lymphoma). However, it is not possible to evaluate the jejunum, and sometimes there can be difficulty accessing the ileum [20]. Careful handling of the endoscopic biopsies is important to minimise artifacts that may hamper histologic evaluation. It is also important to ensure biopsies are placed into formalin immediately after collection. Sample handling should be minimized, and multiple samples need to be taken from each site (6–15 generally advised depending on site and species) [11,20,23,24]. In some cases, full thickness biopsies are preferred, to allow evaluation of all regions, and all layers. This is important for lesions that are transmural, or occupying only deeper layers [20,23,25–27]. Laparotomy or laparoscopy are required to undertake full thickness biopsies, thereby allowing evaluation and sampling of other organs during the same surgery, which may give additional information [20,22,27,28]. However, these procedures are more invasive than endoscopy, with longer surgical times and increased complication risk, particularly for the large intestine due to the risk of surgical dehiscence. They also do not allow visual assessment of the mucosal surface [11,20,23,27–29].

ROUND CELL NEOPLASIA
Intestinal Lymphoma

The gastrointestinal tract (GIT) has a vast population of mucosal associated lymphoid tissue (MALT) and, as a result, is the most common site of extranodal lymphoma. Lymphomas may present as focal/multifocal masses, or diffuse thickening of 1 or more regions of the GIT. Those with a mass effect may result in a functional obstruction, or perforation leading to septic peritonitis. Common clinical signs include anorexia, depression, vomiting, diarrhea, hypoalbuminaemia, and weight loss [30,31]. Classification of GI lymphoma is usually based on the World Health Organization scheme, by determining growth pattern, immunophenotyping (B/T cells), mitotic count, and cell size [32]. The main subtypes are enteropathy-associated T cell lymphoma (EATL), large granular lymphoma (LGL), and diffuse large B cell lymphoma (DLBCL).

Lymphoma is the most common GI neoplasm in cats, with a predominance of EATL (T cells comprise

TABLE 1
Advantages and Disadvantages of Histology Sampling Techniques

Technique	Cytology	Endoscopic Biopsies	Full-Thickness Biopsies
Advantages	• Cheaper • Often requires no anesthesia • Faster turnaround time • Ideal for round cell and good for epithelial neoplasia • Minimal complication risk	• Allows simultaneous assessment of mucosal surface and targeted sampling • Less invasive • Multiple samples, from multiple locations, can easily be taken	• All intestinal layers can be assessed • All locations can be sampled • Other organs can be visualised/sampled
Disadvantages	• Downstream techniques may be limited • Limited utility for some mesenchymal tumors • May not allow subclassification	• Jejunum cannot be sampled • Relatively operator dependant	• More invasive • Increased complication risk • Mucosa cannot be visualised therefore only serosal appearance can be used to select site

90% of the resident intestinal lymphoid population in healthy cats) [33,34]. Small cell, mucosal lymphomas (type 2) comprise the majority, followed by the transmural large cell lymphomas (type 1). The link between chronic lymphoplasmacytic enteritis (LPE) and neoplastic transformation to type 2 EATL is strongly suspected but thus far unproven. Nevertheless, the 2 have been seen to co-exist in the same sample in up to 60% of cases, making a final diagnosis particularly challenging. Despite increases in our understanding of these conditions, some cases remain inconclusive even following IHC and polymerase chain reaction (PCR) for antigen receptor rearrangements (PARR). In cats, EATL is most common in the jejunum, followed by ileum, duodenum, stomach, and colon [33], which is important when deciding sampling method as endoscopy has limited access to some intestinal regions. However, a recent American College of Veterinary Internal Medicine (ACVIM) consensus statement on distinguishing feline low grade lymphoma from inflammation does not recommend full-thickness biopsies over endoscopic [24].

LGL are a specific T cell subtype, more commonly transmural and most easily diagnosed cytologically (Fig. 1A–C). They are more common in cats but have been reported in dogs. In cats EATL type 1 and LGL had a poor prognosis while EATL type 2 (mucosal, small cell) had a median survival time of 29 months [33].

Amongst B cell subtypes, DLBCL neoplasms are the most common in cats, and occur predominantly in the stomach or ileocaecal junction [33,35]. *Helicobacter*-associated gastric lymphomas have been postulated in cats [36].

In dogs, the most frequent site of GI lymphomas is the small intestine, followed by stomach and large intestine [37,38]. T cell lymphomas again dominate [38], but, in contrast to cats, type 1 are more common than type 2 [39]. These have higher mitotic activity, demonstrated by higher Ki67 index than type 2 [30].

Anaplastic large T cell lymphoma (ALTCL) is a rare canine subtype shown to have a rapid progression, it is often associated with necrosis, inflammation, and vascular invasion [40].

Occasionally, more than 1 type of concurrent lymphoid neoplasia has been described in dogs [31].

Cytologic characteristics

Lymphoid cells exfoliate well on cytologic preparation, and cytology can be very useful in the diagnosis of GI lymphoma. Neoplastic lymphoid tissue, characterized by the predominance of a monomorphic population,

needs to be differentiated from reactive lymphoid tissue, characterized by a more heterogeneous lymphoid population. This is not always easy, and advanced diagnostics may be needed, particularly with small cell lymphomas. Cells can be observed in detail in cytology, and, by comparing lymphocytes to erythrocytes and neutrophils, the lymphoid population can be described as composed of small, medium, or large cells. Cells with nuclei that are 1-1.5x an erythrocyte are considered small, 2-2.5x medium, and greater than 3x large [41]. Large lymphocytes often have scant to moderate, deeply basophilic cytoplasm, and a peripheralized, large nucleus with finely stippled chromatin and a variably prominent nucleolus (see Fig. 1A). Large cell lymphomas tend to be more aggressive and have a graver prognosis. Small lymphocytes have scant, basophilic cytoplasm, and a peripheralized round nucleus with denser chromatin. Small cell lymphomas tend to have a more indolent course and better prognosis. Lymphocytes can have characteristics which further aids in the diagnosis. Cytoplasmic granules can be seen in LGL and are particularly evident in cats, in which these neoplastic lymphocytes of cytotoxic T origin [33] need to be differentiated from mast cells (see Fig. 1C). The presence of cytoplasmic round, light basophilic, glassy globules (Russell bodies) indicates Mott cell differentiation of a B cell lymphoma. In young, small breed dogs, GI lymphoma with Mott cell differentiation often has a better prognosis [42,43]. Mitotic figures can be readily recognized and are more numerous in aggressive tumors, and absent or rare in more indolent forms. Tingible body macrophages (containing phagocytized cellular debris) can be seen in increased numbers in high grade lymphomas due to the fast replication rate; however, these can also be seen in lymphoid reactivity and are not pathognomonic for neoplasia. Lymphoglandular bodies (small cytoplasmic fragments) can be seen in the background of FNAs in both reactive and neoplastic conditions; however, noticing their presence may become useful when neoplastic cells are very atypical and their lymphoid origin is uncertain.

Differential diagnoses. Lymphoid reactive hyperplasia, other round cell tumors (if cells are atypical) and poorly cohesive carcinoma.

Histologic characteristics

Large cell lymphomas (B cell or type 1 EATL) are relatively easy to diagnose, assuming accurate biopsy sampling, as aggregates of large lymphocytes are not part of the resident population. When full thickness samples are available, type 1 are also far more likely to invade transmurally than type 2 (see Fig. 1B). In any tumor

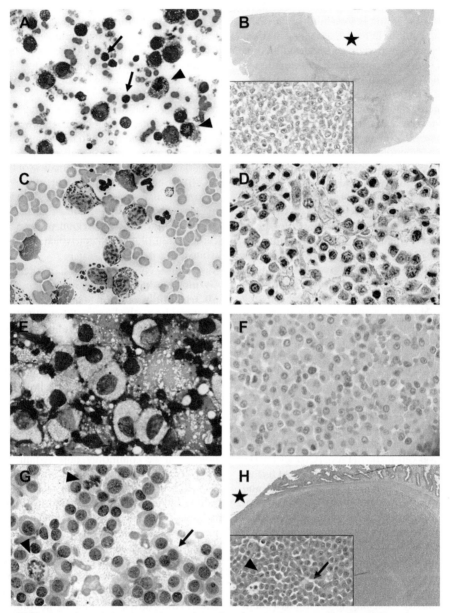

FIG. 1 (**A**) Cytology of gastric lymphoma in a cat. Large lymphocytes (compare size with small lymphocytes, *arrow*) with dark basophilic cytoplasm, punctate vacuoles, and round nucleus with finely stippled chromatin with an evident nucleolus. Mitotic figures are also seen (*arrowhead*). 100X MGG. (**B**) Histology of intestinal large cell lymphoma in a cat; the cellular proliferation completely effaces the mucosa (*star* in lumen) and extends transmurally. Slide overview H&E Inset: monomorphic population of large lymphoid cells with prominent nucleolus. 40X H&E. (**C**) Cytology of intestinal large granular lymphoma (LGL) in a cat. Notice the numerous, purple granules present in the cytoplasm of the large lymphocytes. 100X MGG. (**D**) Histology of ileal LGL in a cat. Cytoplasmic granules are not evident on histology. 100X H&E. (**E**) Cytology of jejunal mast cell tumor (MCT) in a cat. Pleomorphic round cells exfoliating individually and with a highly vacuolated cytoplasm are present. 100X MGG. (**F**) Histology of visceral MCT in a cat. Sheets of round cells with large amounts of cytoplasm and no evident granulation. 40X H&E. (**G**) Cytoloy of rectal plasmacytoma in a dog. Round, individualized plasma cells with mild anisocytosis and anisokaryosis, occasional mitotic figures (*arrowheads*), and rare binucleation (*arrow*) are seen. 100X MGG. (**H**) Histology of rectal plasmacytoma with transmural infiltration by round cells and focal ulceration (*star*). 5X H&E Insert: sheets of round cells with plasmacytoid morphology. Mitotic figure (*arrowhead*) and binucleate cell (*arrow*). 40X H&E.

type this transmural invasion is a useful distinguishing factor from inflammation. In type 2, accurate/sufficient sampling is especially important as single villus tips may sometimes be seen to be affected, with unaffected adjacent villi. Diagnostic algorithms to differentiate feline type 2 EATL from chronic inflammation focus on identifying histologic features more common in neoplasia than inflammation but often require additional testing beyond routine histologic examination as these are not pathognomonic [44].

The monomorphic nature of the infiltrate, despite comprising small lymphocytes, is a key feature, as is epitheliotropism (nests and plaques), found in 50% of small cell lymphomas in cats, versus 5% of LPE [45]. A gradient distribution of lymphocytes from apical villous location to crypts is also associated with lymphoma [45].

ALTCL are characterised by transmural CD3, and frequently CD30 positive, large, pleomorphic cells. ALTCL can be differentiated from EATL type 1 by the lack of villous atrophy, markedly atypical cellular morphology, and vascular invasion [40].

Differential diagnoses. Other round cell neoplasias, lymphocytic inflammation for type 2 EATL.

Additional diagnostic tests

Where diagnosis is equivocal, histology should be complemented by IHC, and if necessary, PARR [44]. Initial IHC choices are laboratory dependant but include T cell (CD3) and a B cell marker (PAX-5/CD20/CD79a). The 2023 ACVIM consensus statement suggested further IHC could include CD56 (natural killer cell marker), and STAT5 (hyperactivation marker which is high in lymphoma) [24]. PARR is a useful adjunct but must be interpreted as part of a whole picture; it is important to note that false positives and negative results can occur. False negatives occur particularly in cases with background inflammation. Precise methodology varies between laboratories. In feline patients, PARR for T cell lymphoma often has a sensitivity exceeding 80%, whereas for B cell tumors it ranges from 34% to 89% [46]. In dogs, sensitivities of 72% to 100% and specificities of 96% to 100% are reported [47]. In the absence of clearly visible granules by routine staining (Fig. 1D), IHC for granzyme B and perforin can be used to confirm LGL.

Mast Cell Tumors

Primary GI mast cell tumors (MCT) are a form of visceral MCT [8,48–50]. They are the third most common GI tumor in cats comprising a reported 4% to 5%, with lower numbers in dogs [8,9,14], in which miniature breeds

appear most commonly affected [8,9,14,50,51]. In both species, they may be focal or part of disseminated disease, with mastocytemia and neoplastic mast cells within abdominal effusions reported [8,9,50,52,53]. While circulating mast cells have been closely associated with visceral MCT in cats [52], mastocytemia in dogs is frequently associated with inflammatory conditions [53]. In cats, intestinal MCT are typically within the distal small intestine and colon; in dogs the small intestine appears to be most commonly affected [9,50,51,54]. There is marked variation in the presentation of these lesions as they may be focal, multifocal or diffuse; eccentric to circumferential; and range from exophytic nodules to plaques, sometimes with surface ulceration [8,51,54]. All result in a thickened region of the GIT, often with compromise of the lumen, which on section may be white to tan or gray.

Cytologic characteristics

MCT generally exfoliate well on cytology and a diagnosis can be reached easily. Pre-treatment with antihistamines is advised prior to aspiration, if MCT is the main diagnostic concern [55]. Cytologically MCT are characterized by a population of round cells exfoliating individually and in aggregates. Cells have distinct cellular borders, moderate cytoplasm with variable amounts of purple-staining granules or vacuoles, and a generally central, round, nucleus. Rapid stains can in some cases under-stain mast cell granules [56]. Non-staining cytoplasmic granules, appearing as empty vacuoles, can be commonly observed in feline visceral MCT (Fig. 1E). Differentiation can vary, with some tumors (eg, sclerosing variant of feline intestinal MCT) exhibiting decreased differentiation and highly atypical features. Eosinophils, mesenchymal cells, and collagen fibers can also be present.

Differential diagnoses. In cats, MCT with marked collagenolysis need to be differentiated from GI eosinophilic sclerosing fibroplasia (FGESF) [57] and from LGL. MCT with poorly staining granules, such as can be seen in cats, must be differentiated from highly vacuolated histiocytic cells.

Histologic characteristics

In both cats and dogs, MCT appear as an unencapsulated proliferation of variably pleomorphic round cells that expand and efface the pre-existing tissue; usually starting in the outer intestinal layers and extending into the mucosa or mesentery (Fig. 1F) [8]. Cells may form sheets with variable amounts of collagenous stroma, or present as packets supported by a small amount of stroma, often with admixed eosinophils. Cytoplasmic granules may be identifiable, but, particularly in cats, they may stain poorly with Toluidine blue or Giemsa; lack of granule staining does not exclude mast cell origin [8,50,51,54,58].

Differential diagnoses. Other round cell tumors. If there is significant collagen deposition (sclerosis) within the MCT, the possibility of FGESF may be considered in cats. If the cells are forming packets, then carcinoid may need to be excluded [8].

Additional diagnostic tests
IHC for c-KIT (CD117) and/or mast cell tryptase may confirm mast cell origin, but the latter may not be readily detected [8,51,54,58]. Evaluation of *c-KIT* mutations may be considered but there is limited information available on these mutations within intestinal neoplasia [8,54].

Gastrointestinal Extramedullary Plasma Cell Tumors/Plasmacytomas
GI extramedullary plasma cell tumors are infrequent in dogs [59–61]. In a study that included 751 canine extramedullary plasmacytomas, 4% were identified within the colorectal region and rare ones were elsewhere within the GIT [59]. Dogs with colorectal plasmacytomas had a median age of 10.7 years; Cocker Spaniels and West Highland White Terriers were predisposed [59]. Progression is usually slow and complete surgical excision is normally curative; however, metastatic cases have been reported [60]. These tumors generally present as single, intramural masses, but multiple masses have been described [59,62]. Lesions may present as variably sized white to red masses, occasionally with associated mucosal ulceration. One case of multiple myeloma involving the GIT of a dog has been reported [63]. Feline GI plasma cell tumors are very rarely reported and appear to have a poor prognosis [9,62,64,65].

Cytologic characteristics
The cellularity of plasma cell lesions is usually good. Cells range from well-differentiated plasma cells to more pleomorphic individualized round cells with generally well-defined cytoplasmic borders and moderate amounts of basophilic cytoplasm, often with a perinuclear clearing (Golgi zone). The nucleus is round to oval and eccentric, with binucleated and multinucleated cells commonly seen. Anisocytosis, anisokaryosis, giant cells, and variable numbers of mitotic figures can be seen, even in neoplasms with benign behavior (Fig. 1G) [61,66].

Plasma cells with "flame cell" morphology, with a peripheral, bright pink cytoplasm, and with intracytoplasmic haemosiderin, have been reported in a case of rectal plasmacytoma [67].

Differential diagnoses. In cases where pleomorphism is marked, histiocytic sarcoma (HS) can be a differential.

Histologic characteristics
As for other round cell tumors, extramedullary plasma cell tumors present as unencapsulated sheets of round to oval cells, some of which are relatively well differentiated with a moderate amount of amphophilic to slightly basophilic cytoplasm, a central to eccentric nucleus and perinuclear halo (Fig. 1H). Well-differentiated cells are usually more readily identified toward the periphery of the lesion and will be admixed with less well differentiated forms including binucleated and multinucleated cells. Cells are supported by a fine fibrovascular stroma and mitoses are generally infrequently seen. Some tumors will also contain amyloid [8,64].

Differential diagnoses. Other round cell tumors are the main differential diagnoses and can be excluded with IHC.

Additional diagnostic tests
Plasma cell origin can be confirmed with IHC for MUM1, monoclonal immunoglobulins (IgA, IgG, or IgM), and kappa or lambda light chains.

Histiocytic Sarcoma
While disseminated histiocytic proliferations may involve the GIT, primary HS of the GIT are rarely reported. There are only 4 cases reported in dogs; 2 gastric and 2 jejunal, some having ulceration or perforation [68–71]. On cytology, many atypical large cells with prominent anisocytosis and anisokaryosis, and occasional multinucleated and markedly atypical cells with occasional erythrophagocytosis were observed in a case [70]. When cells have low pleomorphism, HS must be differentiated from histiocytic inflammation. On histology, cells resemble those described in cytology and are arranged in sheets. Other round cell tumors (eg, lymphoma), or poorly differentiated malignant neoplasia are the main differential diagnoses. Immunohistochemical staining using Iba1 and CD204 may be used to confirm histiocytic origin of the atypical cells but CD18, lysozyme, Mac387 and MHCII may also be utilised.

EPITHELIAL NEOPLASIA

Hyperplastic Polyps, Adenomas and (Adeno) Carcinomas

Benign epithelial proliferations (hyperplastic polyps and adenomas) are recognised throughout the GIT but are generally rare in the stomach and small intestine and more commonly reported in the large intestine (colon and rectum), especially in dogs [6,8,72–77]. A recent study has shown an increased incidence of colorectal polyps in West Highland White Terriers, with increased risk of recurrence [78]. In dogs, carcinomas are the most common gastric tumor and are reported most often in males, 8 years to 10 years old, with a range of predisposed breeds including Rough Collies, Staffordshire Bull Terriers, Belgian Shepherds, Standard Poodle, and Tervuren [5,8,73,79–83]. Intestinal adenocarcinomas are more common in the large intestine than the small intestine in dogs and large intestinal adenocarcinomas are often reported as the predominant form of GI neoplasia [1,23,79,81,84]. In cats, intestinal adenocarcinomas are the second most frequent GI tumor type after lymphoma, often in animals over 10 years old, with male cats, Siamese, and domestic shorthair breeds reportedly predisposed [4,5,7,8,79,85].

At all sites, lesions may present as white to tan or red exophytic/luminal masses with mural thickening or crateriform ulcerated areas often associated with malignant lesions. Associated fibrosis (also known as desmoplasia/scirrhous reaction) may be seen with malignancy and can result in the lesions having a firm texture and/or may result in significant stricture formation, especially in the GIT.

Cytologic characteristics

Depending on the technique used to obtain cytology specimens, gastric and enteric content (bacterial flora and spiral organisms, ingesta, mucinous material) may be present alongside cells from the GIT or lesion [16]. The presence of fibrosis and inflammation may also be confounding factors. Cytologically differentiating between normal, hyperplastic, or adenoma cells can be challenging. In the presence of inflammation some mild dysplastic changes are expected in otherwise normal epithelial cells, posing an additional challenge.

Adenomas usually exfoliate in cohesive clusters, and, while cells might retain some normal characteristics, loss of polarity and mild anisocytosis and anisokaryosis may be present. More marked criteria of malignancy can be seen with adenocarcinomas where cells might lose their cohesiveness (Fig. 2C) [86], and marked anisocytosis/anisokaryosis, macronuclei, prominent nucleoli with anisonucleoliosis, multinucleation, nuclear molding, and cellular cannibalism, may be present. Pseudoacinar formation may be seen. The presence of signet ring cells (which a large vacuole filled with mucin peripheralizing the nucleus) and punctate cytoplasmic vacuolation, often together with poorly cohesive or individualized cells, are often seen in cytologic specimens from gastric adenocarcinomas [19,86] and may indicate a signet ring variant. Large amounts of background eosinophilic material, together with variably cohesive round cells with foamy cytoplasm with eosinophilic material are suspicious of mucinous adenocarcinomas [87], while cells with angular borders and abundant, basophilic cytoplasm would suggest squamous cell differentiation.

Differential diagnoses. Hyperplasia is difficult to distinguish from adenoma. Dysplasia secondary to inflammation should be distinguished from neoplasia. Some adenocarcinomas have poorly cohesive cells and may be difficult to differentiate from round or mesenchymal tumors.

Histologic characteristics

Regardless of tumor location, the histologic features of the lesions are broadly similar, and the advantage of biopsy samples over cytology is that they allow evaluation of tissue architecture (especially if full thickness), which can be essential to differentiate adenomas from well-differentiated carcinomas or in situ carcinomas from adenocarcinomas (see Fig. 2A left). Benign lesions (hyperplastic polyps and adenomas) may be single or multiple and are composed of well-differentiated epithelial cells. In the stomach, polyps often have cystic areas and are associated with inflammation [74–77]. Within the rest of the intestine, epithelial cells form tubular or villous structures (subtyped accordingly) or a combination of both [8,73]. In the colon and rectum (where these lesions are best described), hyperplastic polyps are composed of folds of well-differentiated epithelium but lack crypt branching, whereas adenomas will contain well-differentiated epithelium with branching (see Fig. 2A right) [8]. Lesions with increased cellular dysplasia, but that do not penetrate the basement membrane, are considered as in situ carcinomas.

Carcinomas infiltrate into the submucosa and can range from well to poorly differentiated with various subtypes reported (see Fig. 2B). In the stomach, gastric adenocarcinoma subtypes include tubular, papillary, signet-ring, mucinous, and undifferentiated [8]. Gastric squamous cell carcinomas are uncommon in the dog and not reported in the cat [8,88]. In the GIT, the

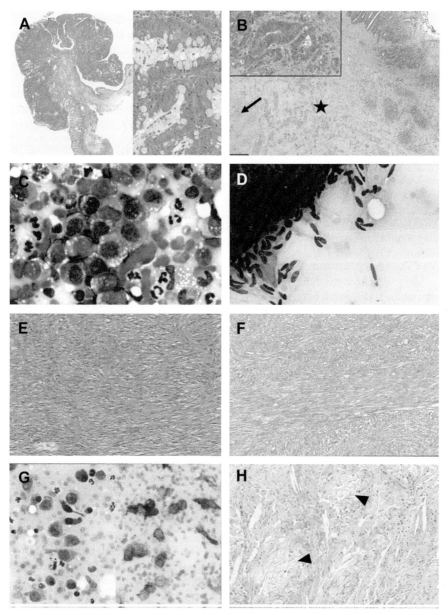

FIG. 2 (**A**) Histology of rectal polypoid mass. Left: full thickness biopsy allows evaluation of the submucosa and muscularis layers. Slide overview H&E Right: cells are well-differentiated with crypt branching consistent with an adenoma. 20X H&E. (**B**) Histology of ileal carcinoma with transmural invasion. Neoplastic cells infiltrate submucosa (*star*) and muscularis (*arrow*) layers. 5X H&E Inset: pleomorphic epithelial cells forming tubuloacinar structures. 40X H&E. (**C**) Cytology of intestinal carcinoma in a dog. Neoplastic cells are highly pleomorphic and poorly cohesive and some neutrophilic inflammation is present. 100X MGG. (**D**) Cytology of duodenal mass in a dog. High numbers of uniform, elongated spindle shaped cells exfoliating in aggregates, compatible with either gastrointestinal stromal tumor (GIST) or leiomyoma. 100X MGG. (**E**) Histology of intestinal GIST. Spindle cell variant with interlacing bundles of elongated cells. 10X H&E. (**F**) Histology of intestinal well-differentiated leiomyosarcoma resembling normal smooth muscle. 10X H&E. (**G**) Cytology of jejunal osteosarcoma in a dog. Left: neoplastic osteoblasts are admixed with neutrophils. 50X MGG Right: Cytoplasm of neoplastic cells is positive for alkaline phosphatase stain, confirming their origin. 50X BCIP/ NBT. (**H**) Histology of gossypiboma with remnants of swab material (*arrow heads*) surrounded by granulomatous inflammation. 10X H&E.

carcinoma subtypes are reported to include adenocarcinoma, signet-ring cell, squamous cell, mucinous, and infrequently medullary carcinomas [8].

Differential diagnoses. Well-differentiated lesions are readily recognised as epithelial though there may be only subtle features distinguishing in situ carcinomas from benign masses. Poorly differentiated lesions may need to be differentiated from mesenchymal and round cell tumors using IHC.

Additional diagnostic tests
Cytokeratin IHC can be used to identify poorly differentiated carcinomas. Glandular secretion within the cells (such as in the signet ring variant) may be highlighted using periodic acid-Schiff (PAS) or Alcian blue [8,86].

Neuroendocrine Tumors (Carcinoids)
Carcinoids are tumors arising from the diffuse enteroendocrine (enterochromaffin) cells, which have been rarely described in the GIT of dogs and cats [8,9,73,89–93]. These are usually non-functional but rare cases with clinical signs associated with hormone production have been reported [89,93]. Carcinoids are often locally invasive and carry a poor prognosis [8,13,73,93]. Although they may be found anywhere within the GIT, duodenum and large intestine are suggested to be the most common sites, and present as lobular, mural lesions occasionally with associated ulceration [73].

Cytologic characteristics
Neuroendocrine neoplasia normally exfoliates well. Cells often appear as free, round to oval nuclei with finely stippled chromatin and one to several nucleoli, in a sea of cytoplasm. When intact, cells are present in cohesive clusters, occasionally forming pseudo-acinar structures. They are round with scant to moderate cytoplasm which can contain small vacuoles or basophilic granules [13,57].

Differential diagnoses. GI metastasis of other neuroendocrine neoplasia such as apocrine gland anal sac adenocarcinoma, adrenal, and thyroid tumors.

Histologic characteristics
Within the lesion, cells are arranged in nests, sheets, rosettes or ribbons and are oval with a moderate to large amount of finely granular cytoplasm, supported by a fine fibrovascular stroma [8,73].

Differential diagnoses. Carcinoma, or possibly a round cell tumor.

Additional diagnostic tests
IHC for chromogranin A and B, neuron specific enolase, synaptophysin and/or PGP9.5 is recommended. Silver stains may also be used to highlight cytoplasmic granules but are considered non-specific [8,73,89]. Electron microscopy can also be used as an additional diagnostic test. Ultrastructurally, cells are characterized by round, membrane-bound, electron-dense, secretory granules with a dense core and atypical mitochondria within the cytoplasm [13].

Non-neoplastic Lesions
Gastric mucosal hypertrophy may be focal or diffuse and a variety of terms have been used to describe the various lesions that occur [8,73,94–97]. Focal mucosal hypertrophy (also known as chronic hypertrophic pyloric gastropathy) is most common in the pylorus of small/terrier breeds [8,94,95]. The mucosal thickening results in pyloric obstruction due to papilliform or polypoid luminal projections. Diffuse gastric mucosal hypertrophy (also known as hypertrophic gastropathy or chronic/giant hypertrophic gastritis) is reported in a range of breeds, including Boxers and Basenjis [8,97,98]. The mucosal thickening forms a cerebriform lesion, the shape of which is unaltered by mucosal stretching.

Differentiating normal epithelial cells from hyperplasia is challenging on cytology; however, increased numbers of mucous-secreting cells or goblet cells with associated globules, may indicate mucosal secretory hyperplasia. Attention should be paid to not confuse lubricant gel contamination with secretory globules [98]. Hyperplasia should be suspected when clusters of cohesive, uniform cells with preserved polarity (nucleus on the basal cellular pole and most of the cytoplasm toward the apex of the cell) and minimal anisocytosis and anisokaryosis are seen [98].

Histologically, focal mucosal hyperplasia results in marked hyperplasia of the surface mucosa with frequent cysts and chronic inflammation [8,94,95]. Diffuse gastric mucosal hypertrophy results in hypertrophy and hyperplasia of the foveolar and glandular tissue, with loss of chief and parietal cells, which are replaced by mucous cells [98].

MESENCHYMAL NEOPLASIA
Gastrointestinal Stromal Tumor
Gastrointestinal stromal tumours (GISTs) fall under the umbrella of non-angiogenic, non-lymphogenic intestinal mesenchymal tumors [99]. They are traditionally thought to originate from Cells of Cajal, pacemaker cells of the gut [100,101]. However, more recent IHC

studies suggest a more primitive mesenchymal cell origin, still capable of multiple lines of differentiation [100,102,103]. GISTs are relatively common in dogs but up until now there have only been 2 case reports in cats [104,105]. They may be found at any level of the GIT as well as in the mesentery. 1 study showed prevalence increased moving distally; location was related to prognosis, with those in the small intestine associated with shorter survival times [100]. GISTs appear grossly as nodular masses which often extend transmurally by the time of detection.

Cytologic characteristics

Although mesenchymal neoplasia often exfoliates poorly on cytology, GIST aspirates are often moderately to highly cellular, and therefore diagnostic on cytology [13,106]. Cells exfoliate individually and in aggregates, occasionally admixed with extracellular pink stroma. Cells are spindle-shaped, have elongated, oval nuclei, and fine, wispy, cytoplasmic tails (see Fig. 2C, D) [13,106]. In the epithelioid variant, cells are more rounded and nuclei are oval and eccentric [13,104]. Bi-nucleation and multi-nucleation can be noted but cells tend to be rather uniform with low criteria of malignancy [13].

Differential diagnoses. Cytologically GISTs are indistinguishable from leiomyomas and leiomyosarcomas and histology (sometimes with IHC) is needed to make the distinction.

Histologic characteristics

The most common histologic subtype by far is the spindle cell variant (see Fig. 2E), comprised of spindloid cells in herringbone to storiform patterns with cigar-shaped nuclei.

Epithelioid variants also occur, though rarely [103]. These are composed of pleomorphic cells, often including frequent multinucleate cells as well as large numbers of lymphocytes and plasma cells. Low numbers of epithelioid cells may also be admixed into spindle cell variant tumors. Both subtypes often show haemorrhage and necrosis.

Differential diagnoses. The main differential is a leiomyosarcoma and these 2 diagnoses have been used relatively interchangeably in the past, before IHC enabled reliable distinction [102,103,107]. Schwannomas may also resemble the spindle-cell variant.

Additional diagnostic tests

IHC for c-KIT (CD117): GISTs will stain positively whilst leiomyoma/leiomyosarcomas will be negative.

GISTs may also show positivity for alpha smooth muscle actin (α-SMA), used traditionally to confirm smooth muscle origin, therefore this should not be used alone as a diagnostic tool.

IHC for DOG-1 (discovered on GI stromal tumors protein 1) has been proven to have increased sensitivity and specificity in differentiating GIST from leiomyoma/leiomyosarcomas [108].

Leiomyoma/Leiomyosarcoma

These tumors of smooth muscle can affect both dogs and cats. Gastric leiomyomas are common in older dogs, and present as single or multiple submucosal nodules that often protrude in the lumen. They are most often localized in the gastric cardia or gastro-oesophageal junction, and tend to grow slowly [48]. Leiomyomas are often indolent and represent incidental findings unless they ulcerate or create obstructions, in which case vomiting or regurgitation may be reported [48]. Leiomyomas producing an insulin-like growth factor II-like peptide and causing hypoglycaemia have been reported [48]. Leiomyosarcomas are more frequently seen in the intestine and occur predominantly in male, older dogs. However, some studies indicated a higher incidence in female German shepherd dogs [48,57]. Gastric pleomorphic leiomyosarcoma is a rare variant with a high mitotic index and pleomorphism, and low expression of usual smooth muscle markers [48,57].

Cytologic characteristics

Smooth muscle tumors often exfoliate poorly on cytology. Additionally, as they are often located in the submucosa, ultrasound guided FNA may be more rewarding than endoscopic sampling. Cells are individualized or in aggregates, have an oval, often elongated and "cigar-shaped," central nucleus, and thin, light basophilic, cytoplasmic tails (see Fig. 2D) [57]. The presence of increased anisocytosis and anisokaryosis, mitotic figures, and necrosis raise the possibility of leiomyosarcoma [57]. However, well-differentiated leiomyosarcomas can be difficult to differentiate on cytology from their benign counterpart, and caution should be used [13].

Differential diagnoses. Benign and well-differentiated malignant forms can be difficult to differentiate from each other and from GIST, and histology and IHC are necessary to confirm the diagnosis.

Histologic characteristics

Leiomyomas are unencapsulated and non-invasive, often closely resembling normal smooth muscle and in some cases only distinguishable from normal tissue by a mass effect [8]. They have a typical cigar-shaped nucleus and are often arranged in interlacing fascicles with a herringbone pattern, though this feature is not always observed. They therefore tend not to prove a diagnostic challenge [73]. Leiomyosarcomas exhibits a range of differentiation from those resembling smooth muscle to the pleomorphic form with anaplastic spindle cells (see Fig. 2F).

Differential diagnoses. As above, IHC is required in less well-differentiated cases to definitively distinguish smooth muscle neoplasms from GISTs. In the case of pleomorphic neoplasms, the differential list may expand to include other poorly differentiated sarcomas.

Additional diagnostic tests

Leiomyoma/leiomyosarcomas are vimentin and α-SMA positive. Approximately two-thirds are desmin positive. However, pleomorphic variants can express decreased immunoreactivity for those markers [48,57].

Other Uncommon Mesenchymal Neoplasms

The GIT can be the site of almost any stromal neoplasm but all except those described above are rare, with only case series or individual case reports.

Primary extraskeletal osteosarcomas of the GIT are exceedingly rare [109,110]. Association with retained surgical swabs has also been reported. They may be identified cytologically by variable amounts of extracellular, pink, osteoid, in association with osteoblasts, and large multinucleated cells with uniform nuclei and marked cytoplasmic eosinophilic dusting (osteoclasts) [109]. Neoplastic osteoblasts often have mid-basophilic cytoplasm which can have few punctate vacuoles and some eosinophilic dusting, and a peripheralized round to oval nucleus giving the cells a plasmacytoid appearance (see Fig. 2G left). As such, plasma cell tumors are often one of the main differentials along with other mesenchymal neoplasms. For equivocal cases, cytology has the advantage as 5-bromo, 4-chloro, 3-indolyl phosphate/nitroblue tetrazolium (BCIP/NBT) can be applied to stained or unstained slides to highlight the expression of alkaline phosphatase typical of osteoblasts, aiding in the diagnosis (see Fig. 2G right) [111].

Angiosarcomas include lymphangiosarcoma and hemangiosarcoma, deriving from lymphatic and blood vessels, respectively. GI forms are extremely rare, with a case series of 4 hemangiosarcomas reported in cats; these had no apparent site predilection. This small series reported metastasis to regional lymph nodes and dissemination within the omentum. Grossly they can appear as thickened, dark red tissue causing luminal occlusion in the intestine [112]. Cytologically, plump, atypical, occasionally erythrophagocytic spindle cells, or small aggregates of epitheliod cells can be seen, occasionally in association with extramedullary hematopoiesis [113,114]; however, histology is usually needed for a definitive diagnosis. Histologically the described feline GI hemangiosarcomas all had areas of differentiation to vascular channel formation but solid regions were also present. The latter were less likely to stain positively with endothelial markers such as factor VIII-related antigen (FVIII-ra), making morphology the more useful feature [112]. On the contrary, in a case report of lymphangiosarcoma in the jejunum of a dog (seemingly the only reported GI example of this entity in dogs or cats), IHC was vital in making the final diagnosis [115]. Various subtypes of peripheral nerve sheath tumors (PNST), including neurofibromas and malignant PNST have been reported, in low numbers, predominantly in dogs [109,110,116,117]. Fibrosarcomas have been reported secondary to retained surgical swabs in both cats and dogs (see gossypiboma below) [118,119].

NON-NEOPLASTIC TUMOR-LIKE LESIONS

Gossypiboma

Also known as textiloma, muslinoma, or gauzoma, this is an iatrogenic entity comprising a granulomatous/pyogranulomatous reaction to a retained surgical swab. They are exceedingly rare but more common in dogs than cats [120]. A handful of case reports show the potential for fibrosarcoma or osteosarcoma to develop secondarily in both species [118,119,121,122]. The key cytologic and histologic feature is of inflammation surrounding foreign material, along with a relevant clinical history (see Fig. 2H). In the absence of observed foreign material, infectious agents are the primary differential, including fungi and, in cats, feline infectious peritonitis (FIP) should be considered (see below). Foreign material can often be highlighted using polarized light [118] as well as special stains such as PAS. Special staining can also help distinguish foreign material from fungal agents.

Feline Infectious Peritonitis

Intestinal feline coronavirus infection (FCoV) is usually a self-limiting enteric disease whilst FIP, caused by host interaction with a pathogenic form of FCoV, is commonly multisystemic. However, there are rare cases in which FIP presents as a solitary intestinal mass caused by mural pyogranulomatous inflammation [123]. Macrophagic inflammation should be differentiated from HS in cytology. FCoV IHC is useful for confirmation.

Feline Gastrointestinal Eosinophilic Sclerosing Fibroplasia

Feline gastrointestinal eosinophilic sclerosing fibroplasia (FGESF) is a unique inflammatory entity of unknown cause which frequently masquerades both grossly and histologically as neoplasia [124]. Grossly it may be mistaken for any focal neoplastic mass (eg, lymphoma, adenocarcinoma), whilst histologically sclerosing MCT is the main differential [49]. There is some debate whether sclerosing MCT and FGESF are distinct processes [8].

The pyloric sphincter is the most common location, followed by ileocecocolic junction or colon, and small intestine [124]. A significant minority are accompanied by eosinophilic lymphadenitis [124].

SUMMARY

Cytology and histology for GI neoplasia have advantages and disadvantages which are important to understand when planning clinical work-ups. Although the least invasive techniques should be considered first, awareness of their limitations is crucial. More invasive methodologies often allow more in-depth characterization of the lesion. However, it is important to consider what level of characterization will be of benefit in tailoring an appropriate treatment plan.

CLINICS CARE POINTS

- Least invasive techniques should be used first to try and reach a diagnosis or refine the differential list.
- More invasive techniques need to be planned carefully depending on the area to be sampled and the list of differential diagnoses for the lesion.
- Additional diagnostic tests are required in some cases to reach a final diagnosis, resulting in extra reporting time and expense.

DISCLOSURE

The author(s) declared no potential conflicts of interest with respect to the research, authorship, and/or publication of this article. The author(s) received no financial support for the research, authorship, and/or publication of this article.

REFERENCES

[1] Adamovich-Rippe KN, Mayhew PD, Marks SL, et al. Colonoscopic and histologic features of rectal masses in dogs: 82 cases (1995-2012). J Am Vet Med Assoc 2017;250(4):424–30.

[2] Bastianello SS. A survey on neoplasia in domestic species over a 40-year period from 1935 to 1974 in the Republic of South Africa. VI. Tumours occurring in dogs. Onderstepoort J Vet Res 1983;50(3):199–220.

[3] Cotchin E. Some tumours of dogs and cats of comparative veterinary and human interest. Vet Rec 1959;71:1040–50.

[4] Cribb AE. Feline gastrointestinal adenocarcinoma: a review and retrospective study. Can Vet J = La Rev Vet Can 1988;29(9):709–12.

[5] Gualtieri M, Monzeglio MG, Scanziani E. Gastric neoplasia. Vet Clin North Am - Small Anim Pract 1999;29(2):415–40.

[6] Holt PE, Lucke VM. Rectal neoplasia in the dog: a clinicopathological review of 31 cases. Vet Rec 1985;116(15):400–5.

[7] Bastianello SS. A survey on neoplasia in domestic species over a 40-year period from 1935 to 1974 in the Republic of South Africa. V. Tumours occurring in cats. Onderstepoort J Vet Res 1983;50(3):110–50.

[8] Munday J, Löhr C, Kiupel M. Tumors of the Alimentary Tract. In: Meuten D, editor. Tumors in domestic animals. Fifth. Ames: Wiley Blackwell; 2017. p. 499–601.

[9] Rissetto K, Villamil JA, Selting KA, et al. Recent trends in feline intestinal neoplasia: an epidemiologic study of 1,129 cases in the veterinary medical database from 1964 to 2004. J Am Anim Hosp Assoc 2011;47(1):28–36.

[10] Stidworthy M, Priestnall S. Getting the best results from veterinary histopathology. In Pract 2011;33(6):252–60.

[11] Veiga-Parga T, Palgrave C. CPD article Histopathology : how to get the best from gastrointestinal biopsies. Companion Anim 2021;26(3):43–50.

[12] Moore AR. Preparation of Cytology Samples: Tricks of the Trade. Vet Clin North Am - Small Anim Pract 2017;47(1):1–16.

[13] Bonfanti U. Intestines and rectum. In: Sharkey LC, Radin JM, Seelig DM, editors. Veterinary Cytology. 1st edition. Hoboken: Wiley; 2020. p. 394–406.

[14] Bonfanti U, Bertazzolo W, Bottero E, et al. Diagnostic value of cytologic examination of gastrointestinal tract tumors in dogs and cats: 83 Cases (2001-2004). J Am Vet Med Assoc 2006;229(7):1130–3.

[15] Marrinhas C, Oliveira LF, Sampaio F, et al. Needle rinse cell blocks as an ancillary technique: Diagnostic and clinical utility in gastrointestinal neoplasia. Vet Clin Pathol 2022;50(S1):47–54.

[16] Jergens AE, Andreasen CB, Hagemoser WA, et al. Cytologic Examination of Exfoliative Specimens Obtained during Endoscopy for Diagnosis of Gastrointestinal Tract Disease in Dogs and Cats. J Am Vet Med Assoc 1998;213(12):1755–9.

[17] Jergens AE, Andreasen CB, Miles KG. Gastrointestinal Endoscopic Exfoliative Cytology: Techniques and Clinical Application. Compend Continuing Educ Pract Vet 2000;22(10):941–52.

[18] Maeda S, Tsuboi M, Sakai K, et al. Endoscopic Cytology for the Diagnosis of Chronic Enteritis and Intestinal Lymphoma in Dogs. Vet Pathol 2017;54(4):595–604.

[19] Riondato F, Miniscalco B, Berio E, et al. Diagnosis of canine gastric adenocarcinoma using squash preparation cytology. Vet J 2014;201(3):390–4.

[20] Jergens AE, Willard MD, Allenspach K. Maximizing the diagnostic utility of endoscopic biopsy in dogs and cats with gastrointestinal disease. Vet J 2016;214:50–60.

[21] Fernandez JR-R, Dawson L. CPD article: Histopathology: how to maximise sample submission. Companion Anim 2020;25(9):1–5.

[22] Hall EJ. Small intestinal disease - is endoscopic biopsy the answer? J Small Anim Pract 1994;35:408–14.

[23] Rychlik A, Kaczmar E. Endoscopic Biopsies and Histopathological Findings in Diagnosing Chronic Gastrointestinal Disorders in Dogs and Cats. Vet Med Int 2020; 2020:8827538.

[24] Marsilio S, Freiche V, Johnson E, et al. ACVIM consensus statement guidelines on diagnosing and distinguishing low-grade neoplastic from inflammatory lymphocytic chronic enteropathies in cats. J Vet Intern Med 2023;37(3):794–816.

[25] Evans SE, Bonczynski JJ, Broussard JD, et al. Comparison of endoscopic and full-thickness biopsy specimens for diagnosis of inflammatory bowel disease and alimentary tract lymphoma in cats. J Am Vet Med Assoc 2006;229(9):1447–50. Available at: http://avmajournals.avma.org/doi/abs/10.2460/javma.229.9.1447.

[26] Gieger T. Alimentary Lymphoma in Cats and Dogs. Vet Clin North Am - Small Anim Pract 2011;41(2):419–32.

[27] Kleinschmidt S, Harder J, Nolte I, et al. Chronic inflammatory and non-inflammatory diseases of the gastrointestinal tract in cats: diagnostic advantages of full-thickness intestinal and extraintestinal biopsies. J Feline Med Surg 2010;12(2):97–103.

[28] Swinbourne F, Jeffery N, Tivers MS, et al. The incidence of surgical site dehiscence following full-thickness gastrointestinal biopsy in dogs and cats and associated risk factors. J Small Anim Pract 2017;58(9):495–503.

[29] Kleinschmidt S, Meneses F, Nolte I, et al. Retrospective study on the diagnostic value of full-thickness biopsies from the stomach and intestines of dogs with chronic gastrointestinal disease symptoms. Vet Pathol 2006; 43(6):1000–3.

[30] Wolfesberger B, Burger S, Kummer S, et al. Proliferation Activity in Canine Gastrointestinal Lymphoma. J Comp Pathol 2021;189:77–87.

[31] Lane J, Price J, Moore A, et al. Low-grade gastrointestinal lymphoma in dogs: 20 cases (2010 to 2016). J Small Anim Pract 2018;59(3):147–53.

[32] Valli VE, Myint M, Barthel A, et al. Classification of canine malignant lymphomas according to the world health organization criteria. Vet Pathol 2011;48(1): 198–211.

[33] Moore PF, Rodriguez-Bertos A, Kass PH. Feline Gastrointestinal Lymphoma: Mucosal Architecture, Immunophenotype, and Molecular Clonality. Vet Pathol 2012; 49(4):658–68.

[34] Roccabianca P, Woo JC, Moore PF. Characterization of the diffuse mucosal associated lymphoid tissue of feline small intestine. Vet Immunol Immunopathol 2000; 75(1–2):27–42.

[35] Kariya K, Konno A, Ishida T. Perforin-like immunoreactivity in Four Cases of Lymphoma of Large Granular Lymphocytes in the Cat. Vet Pathol 1997;34(2):156–9.

[36] Bridgeford EC, Marini RP, Feng Y, et al. Gastric Helicobacter species as a cause of feline gastric lymphoma: A viable hypothesis. Vet Immunol Immunopathol 2008; 123(1–2):106–13.

[37] Coyle KA, Steinberg H. Characterization of lymphocytes in canine gastrointestinal lymphoma. Vet Pathol 2004; 41(2):141–6.

[38] Frank JD, Reimer SB, Kass PH, et al. Clinical outcomes of 30 cases (1997-2004) of canine gastrointestinal lymphoma. J Am Anim Hosp Assoc 2007;43(6):313–21.

[39] Carrasco V, Rodríguez-Bertos A, Rodríguez-Franco F, et al. Distinguishing Intestinal Lymphoma From Inflammatory Bowel Disease in Canine Duodenal Endoscopic Biopsy Samples. Vet Pathol 2015;52(4):668–75.

[40] Stranahan LW, Whitley D, Thaiwong T, et al. Anaplastic Large T-Cell Lymphoma in the Intestine of Dogs. Vet Pathol 2019;56(6):878–84.

[41] Raskin RE. Lymphoid System. In: Raskin RE, Meyer DJ, editors. Canine and feline cytology: a color atlas and interpretation guide. 2nd edition. St Luis: Saunders Elsevier; 2010. p. 77–122.

[42] Rimpo K, Hirabayashi M, Tanaka A. Lymphoma in Miniature Dachshunds: A retrospective multicenter study of 108 cases (2006-2018) in Japan. J Vet Intern Med 2022;36(4):1390–7.

[43] Ohmi A, Tanaka M, Rinno J, et al. Clinical characteristics and outcomes of Mott cell lymphoma in nine miniature dachshunds. Vet Med Sci 2023;9(2):609–17.

[44] Kiupel M, Smedley RC, Pfent C, et al. Diagnostic algorithm to differentiate lymphoma from inflammation in feline small intestinal biopsy samples. Vet Pathol 2011;48(1):212–22.

[45] Freiche V, Paulin MV, Cordonnier N, et al. Histopathologic, phenotypic, and molecular criteria to discriminate low-grade intestinal T-cell lymphoma in cats from lymphoplasmacytic enteritis. J Vet Intern Med 2021;35(6):2673–84.

[46] Rout ED, Burnett RC, Yoshimoto JA, et al. Assessment of immunoglobulin heavy chain, immunoglobulin light chain, and T-cell receptor clonality testing in the diagnosis of feline lymphoid neoplasia. Vet Clin Pathol 2019;48(S1):45–58.

[47] Ehrhart EJ, Wong S, Richter K, et al. Polymerase chain reaction for antigen receptor rearrangement: Benchmarking

performance of a lymphoid clonality assay in diverse canine sample types. J Vet Intern Med 2019;33(3): 1392–402.

[48] Amorim I, Taulescu MA, Day MJ, et al. Canine Gastric Pathology: A Review. J Comp Pathol 2016;154(1): 9–37.

[49] Halsey CHC, Powers BE, Kamstock DA. Feline intestinal sclerosing mast cell tumour: 50 cases (1997-2008). Vet Comp Oncol 2010;8(1):72–9.

[50] Takahashi T, Kadosawa T, Nagase M, et al. Visceral mast cell tumors in dogs: 10 cases (1982-1997). J Am Vet Med Assoc 2000;216(2):222–6.

[51] Ozaki K, Yamagami T, Nomura K, et al. Mast Cell Tumors of the Gastrointestinal Tract in 39 Dogs. Vet Pathol 2002;39(5):557–64.

[52] Piviani M, Walton RM, Patel RT. Significance of mastocytemia in cats. Vet Clin Pathol 2013;42(1):4–10.

[53] McManus PM. Frequency and severity of mastocytemia in dogs with and without mast cell tumors: 120 cases (1995-1997). J Am Vet Med Assoc 1999; 215(3):355–7.

[54] Sabattini S, Giantin M, Barbanera A, et al. Feline intestinal mast cell tumours: clinicopathological characterisation and KIT mutation analysis. J Feline Med Surg 2016;18(4):280–9.

[55] Henry C, Herrera C. Mast Cell Tumors in Cats: Clinical update and possible new treatment avenues. J Feline Med Surg 2013;15(1):41–7.

[56] Sabattini S, Renzi A, Marconato L, et al. Comparison between May-Grünwald-Giemsa and rapid cytological stains in fine-needle aspirates of canine mast cell tumour: Diagnostic and prognostic implications. Vet Comp Oncol 2018;16(4):511–7.

[57] Taulescu M, Amorim I, Washabau R. Esophagus and stomach. In: Veterinary Cytology. Hoboken: Wiley; 2020. p. 380–93.

[58] Alroy J, Leav I, DeLellis R, et al. Distinctive intestinal mast cell neoplasms of domestic cats. Lab Invest 1975;33(2):159–67.

[59] Kupanoff PA, Popovitch CA, Goldschmidt MH. Colorectal plasmacytomas: A retrospective study of nine dogs. J Am Anim Hosp Assoc 2006;42(1):37–43.

[60] Trevor PB, Saunders GK, Waldron DR, et al. Metastatic extramedullary plasmacytoma of the colon and rectum in a dog. J Am Vet Med Assoc 1993;203(3):406–9.

[61] Caruso KJ, Meinkoth JH, Cowell RL, et al. A distal colonic mass in a dog. Vet Clin Pathol 2003;32(1):27–30.

[62] Zikes CD, Spielman B, Shapiro W, et al. Gastric extramedullary plasmacytoma in a cat. J Vet Intern Med 1998;12(5):381–3.

[63] Roberts E, Shirlow A, Cox A, et al. Multiple myeloma involving the gastrointestinal tract in an English Springer Spaniel. Vet Med Sci 2022;8(6):2273–6.

[64] Tamura Y, Chambers JK, Neo S, et al. Primary duodenal plasmacytoma with associated primary (amyloid light-chain) amyloidosis in a cat. J Feline Med Surg Open Reports 2020;6(2). https://doi.org/10.1177/2055116920957194.

[65] Mellor PJ, Haugland S, Smith KC, et al. Feline Myeloma-Related Disorders : Further Evidence for Primary Extramedullary Development in the Cat. Vet Pathol 2008;45(2):159–73. Available at: http://vet. sagepub.com/content/45/2/159.

[66] Rakich PM, Latimer KS, Weiss R, et al. Mucocutaneous plasmacytomas in dogs: 75 cases (1980-1987). J Am Vet Med Assoc 1989;194(6):803–10.

[67] Rannou B, Hélie P, Bédard C. Rectal plasmacytoma with intracellular hemosiderin in a dog. Vet Pathol 2009;46(6):1181–4.

[68] Kojimoto A, Itoh T, Uchida K, et al. Primary Jejunal Histiocytic Sarcoma with Spontaneous Perforation in a Dog. Jpn J Vet Anesth Surg 2017;48(1+2):9–13.

[69] Hoffeld EH, Shriwise GB, Aschenbroich SA. Pathology in Practice. J Am Vet Med Assoc 2021;259(S2):1–4.

[70] Fant P, Caldin M, Furlanello T, et al. Primary gastric histiocytic sarcoma in a dog - a case report. J Vet Med A Physiol Pathol Clin Med 2004;51(7–8):358–62.

[71] Elliott J. Gastric histiocytic sarcoma in a dog. J Small Anim Pract 2016;57(12):719.

[72] Uneyama M, Chambers JK, Nakashima K, et al. Histological Classification and Immunohistochemical Study of Feline Colorectal Epithelial Tumors. Vet Pathol 2021;58(2):305–14.

[73] Uzal FA, Plattner BL, Hostetter JM. Alimentary system. In: Jubb, Kennedy and Palmer's Pathology of Domestic AnimalsVol. 2, 6th edition. New York: Elsevier Saunders; 2016. p. 1–257.e2.

[74] Kuan SY, Kl H, Tisdall PLC. Ultrasonographic and surgical findings of a gastric hyperplastic polyp resulting in pyloric obstruction in an 11-week-old French Bulldog. Aust Vet J 2009;87(6):253–5. Available at: https://api. semanticscholar.org/CorpusID:41905814.

[75] Diana A, Penninck DG, Keating JH. Ultrasonographic appearance of canine gastric polyps. Vet Radiol Ultrasound 2009;50(2):201–4.

[76] Kim K, Jun B, Han S, et al. Gastric Hyperplastic Polyp Causing Upper Gastrointestinal Hemorrhage and Severe Anemia in a Dog. Vet Sci 2022;9(12):1–6.

[77] Taulescu M, Valentine B, Amorin I, et al. Histopathological features of canine spontaneous non-neoplastic gastric polyps - a retrospective study of 15 cases. Histol Histopathol 2014;29:65–75.

[78] Méric T, Issard J, Maufras T, et al. Recurrence and survival in dogs with excised colorectal polyps: A retrospective study of 58 cases. J Vet Intern Med 2023;37(6):2375–84.

[79] Birchard SJ. Nonlymphoid intestinal neoplasia in 32 dogs and 14 cats. J Am Anim Hosp Assoc 1986;22: 533–7. Available at: https://api.semanticscholar.org/ CorpusID:222269076.

[80] Scanziani E, Giusti AM, Gualtieri M, et al. Gastric carcinoma in the Belgian shepherd dog. J Small Anim Pract 1991;32(9):465–9.

[81] Patnaik AK, Hurvitz AI, Johnson GF. Canine Gastrointestinal Neoplasms. Vet Pathol 1977;14(6):547–55.

[82] Seim-Wikse T, Jörundsson E, Nødtvedt A, et al. Breed predisposition to canine gastric carcinoma–a study based on the Norwegian canine cancer register. Acta Vet Scand 2013;55:25.

[83] Sullivan M, Lee R, Fisher EW, et al. A study of 31 cases of gastric carcinoma in dogs. Vet Rec 1987;120(4):79–83.

[84] Patnaik AK, Hurvitz AI, Johnson GF. Canine intestinal adenocarcinoma and carcinoid. Vet Pathol 1980; 17(2):149–63.

[85] Turk MAM, Gallina AM, Russell TS. Nonhematopoietic gastrointestinal neoplasia in cats: A retrospective study of 44 cases. Vet Pathol 1981;18(5):614–20.

[86] Miller Z, Longue C, Nerhagen S, et al. What is your diagnosis? Gastric wall thickening in a dog. Vet Clin Pathol 2023;52(S2):116–8.

[87] Dell'Orco M, Bertazzolo W, Vergine M, et al. Gastric mucinous adenocarcinoma with cutaneous metastases in a dog: diagnosis by fine-needle aspiration cytology. J Small Anim Pract 2005;46(9):449–53.

[88] Patnaik AK, Lieberman PH. Gastric squamous cell carcinoma in a dog. Vet Pathol 1980;17(2):250–3.

[89] Kiupel M, Capen C, Miller M, et al. Histological classification of tumors of the endocrine system of domestic animals. Second ser. Washington DC: Armed Forces Institute of Pathology; 2008. Available at: https://api.semanticscholar.org/CorpusID:83297889.

[90] Nabeta R, Kanaya A, Ikeda N, et al. A case of feline primary duodenal carcinoid with intestinal hemorrhage. J Vet Med Sci 2019;81(8):1086–9.

[91] Qvigstad G, Kolbjørnsen Skancke E, Waldum HL. Gastric Neuroendocrine Carcinoma Associated with Atrophic Gastritis in the Norwegian Lundehund. J Comp Pathol 2008;139(4):194–201.

[92] Rossmeisl JH, Forrester SD, Robertson JL, et al. Chronic Vomiting Associated With a Gastric Carcinoid in a Cat. J Am Anim Hosp Assoc 2002;38(1):61–6.

[93] Sako T, Uchida E, Okamoto M, et al. Immunohistochemical evaluation of a malignant intestinal carcinoid in a dog. Vet Pathol 2003;40(2):212–5.

[94] Biller BS, Partington B, Miyabayashi T, et al. Ultrasonographic Appearance of Chronic Hypertrophic Pyloric Gastropathy in the Dog. Vet Radiol UltrasoundUltrasound 1994;35(1):30–3.

[95] Leib MS, Saunders GK, Moon ML, et al. Endoscopic Diagnosis of Chronic Hypertrophic Pyloric Gastropathy in Dogs. J Vet Intern Med 1993;7(6):335–41.

[96] Van Der Gaag I, Happé RP, Wolvekamp WTC. A Boxer Dog with Chronic Hypertrophic Gastritis Resembling Menetrier's Disease in Man. Vet Pathol 1976;13(3):172–85.

[97] Van Kruiningen HJ. Giant hypertrophic gastritis of Basenji dogs. Vet Pathol 1977;14(1):19–28.

[98] Andersen CB, Jergens AE, Meyer DJ. Oral cavity, gastrointestinal tract, and associated structures. In: Raskin R, Meyer D, editors. Canine and feline cytology: a color Atlas and interpretation guide. Missouri: Sanders El. St Louis; 2010. p. 192–214.

[99] Hayes S, Yuzbasiyan-Gurkan V, Gregory-Bryson E, et al. Classification of Canine Nonangiogenic, Nonlymphogenic, Gastrointestinal Sarcomas Based on Microscopic, Immunohistochemical, and Molecular Characteristics. Vet Pathol 2013;50(5):779–88.

[100] Irie M, Tomiyasu H, Tsujimoto H, et al. Prognostic factors for dogs with surgically resected gastrointestinal stromal tumors. J Vet Med Sci 2021;83(9):1481–4.

[101] Streutker CJ, Huizinga JD, Driman DK, et al. Interstitial cells of Cajal in health and disease. Part II: ICC and gastrointestinal stromal tumours. Histopathology 2007;50(2):190–202.

[102] Bettini G, Morini M, Marcato PS. Gastrointestinal spindle cell tumours of the dog: Histological and immunohistochemical study. J Comp Pathol 2003;129(4):283–93.

[103] Frost D, Lasota J, Miettinen M. Gastrointestinal Stromal Tumors and Leiomyomas in the Dog: A Histopathologic, Immunohistochemical, and Molecular Genetic Study of 50 Cases. Vet Pathol 2003;40(1):42–54.

[104] Suwa A, Shimoda T. Intestinal gastrointestinal stromal tumor in a cat. J Vet Med Sci 2017;79(3):562–6.

[105] McGregor O, Moore AS, Yeomans S. Management of a feline gastric stromal cell tumour with toceranib phosphate: a case study. Aust Vet J 2020;98(5):181–4.

[106] Morini M, Gentilini F, Pietra M, et al. Cytological, Immunohistochemical and Mutational Analysis of a Gastric Gastrointestinal Stromal Tumour in a Cat. J Comp Pathol 2011;145(2–3):152–7.

[107] Maas CPHJ, Ter Haar G, Van Der Gaag I, et al. Reclassification of Small Intestinal and Cecal Smooth Muscle Tumors in 72 Dogs: Clinical, Histologic, and Immunohistochemical Evaluation. Vet Surg 2007;36(4):302–13.

[108] Dailey DD, Ehrhart EJ, Duval DL, et al. DOG1 is a sensitive and specific immunohistochemical marker for diagnosis of canine gastrointestinal stromal tumors. J Vet Diagn Invest 2015;27(3):268–77.

[109] Urbiztondo R, Chapman S, Benjamino K. Primary mesenteric root osteosarcoma in a dog. Vet Clin Pathol 2010;39(3):377–80.

[110] Delisser PJ, Burton NJ. What is your diagnosis? J Am Vet Med Assoc 2012;240(11):1289–90.

[111] Ryseff JK, Bohn AA. Detection of alkaline phosphatase in canine cells previously stained with Wright-Giemsa and its utility in differentiating osteosarcoma from other mesenchymal tumors. Vet Clin Pathol 2012;41(3):391–5.

[112] Sharpe A, Cannon MJ, Lucke VM, et al. Intestinal haemangiosarcoma in the cat: clinical and pathological features of four cases. J Small Anim Pract 2000;41:411–5.

[113] Barger AM, Skowronski MC, Macneill AL. Cytologic identification of erythrophagocytic neoplasms in dogs. Vet Clin Pathol 2012;41(4):587–9.

[114] Bertazzolo W, Dell'Orco M, Bonfanti U, et al. Canine angiosarcoma: Cytologic, histologic, and immunohistochemical correlations. Vet Clin Pathol 2005;34(1):28–34.

[115] Ballarini L, Stewart J, Fleming K, et al. Primary small intestinal lymphangiosarcoma in a dog presenting with a

segmental partial mesenteric volvulus. J Comp Pathol 2024;208(Jan):37–41.

[116] Schöniger S, Summers BA. Localized, plexiform, diffuse, and other variants of neurofibroma in 12 dogs, 2 horses, and a chicken. Vet Pathol 2009;46(5):904–15.

[117] Ahn H, Song W, Choi S, et al. A rare case of cecal malignant peripheral nerve sheath tumor in a dog. J Vet Med Sci 2022;84:1051–5.

[118] Haddad JL, Goldschmidt MH, Patel RT. Fibrosarcoma arising at the site of a retained surgical sponge in a cat. Vet Clin Pathol 2010;39(2):241–6.

[119] Rayner EL, Scudamore CL, Francis I, et al. Abdominal Fibrosarcoma Associated with a Retained Surgical Swab in a Dog. J Comp Pathol 2010;143(1):81–5.

[120] Reed N, Gosling M. Intra-thoracic gossypiboma (textiloma) in a 6-year-old cocker spaniel. Aust Vet J 2021; 99:6–10.

[121] Miller MA, Aper RL, Fauber A, et al. Extraskeletal osteosarcoma associated with retained surgical sponge in a dog. J Vet Diagn Invest 2006;18(2):224–8.

[122] Pardo A, Adams W, McCracken M, et al. Primary jejunal osteosarcoma associated with a surgical sponge in a dog. J Am Vet Med Assoc 1990;196(6):935–8.

[123] Harvey CJ, Lopez JW, Hendrick MJ. An uncommon intestinal manifestation of feline infectious peritonitis: 26 cases (1986-1993). J Am Vet Med Assoc 1996; 209(6):1117–20. Available at: http://www.ncbi.nlm.nih.gov/pubmed/8800260. [Accessed 1 October 2014].

[124] Craig LE, Hardam EE, Hertzke DM, et al. Feline Gastrointestinal Eosinophilic Sclerosing Fibroplasia. Vet Pathol 2009;46:63–70.

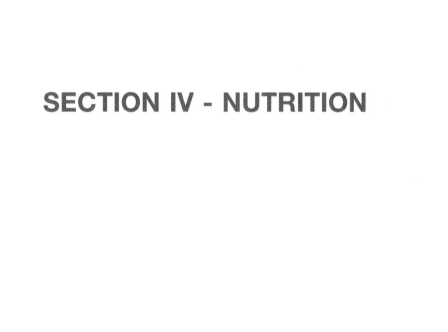

SECTION IV - NUTRITION

Advances in Small Animal Care 5 (2024) 151–164

ADVANCES IN SMALL ANIMAL CARE

Conversations and Considerations Relevant to Nutrition for Senior Pets

Jonathan Stockman, DVM, DACVIM (Nutrition)[a,b,*], Tammy Jane Owens, DVM, MS, DACVIM (Nutrition)[c]

[a]Department of Veterinary Clinical Sciences, College of Veterinary Medicine, Long Island University, Old Brookville, NY 11548, USA; [b]Department of Clinical Sciences, College of Veterinary Medicine & Biomedical Sciences at Colorado State University, Fort Collins, CO 80523, USA; [c]Department of Small Animal Clinical Sciences, Western College of Veterinary Medicine, University of Saskatchewan, Saskatoon, Saskatchewan S7N4M3, Canada

KEYWORDS

• Dog   • Cat   • Aging   • Senior   • Omega-3 fatty acids   • Medium chain triglycerides   • Prebiotic fiber
• Phosphorous

KEY POINTS

- The aging process is influenced by interactions between genetics, lifestyle, and environmental factors; therefore, individuals do not age at the same rate.
- Nutritional modifications may help mitigate age-related concerns; however, relatively few have robust data to support efficacy. Veterinarians should help guide and educate pet owners to make informed decisions regarding evidence-based options.
- Pets with excess adiposity age more quickly compared to lean counterparts and have an increased incidence of disease and reduced lifespans.
- Supplementation of long-chain omega-3 fatty acids, outlined by various dosing guidelines, modulates inflammation, supports maintenance of lean body mass, and supports the management of various disease processes. Both long-chain omega-3 fatty acids and medium-chain triglycerides benefit age-related cognitive decline.
- "Senior diets" are a marketing category without senior-specific nutritional guidelines; therefore, nutrient contents and features vary and each product must be assessed regarding appropriateness for individual pets.

INTRODUCTION

Nutrition is vital for normal development and function, but nutritional needs change throughout life. For example, requirements for growth and reproduction are higher than for maintenance of adult animals, reflecting increased demand for protein and essential amino acids, fats, and altered mineral requirements required for skeletal growth and maturation [1]. As animals age, many notable changes in physiology and metabolism are likely to result in altered nutritional demand. Certain age-related diseases also impact dietary requirements and tolerance. Very little research is available regarding aging and senior-specific nutritional requirements in dogs and cats, although some age-related changes appear conserved between pets and humans. This article reviews current information about aging in dogs and cats to assist veterinarians in making nutritional recommendations and helping pet owners evaluate products marketed for "senior" pets.

SIGNIFICANCE

Pet ownership trends shifted over the past decade in response to increased lifespan of dogs and cats, with pets ≥7 years of age in more than half of US dog and cat-owning households [2]. Most pet owners believe

---

*Corresponding author, E-mail address: Jonathan.stockman@liu.edu

https://doi.org/10.1016/j.yasa.2024.06.009
2666-450X/24/

senior pets have different nutritional needs compared to younger adults [3] and are more likely to use "high-protein," "high-omega," and "senior/mature" pet foods, or those intended to manage weight, mobility, or digestive concerns [2]. As a result, there are more commercial options for "functional products," including various nutraceuticals and pet foods; however, research indicates a disconnect between pet owner and veterinarian assumptions regarding features of "senior" diets compared to the actual composition of these diets, as well as wide variations in nutrient profiles between diet options [3,4]. Veterinarians remain a preferred source of information on pet nutrition and health for many pet owners [5]; therefore, veterinarians need to understand the physiology and effects of aging so they can anticipate and explain changes to pet owners, respond to their concerns, and be prepared to offer guidance and evidence-based recommendations for aging dogs and cats.

THE PROCESS OF AGING: WHAT IS HAPPENING?

After animals mature, aging results in ongoing declines in cellular function and increasing populations of senescent cells. Senescence is the irreversible inability of cells to proliferate, or cell cycle arrest [6], following chronic, progressive loss of regenerative and bio-protective mechanisms over time [7]. As senescent cells increase, overall cellular proliferation progressively decreases, eventually affecting tissue and organ function. Various cellular changes herald this process, including dysfunction of the ubiquitin system (responsible for removing defective proteins) and accumulation of less efficient or defective proteins. If cells also acquire changes that increase resistance to apoptosis, proliferation continues and increases the risk for neoplasia or other pathologies [7].

Telomere shortening is a biomarker of cellular senescence, acting as a "molecular clock" [8]. Telomere shortening is an age-related process with similarities between humans, cats, and dogs [9,10]. Genetics are partially responsible for initial telomere length; however, multiple factors affect the function of telomerase, an enzyme responsible for maintaining telomere length, and rate of attrition over time. Chronic inflammation and oxidative stress are associated with accelerated shortening of telomeres [11].

Even in the absence of disease, the normal aging process increases inflammation—known as "inflamm-aging"—and decreases immune function, tissue regeneration, and neuronal flexibility. Aging also changes body composition (sarcopenia), alters gut microbiota, and increases the risk for age-related diseases. Age-associated inflammation also reduces resilience to disease and the ability to cope with environmental changes. Sensory acuity typically decreases with age and can affect vision, hearing, olfaction, and taste, which can also impact desire or ability to consume food. Deteriorating senses and a decrease in neural flexibility contribute to cognitive decline, which can lead to cognitive dysfunction and behavioral changes ranging in severity [12]. Accumulated cellular dysfunctions and senescence contribute to physical and metabolic changes associated with aging; however, various factors determine the rate at which this process occurs. Contributing factors that are potentially modifiable are of clinical interest. Increased client education regarding the aging process, with discussion of their expectations, in addition to available preventative or interventional options should be part of comprehensive wellness planning for aging companion pets.

WHEN IS MY PET CONSIDERED "SENIOR"?

Discrepancies between terminology, informal guidelines, and pet wellness marketing may confuse pet owners and they may seek guidance from veterinarians. Additionally, individual pets will vary widely in presentation, severity, and progression of age-related changes due to differences in genetics, lifestyle, and environmental influences, such that chronologic and "biological" ages diverge. When trying to define "senior," a primary consideration is the ability to recognize when the increased frequency of wellness examinations and other monitoring for early disease detection is warranted. Senior pet health care should include proactive client education regarding common aging sequelae, signs to monitor for, and supportive lifestyle changes, such as avoiding high-impact activities and using ramps to maintain ease of access to resources and decrease joint wear-and-tear. Even with the development of age-related changes, pets can be "healthy seniors" for considerable portions of their lifespan and maintain an overall good quality of life. As age increases, however, so does the likelihood of developing age-related disease, which affects overall wellness, accelerates the aging process, and alters life expectancy.

Many pet owners may be familiar with the term "dog-years," in which 1 year in a dog's life is equivalent to 7 years for a human, alluding to the faster rate at which dogs age compared to people; however, this conversion is inaccurate. Although there is some equivalence between canine and human aging, there are known differences in expected lifespan and aging not only between different species but also between different breeds and individuals. Mechanisms of aging are often conserved between species, such as similar DNA methylation patterns of aging humans, dogs, and cats, which could eventually become useful tools to better describe the relationship between aging humans and pets [13–15].

Unfortunately, the terms '"senior," "geriatric," "old," and "elderly" are often used interchangeably due to a lack of consensus regarding definitions. "Senior" pet foods and "senior profiles" were marketed, historically, for dogs and cats once they were 7 years old; however, given significant differences in maturation and longevity between individuals, this age is somewhat arbitrary and does not fall within the "senior" portion of lifespan. For example, although skeletal maturation is completed at a younger age in small breed dogs compared to large and giant breeds, they tend to develop age-related changes later in life and have increased lifespans compared to larger breeds [16,17].

Recent guidelines define 3 to 4-year-old dogs as "mature adults," while "senior" starts when reaching the last 25% of life expectancy [18] which will vary by breed and individual factors that accelerate or slow aging processes. There is less variation between cats; therefore, cats are "mature adults" at 7 to 10 years old, "senior" at 11 to 14 years, and "geriatric" at 15+ years [19]. It is important to note, however, that even individuals of the same breed and genetic background (eg, litter-matched puppies) may not age at the same rate if lifestyle and environment are different; therefore, estimating life expectancy or "biological age" is complex and individual aging phenotypes should also be taken into consideration when estimating life expectancy.

WHAT CAN BE DONE TO SLOW THE AGING PROCESS OR SUPPORT "HEALTHY" AGING FOR MY PET?

Increased nutraceutical and food options marketed for aging pets reflect increased pet-owner concern for their aging dogs and cats, but it can be difficult to discern evidence-based information from marketing propaganda. Although several studies indicate nutritional modification may benefit senior pets, only a few nutritional interventions have relatively robust data to support their benefits. Diet, lifestyle, and environment are known to interact with individual genetics to determine the aging process. For example, dogs living with smokers suffer reactive oxygen species-related DNA damage, lose telomere length more quickly, and likely die younger [20]. Chronic psychological stress is also

detrimental, as demonstrated by accelerated telomere shortening in socially isolated African Gray Parrots [21]. Numerous studies into telomere length and aging in humans indicate positive correlations with specific antioxidants (eg, zeaxanthin), nutrients (eg, omega-3 PUFAs), and lifestyle habits (eg, exercise/activity), and negative correlation with chronic oxidative stress and inflammation, such as with low activity, increased body mass index or obesity, smoking, chronic psychological stress, and chronic diseases such as diabetes mellitus and inflammatory bowel disease [11].

The best documented factor affecting both lifespan and development of disease in dogs and cats is body composition. Excess adiposity (body fat) resulting from increased energy consumption is associated with accelerated aging and reduced lifespan in multiple species; whereas, modest energy restriction is associated with increased lifespan. The relationship between body condition score (BCS) and lifespan may be partially explained by adipose tissue's influence on relative risk for various diseases. Like humans, obesity in dogs and cats increases the risk of developing myriad complications, including cardiovascular, renal, joint, and dermatologic diseases, certain neoplasias, and metabolic abnormalities including dyslipidemia and insulin resistance [22,23]. Lifespan was retrospectively correlated to BCS for 12 breeds of neutered dogs. As expected, overweight dogs had shorter median lifespans and increased risk of acute death; however, the degree of difference changed relative to breed, ranging from 0.4 months (German Shephard Dogs) to 2.5 years (Yorkshire Terriers) [24]. Similarly, excess adiposity is associated with reduced lifespan in cats[23] and laboratory rodents [25].

However, even without obesity, excess adipose tissue negatively affects aging and lifespan. In a 14-year prospective study of paired, litter-matched Labrador Retriever puppies, one group was fed ~25% fewer Calories to maintain BCS of 4.6 (± 0.2) and lived, on average, 21.5 months longer than the group of overweight, but not obese, dogs with BCS of 6.7 (± 0.2). In addition to living significantly longer, the incidence of osteoarthritis was only 50% in the lean group (vs 83%) and onset of related clinical signs, and development of other chronic diseases, was delayed by 2 years [26]. Thus, achieving and maintaining ideal body fat, or BCS, supports healthy aging and reduces disease development and progression. It is the key to recognize, however, that BCS primarily estimates body fat stores. Muscle condition plays a vital role in healthy aging and stalling age-related frailty; therefore, it also needs to be assessed.

SARCOPENIA AND FRAILTY

Body composition changes during the aging process. Reduction in lean body mass (LBM) over time, with reduced total body protein and muscle mass, is termed "sarcopenia." This process is expected to occur with aging and differs from cachexia, which is wasting attributed to disease; however, sarcopenia is a complex, multifactorial process that becomes pathologic when it severely impacts well-being and physical activity. Cumulative research indicates that the progression of sarcopenia is likely multifactorial with contributions from diet, activity type and level, metabolism, genetic factors, and disease.

An important site for various metabolic processes (eg, fatty acid oxidation & carbohydrate metabolism), muscle is integral to thermoregulation and important for strength, mobility, and balance. Declining immune function correlates with decreasing LBM, cumulatively termed "frailty," and predictive of increased morbidity and all-cause mortality in elderly people and pets. More research is needed into pet-specific mechanisms of sarcopenia; however, etiology is suspected to be similar to humans, as histologic changes documented in elderly dogs are the same as in people. As muscles age, hypoplasia and decreased metabolic function results in atrophy, accumulation of intramyocellular lipid, and accumulation of damage and abnormalities [27].

In the lifetime study of Labrador Retrievers, progressive muscle loss of ~ 10% with corresponding increased fat mass started around 8 to 9 years of age, but the onset was delayed in the lean group and the longest-lived dogs were those with the slowest loss of LBM [26,28]. Similar results were also observed in cats [29].

Important to clinical practice, decreasing LBM or the relative amount of lean-to-fat mass can be highly predictive of disease or death. Lean dogs have lower fasted circulating levels of triglycerides, triiodothyronine, insulin, and glucose; as well as lower peak response to IV glucose tolerance testing, compared to overweight dogs [30]. In dogs, either declining LBM or high static body fat mass were associated with changes in metabolic response and predicted death within a year [30]. Other predictors of earlier death included lower lymphoproliferative responses and increasing insulin resistance associated with fat mass above 25% [28]. In cats, weight and muscle loss may be observed up to 3 years before the diagnosis of chronic kidney disease (CKD) or hyperthyroidism [31], and healthy cats may lose almost one-third LBM between 10 to 15 years of age, which is highly significant given that similar loss can be correlated with increased risk for mortality in people [32].

Age-related factors contributing to sarcopenia include increased pro-inflammatory cytokines (eg, interleukin [IL]-1, IL-6, tumor necrosis factor [TNF]-alpha) and chronic inflammation, changes in hormonal activity, decreased protein synthesis, and impaired uptake of amino acids and response to insulin in muscle, despite increased protein turnover [33,34]. Coupled with altered denervation/reinnervation of muscle with advancing age, overall muscle regeneration decreases with age.

Changes in body composition result from complex, multifactorial processes; however, decreased activity is an important contributor to reduced energy requirement and muscle loss in many aging pets. In aging dogs and cats, reduced vascular compliance and cardiovascular changes, and increased lung fibrosis or degenerative changes in the respiratory tract also contribute. Decreased LBM and degenerative skeletal changes are common features of aging that contribute to decreased strength, mobility, and exercise tolerance, with increased frailty; however, diet and lifestyle can modulate this process.

Other common features of aging include decreased thickness and protective function of the dermal barrier, decreased functional nephrons and glomerular filtration even in the absence of clinical CKD, and accumulation of fibrosis or pathology in other organs. Of particular interest when considering nutrition for senior pets is how age affects gastrointestinal tract function, since structural changes or altered motility may affect digestion and absorption of nutrients. It appears that some aging pets develop dietary intolerances [35]; however, the overall significance relative to age remains unclear.

WILL ENERGY REQUIREMENTS CHANGE AS DOGS OR CATS BECOME "SENIOR"?

Due to the complexity of factors influencing the energy input and output of individuals, it is important to remember that daily maintenance energy requirements (MER) may increase, decrease, or stay the same throughout an individual pet's lifespan; therefore, no absolute rule applies to all dogs or cats. There are, however, trends that may be anticipated. As dogs age, MER often decreases by 18% to 24% [36]. This is contributed by the lower basal metabolic rate stemming from a decreased lean-to-fat mass ratio. This and other age-related factors (eg, osteoarthritis) may also contribute to decreased energy demands. In the authors' experience, the MER of many overweight, aging adult dogs becomes less than their estimated resting energy requirement (RER).

The energy requirements of aging cats appear less consistent. Research indicates energy demand tends to decrease in cats around 8 to 10 years of age but may then re-increase around 10 to 12 years of age [37] and could continue to further increase in some cats past 11 to 12 years old [38]. This is somewhat counter to expectations since LBM inversely correlates with advancing age in cats; therefore, it is unclear if increased energy requirements in (some) older cats result from altered metabolic rates preceding disease such as hyperthyroidism, or if reduced digestive capacity reduces accessibility of a portion of the consumed calories, or both. The "obesity paradox," is the observation that some overweight pets with certain chronic diseases tend to live longer than those in an ideal body condition or lower; therefore, some feline BCS charts (World Small Animal Veterinary Association [WSAVA]) note that mild excess body weight can be as beneficial for some senior cats and those with a specific disease.

SHOULD AGING PETS EAT MORE OR LESS? CONTROVERSIES AROUND DIETARY PROTEIN AND FAT

Protein digestibility and protein synthesis both decline with age in people contributing to sarcopenia [39]. Sarcopenia may also be exacerbated by decreased intake or decreased protein quality in aging individuals.

Conflicting data exist regarding protein, fat, and total energy digestibility in aging dogs and cats. This is likely because digestive function does not change uniformly in dogs and cats over time. An increased incidence of intestinal diseases in aging pets may contribute to poor digestion in some animals. Although many functions typically appear intact in healthy aging pets, there may be changes in gut structure, microbial populations, and motility [40–42].

Although protein digestibility decreased to ∼77% in cats ≥14 years old, compared to 85% to 90% in younger cats [43], this may apply to only a subset of cats [44]. The impact of reduced fat digestion on the absorption of other nutrients such as fat-soluble vitamins is unclear. Despite previous findings, a recent study evaluating diet digestibility in dogs and cats failed to find an age-associated difference for most of the diets studied [45]; thus, it appears there is variation in whether aging impacts digestive function or whether the effect is diet-dependent. Although highly digestible diets are often recommended to address potential age-related changes in digestive physiology [35], they appear unnecessary for every aging dog or cat.

Exercise and resistance training are vital to mitigating sarcopenia in humans, with similar expectations for our companion pets; however, the effect of diet or nutritional supplementation on increasing response to exercise is still of great interest. Results from human studies have been conflicting and sometimes complicated by trends indicating increased strength even in the absence of measurable increases in muscle mass. It is known that protein synthesis decreases and muscles become less responsive to protein intake in aging people; however, whether increasing protein intake can help overcome this, either combined with exercise or not, remains controversial.

In people, rapidly absorbed proteins, and increased concentrations of specific amino acids (eg, Leucine and Lysine) may support protein synthesis better than increasing total protein intake; however, research in pets is limited. In young dogs, lysine intake was correlated with LBM [46]; however, its significance to older dogs is unknown. In a study, lysine appeared to protect LBM of geriatric cats, independent of total protein intake [47], so further investigation is needed.

Once protein synthesis capacity is saturated, however, increased intake cannot further increase total body protein or muscle anabolism. Excess protein is then used for energy, with increased byproducts of digestion and metabolism for excretion (eg, nitrogen → ammonia → urea). Aging muscle also becomes more resistant to anabolic signals and less effective at suppressing catabolic muscle breakdown; therefore, maximal protein synthesis is eventually unable to overcome the shift toward muscle loss.

Although a reduction of protein intake is needed to manage some diseases (eg, CKD and proteinuria), overly reducing protein consumption may be harmful. Restricting protein intake does not benefit healthy aging pets or prevent the development of CKD in dogs and cats; whereas, protein malnutrition leads to reduced LBM, reduced skin thickness, decreased wound healing, and ability to respond to infection.

Since most pets eat complete and balanced commercial diets, inadequate protein intake is primarily a concern when pets fail to consume sufficient calories to meet daily energy requirements. This happens during times of significantly decreased food intake but also when too many daily calories are provided by food(s) with insufficient protein, which can occur if the diet is unbalanced by excessive lower protein "treats." Negative protein balance would be further exacerbated by feeding lower protein and/or unbalanced diets, particularly if amino acid deficiency further limits protein utilization.

Aging and chronic disease likely affect daily protein requirements, although exactly how remains unknown. One study indicates protein demand to maintain LBM in aging cats exceeds demands for traditional nitrogen balance [48], historically used as a marker for dietary protein adequacy. Although increasing protein intake could help reduce sarcopenia in some aging dogs and cats [49–51], there are also concerns with arbitrarily increasing protein intake as it may be contraindicated in some animals with compromised renal function and even in healthy animals where excess protein fermentation is undesirable. Increasing protein quality, therefore, is an important consideration before increasing intake.

A negative energy balance could divert protein for energy metabolism; therefore, fat and overall diet digestibility must be considered as potential contributors to loss of body and muscle condition. Digestibility can be affected by factors such as protein quality and fat ingredients, processing methods of diet, and dietary fiber.

OMEGA-3 FATTY ACIDS

Dogs and cats cannot de-novo synthesize omega-3 fatty acids; therefore, these must be consumed pre-formed. Alpha-linolenic acid (ALA) can be consumed via many plant-derived sources, being particularly concentrated in flaxseeds, walnuts, and hemp. Omega-6 and omega-3 fats compete for the same mammalian desaturase and elongase enzymes to create longer-chain polyunsaturated fatty acids (PUFAs), including eicosapentaenoic acid (EPA) and docosahexaenoic acid (DHA). Conversion is inefficient in adult animals, with less than 2% to 5% of ingested ALA converted to EPA in cats and dogs [1].

Long-chain omega-3 PUFAs, specifically EPA and DHA, are helpful in the therapeutic management of multiple diseases because of their effects on modulating inflammation and other processes. For example, EPA (20 carbon omega-3) competes with arachidonic acid (AA; 20 carbon omega-6) for incorporation into cellular membranes and as a substrate for cyclooxygenase and 5-lipoxygenase enzymes. These enzymes create highly inflammatory prostaglandin E_2 (PGE_2) and leukotriene B_4 (LTB_4) from AA, but less inflammatory PGE_2 and LTB_5 from EPA. 15-lipooxygenase also utilizes EPA to form hydroxyl fatty acids, a potent inhibitor of LTB_4 [1]. Thus, the overall effect of increased EPA and other omega-3 PUFA is anti-inflammatory. High intakes of EPA + DHA are required to achieve significant anti-inflammatory effects. Marine-based fats (eg, fish or algae oils) can typically provide sufficiently high concentrations while terrestrial-based oils cannot, even those with high total omega-3s (eg, flaxseed) because they contain mostly ALA.

Given the increased risk for developing age-related pathologies, increased EPA + DHA intakes can benefit many senior dogs and cats and may also help mitigate sarcopenia and other age-related changes even in healthy aging pets. Increased markers of inflammation are common in sarcopenia and associated with declining strength and mobility in people, while consumption of EPA + DHA is associated with reductions in inflammatory mediators such as C-reactive protein, IL-6, and TNF-alpha and stimulation of muscle protein synthesis. Specifically, EPA and DHA have an anabolic effect on muscle by promoting mTOR signaling, may reduce insulin resistance [52], and EPA may reduce muscle breakdown mediated by the ubiquitin-proteosome-proteolytic pathway. Supplementation is also associated with reduced cardiac cachexia in dogs [53]. Thus, providing therapeutic anti-inflammatory doses of EPA + DHA to senior dogs and cats is generally recommended, either via diets providing sufficiently high concentrations of EPA + DHA per kilocalorie intake or by appropriate supplemental doses; however, several precautions must be noted.

Oils are fats and are concentrated sources of energy (calories), which may be unwanted. Situations requiring moderation include fat intolerance (eg, pancreatitis, hypertriglyceridemia, lymphangiectasia) and/or overweight pets. Additionally, sources should be evaluated for quality and safety. Fat oxidizes over time and with exposure to heat or oxygen. Oxidized or rancid fats are pro-inflammatory; therefore, freshness, appropriate storage, and antioxidants (eg, vitamin E) are important. Marine oil supplements should be pure and fat-soluble vitamins A and D (high in salmon and cod liver oils) should not be present in high amounts because excess intake is toxic to dogs and cats (human doses are unsafe). Fish oil supplements (or similar products from krill, algae, green-lipped mussels, or seal fat) also differ widely in potency, providing variable concentrations of EPA + DHA. It is recommended to select products with routine third-party testing (eg, accredited independent laboratory) from manufacturers willing to provide recent certificates of analysis. An alternative for supplementation is using diets already containing higher concentrations of EPA + DHA, from reputable manufacturers with good quality control.

It is important to account for the total daily intake of EPA + DHA (not just total omega-3s), from both diet and supplements, to ensure appropriate therapeutic dosing while avoiding excess. This requires manufacturers to provide specific typical/average dietary concentrations of EPA and DHA in each diet. It is important not to exceed the safe upper limit for EPA + DHA intake of adult dogs [body weight (BW) (kg)$^{0.75}$ × 370 mg] to avoid negative side effects, such as diarrhea, vomiting, and inhibition of platelet function [1]. A safe upper limit is not yet established for cats. Daily intakes below BW(kg)$^{0.67}$ × 75 mg per day appear safe; however, it can be noted that cats consuming veterinary feline mobility diets routinely exceed this intake without apparent issues, but caution should be used with supplemental dosing.

DIETARY FIBER, PROBIOTICS, AND THE GUT MICROBIOME

There is increasing awareness regarding the importance of healthy gut microbiota populations in humans and animals. Gut microbial diversity is considered a general indicator of good health, but gut populations shift with age. Data from older people indicate gut microbiome reflects health and changes are associated with age-related disease [54]. Gut microbial diversity decreased in aging colony-housed Shiba-Inu dogs [55]. In aging dogs, these changes shift fecal fermentation products and correlate with declining lymphocyte counts [41] similar to known correlations between gut microbiota and metabolite production, such as decreased short-chain-fatty-acids, that correspond with increased frailty in humans.

Supplements providing live cultures are now commonplace for both healthy and diseased pets. Although the intention is to supplement aging dogs and cats with various strains of beneficial bacteria, particularly bifidobacteria and lactobacilli, true probiotics provide "live microorganisms that, when administered in adequate amounts confer health benefit' to the host" [56]; however, many supplements labeled as probiotic contain microorganisms with no proven health benefit to species intended. Other common issues include the use of "correct" genera and/or species but incorrect strains for proven benefit, containing inadequate microorganisms to confer benefits, and/or providing nonviable microorganisms.

There is some evidence that a specific strain, *Enterococcus faecium* SF68 (Purina Fortiflora, Nestle Purina, Allentown, PA), may support immune response and function in dogs and cats; however, these studies looked at response to vaccination in young dogs [57], response to therapy and dosing of oclacitinib in dogs with atopic dermatitis [58], and effect on morbidity of chronic

herpes virus in cats [59]. How these findings might apply to aging dogs and cats is unclear. Similarly, *Bifidobacterium longum* BL999 (Purina Calming Care, Nestle Purina, Allentown, PA), was evaluated to help humans [60] and dogs displaying anxious behaviors [61]. *Lactiplantibacillus plantarum* PS128 appeared to help dogs with aggression and separation anxiety behaviors [62], but whether either of these strains (or others) are helpful for behaviors related to cognitive decline and dysfunction is unknown.

Dietary fiber impacts energy density, palatability, digestion, and gut function. Effects vary depending on types and concentrations of fiber and individual variability; the effects and applications of which cannot be fully detailed here. Dietary fiber blends can be useful for the management of various chronic diseases of aging dogs and cats, such as diabetes mellitus, dental disease, and gastrointestinal concerns; however, effects are not uniform and depend on interactions with other dietary components and within the individual.

Fermentable prebiotic fibers can be supplemented to the diet of senior pets for several reasons. These can support the normal microbial populations and the production of metabolites with associated with health benefits, such as the production of short-chain fatty acids, and a healthier gut microbiome.

MANAGING AGE-RELATED DECLINES IN COGNITION & BEHAVIOR, OSTEOARTHRITIS, OR OTHER DISEASES

The development of many diseases is somewhat age-dependent; however, the disease itself, or its effects can accelerate the aging process, creating a vicious cycle. Nutritional management of specific diseases is outside the scope of this article; however, nutritional interventions that may prevent or delay the onset of common age-related issues are briefly reviewed.

BEHAVIOR AND COGNITION

Cognitive decline is estimated to affect 20% to 68% of senior dogs [63], 28% of 11 to 14-year-old cats, and >50% of cats 15 years old or older [64–66]. Impairment is detectable in apparently healthy dogs and cats as early as 6 to 7.7 years, however, disease progress is highly variable and early signs are subtle and may be missed by pet owners, who are more likely to become concerned by overt behavioral changes such as disturbed sleep patterns, vocalization, aggression, or pacing, which can negatively impact the human-animal bond. Nutritional modifications, exercise, and mental stimulation can support measurable improvements in the cognitive function of older pets. It is important to ensure these pets receive, at minimum, a complete and balanced diet to avoid deficiencies negatively impacting energy metabolism and brain function. In addition, antioxidant blends, EPA + DHA, MCTs, and mitochondrial co-factors such as L-carnitine and alpha-lipoic acid (dogs only) have been investigated. Antioxidants may help counteract the effects of oxidative stress and associated damage; however, various studies trialed specific diets or nutraceutical blends rather than a specific modification or supplement that differ in antioxidant blend provided, and/or added EPA + DHA; therefore, although positive improvements in cognitive function were noted in aging dogs and cats with some products, it is difficult to discern which antioxidants or amounts are needed to achieve benefits, if other nutrients act synergistically, or whether antioxidants even contribute to the benefits. The same is true of various supplements and diets used for anxiety, fear, and sleep disturbances, which may accompany cognitive decline.

Combined supplementation of EPA + DHA with various antioxidants was demonstrated to improve cognitive function and memory in senior dogs [67]. EPA + DHA may positively impact cognitive function through several mechanisms, such as mitigating inflammation that is implicated in age-related cognitive decline. Additionally, DHA is metabolized to a neurotransmitter called phosphatidylserine.

Increased intake of medium-chain triglycerides (MCT), 6 to 12-carbon fatty acids, shows promise in supporting neurologic function in dogs, both for epilepsy and cognitive decline or canine cognitive dysfunction. MCTs are absorbed and metabolized quickly leading to increased production of ketone bodies to serve as an alternative energy source for neurons in the central nervous system [68] and circumvent impaired glucose utilization of aged neurons.

When senior beagles with age-related cognitive decline received diets containing 5.5% (as-fed) of a specific MCT blend, cognitive trial results improved significantly [69]. Based on this study, and those in epileptic dogs, commercial diets to support cognitive and neural function were formulated to include increased MCTs in combination with antioxidants and EPA + DHA.

MCT oils are also available as supplements for use; however, the response may not replicate the results with commercial diets. Given the variability in nutrient profiles of diets fed to aging dogs, dietary interactions may explain potential variations in responding to MCT-oil supplements. Additionally, concentrations of C-8, C-10, and C-12 MCTs vary between available MCT oils, which likely also contribute to discrepancies between positive results of diet trials compared to more varied responses reported with supplementing MCT oil to other diets. MCT oil supplementation can also have adverse effects as it may affect diet palatability and can cause vomiting and diarrhea in high intake. Low palatability is largely why diets containing MCTs have not been extensively trialed in cats. Coconut oil is a popular food for its perceived health benefits; however, whole coconut oil is not a good source of MCTs for therapeutic purposes. MCTs are naturally present in coconut oil, milk fat, and palm oil, but these are impractical for therapeutic use because concentrations are too low.

S-adenosyl–L-methionine (SAMe), commonly used in pets with liver disease, helps maintain cell membrane fluidity, is important to 1-carbon metabolism (encompassing methionine and folate cycles & trans-sulfuration pathways), and is a methyl-donor for most methylation reactions in the body [70]. This supports glutathione production and all DNA/RNA methylation reactions which are associated with aging and neoplasia. In humans, low SAMe was associated with an increased risk of CKD, cardiovascular disease, and some carcinogenesis [71–73]. SAMe improved cognitive test results in elderly cats, but effects were most evident in cats with only mild cognitive decline; therefore, earlier supplementation is more beneficial. A combination of SAMe, L-carnitine, and alpha-lipoic acid appeared beneficial for canine cognitive decline [69]; however, the benefit of individual supplementation remains unknown. Alpha-lipoic acid is toxic to cats and not recommended in this species. Other nutrients and nutraceuticals are often studied as pre-formulated blends in limited patient populations, making it difficult to draw conclusions.

OSTEOARTHRITIS AND IMPAIRED MOBILITY

The most important intervention to help prevent, delay, and mitigate signs of osteoarthritis in dogs and cats is the maintenance of ideal BCS and LBM. In those at risk or already displaying signs of osteoarthritis, avoiding repetitive high-impact activities and interventions to support mobility and avoid unnecessary joint strain, such as ramps and flooring materials to provide traction and avoid slips or falls, is recommended [74]. The nutritional intervention most strongly supported is the provision of EPA + DHA via diet or supplements for reasons described above.

Oral supplementation of glucosamine and chondroitin is common in dogs suffering from osteoarthritis and in senior dogs; however, there is a lack of evidence for the therapeutic efficacy of these supplements. A recent scientific analysis found that across many studies these compounds do not appear beneficial in dogs and cats [75]. Other nutraceuticals and nutraceutical combinations have shown some promise; however, studies are mostly focused on dogs, and are limited in number and scope. Only nutraceuticals that have dog or cat-specific safety data should be recommended, provided they come from reputable manufacturers, are administered in dosages consistent with studies demonstrating positive intended effects, can be easily administered to pets, and are neither cost-prohibitive to clients nor preclude the use of strongly supported interventions (eg, weight management; EPA + DHA).

DIETARY CONSIDERATIONS FOR SENIOR PETS AND PET FOOD

Dietary modifications for pets as they age are aimed to prevent or slow age-related changes, manage disease when needed, and enhance the quality of life or "health span." Initial signs of age-related disease are often subtle and may be overlooked or perceived as "normal"; however, early intervention is most beneficial. It is, therefore, important to educate pet owners regarding signs to watch for and supportive modifications to consider proactively.

SUPPORTING FOOD INTAKE

Decreased sense of taste and smell, cognitive impairment, and chronic disease or pain are all potential age-related problems that may impact appetite and food intake [76,77]. Decreased food intake may result in malnutrition leading to poor body composition with increased frailty. Various interventions may help pets meet nutritional requirements, although an individualized trial-and-error approach is often required. Most importantly, potential underlying reasons for declining food intake must be addressed, including pain, medication side-effects or polypharmacy interactions, disease progression, oral discomfort or pain, psychological stress, discomfort associated with accessing food, and cognitive decline affecting memory or appetite. Depending on the underlying issues, various interventions may improve appetite and intake.

The frequency of feeding and access to food should be considered first. Many pets are fed twice daily; however, this may be insufficient for aging pets or those with chronic diseases. Increased opportunity to consume smaller portions of food may be more acceptable to the pet, help with issues related to cognitive decline, and reduce digestive workload. Conversely, free feeding without tracking daily food intake (eg, weighing food every 12–24 hours) may mask changes in food intake, especially in multi-pet households. Competition for access to food can become an issue and offering separate locations accessible only to pets of concern may help. For example, microchip or radio frequency identification pet doors, feeding boxes, or feeders are available. Automatic, timed meal feeders can also help provide additional meals of kibble or canned foods.

Transitioning to appropriate energy-dense foods can also help meet daily requirements more easily. Sometimes novelty or improved palatability can also re-increase interest in food. Food form, texture, palatability, and presentation are additional considerations, particularly in smaller dogs and cats. Senior cats show a preference for food served warm, ideally close to "prey" body temperature [78], which can be accomplished by adding hot water or using hot water baths, baby bottle warmers, or specialized food warming plates for canned-type foods.

Adding moist foods may also be helpful as these are often highly palatable. Additions to enhance or introduce new aromas or flavors can also be trialed if no medical contraindications are present, and foods can be kept to <10% of total daily intake, to minimize the risk of unbalancing diets. Examples include storing small portions of kibble with a few drops of liquid smoke on a cotton pad (food allergy safe), pet-safe broths, gravies, and/or pastes, using (cooked) liver powder sprinkled onto food, or other favorite foods/treats.

Presentation of food can also become more important to older pets. Osteoarthritis, spondylosis, and decreased muscle mass make it more difficult to maintain the postures required to eat from the floor level or use stairs to access food or other resources. Keeping food close to pets' preferred resting location and elevating food dishes, such as using raised angled platforms to improve cervical posture is helpful. Alternate feeding locations and different types and sizes of food dishes should be trialed, as preferences may change. For example, cats may prefer larger shallow or flat dishes to avoid vibrissae contact.

SENIOR DIETS FOR DOGS & CATS AND NUTRIENT CONSIDERATIONS

Nutrient requirement guidelines for dogs and cats during growth, reproduction, and general adult maintenance exist, but there is no specific category for senior pets. Therefore "senior" diets lack uniformity in dietary formulation and meaning. In North America, diets marketed for senior pets typically have nutritional adequacy statements for adult maintenance and their nutrient profiles often do not differ from adult maintenance diets. When amounts of crude protein, crude fat, crude fiber, calcium, phosphorus or sodium contents were compared between adult maintenance and senior pet diets, there was no significant difference between categories [3,4]. There is, however, wide variation within each category. This exemplifies the importance of evaluating individual diet nutrient profiles for comparison with a pet's current diet, particularly for nutrients of concern or interest.

Although the lack of uniformity in formulation or meaning for senior diets can create confusion for pet owners and veterinarians, the wide variety of diets can be leveraged to meet the non-uniform and varying demands of aging pets. The downside is dietary characteristics cannot be assumed based on the term "senior" and diets marketed for senior pets may be contraindicated or inappropriate for some senior pets, particularly for specific age-related concerns. Additionally, "senior" diets may only be modified relative to a particular adult maintenance diet, and different options or companies may target different feeding philosophies or goals; therefore, a "senior" diet may contain either more or less protein, fat, fiber, calories, and more or less of individual nutrients, or be more or less digestible relative to a pet's current diet.

Some pet food companies now market multiple foods to more specific age categories, differentiating age brackets based on species or size. In contrast, others do not make similar differentiations and may continue using the more antiquated pet food marketing guidelines of only targeting age 7+. Although many senior diets provide EPA + DHA, concentrations vary. Therefore, if the diet is otherwise appropriate for that pet but increased EPA + DHA is recommended, it can be supplemented with additional expense, and this may reduce client compliance compared to transitioning to diets providing EPA + DHA. Other specific nutritional factors to consider when evaluating diets for individual pets may include ingredient quality, overall digestibility, and amounts of protein, fat, phosphorus, calcium, and electrolytes such as sodium or potassium. For example, if calorie intake needs to decrease to avoid weight gain in pets with reduced activity and energy demand, then protein content may need to increase to ensure daily intake remains adequate and to support maintenance of LBM. Conversely, if there are contraindications to increasing protein intake (eg, proteinuria),

dietary protein content needs to decrease, and to have high quality and enough to meet the requirements.

Although many, if not most, senior pets retain adequate digestive capacity, some may not. Anecdotally, the authors experienced a clinical improvement in patients with generalized muscle wasting with a change from a high-fiber diet to a diet with improved digestibility.

The dietary concentration of phosphorus is also important in pets as they age, particularly cats. Phosphorus is an essential mineral; however, intake may affect the progression or delay of renal disease in cats. The lack of consensus regarding dietary phosphorus in stage 1 CKD is likely due to the lack of research data, rather than evidence that it lacks importance. Importantly, evidence suggests high dietary phosphorus may induce kidney disease in a subset of soluble or inorganic forms of phosphorus potentially more detrimental compared to organic phosphorus [79]. Dietary phosphorus content can be challenging to evaluate. Pet foods are not required to report dietary phosphorus. Moreover, when voluntarily reported on labels, it is usually only as a guaranteed minimum value, which is not as useful as typical or maximum values. Additionally, declared label amounts do not differentiate contributions from different sources, solubility, or bioavailability.

It can be challenging to evaluate nutrient amounts in pet foods using the guaranteed analysis from labels, which are currently only required to report minimum protein and fat and maximum crude fiber and moisture as percentages "as fed" (equivalent to grams per 100 g of food). These values can be used to estimate daily protein intake if the amounts of food consumed are known, however, no information regarding digestibility or quality of protein is provided. It is possible to contact manufacturers directly, and some are able and willing to provide additional information such as typical nutrient profiles. Diets with longer-term clinical trials demonstrating efficacy may also be preferred when available, provided nutrient profiles are otherwise appropriate for an individual.

FUTURE AVENUES FOR RESEARCH

Senior pets have unique nutritional concerns and further research is needed to establish aging-specific dietary guidelines. The relationship between nutrition and health in senior pets is complex, multifactorial, and insufficiently understood. Options to mitigate sarcopenia and frailty are important and investigation into specific nutritional interventions, exercise, and potential utility of myostatin antagonists is needed. Further understanding protein metabolism in aging pets and the effects of changing protein quantity, digestibility, and/or amino acid profile is highly relevant. Newer research methods such as metabolomics, proteomics, and microbiome analysis will also help define the effects of specific nutritional interventions on health and disease. Specialized diets, functional foods, nutraceuticals, or other supplements may be leveraged to tailor nutritional plans to individual patients; however, many supplements have limited to no data supporting efficacy and it is important supplements have safety data for dogs and cats and come from reputable manufacturers testing for contaminants and concentrations, to avoid harm.

CLINICS CARE POINTS

- Aging is not a uniform process. Individuals age differently with varying health spans relating to different interactions between genetics and lifestyle. This is highlighted by the relation between body size rates of aging in dogs. Diseases also affect the aging process.

- Energy intake influences the aging process and the development of disease. Maintaining BCS above ideal is associated with accelerated aging, earlier onset and faster progression of age-related diseases, and decreased longevity.

- It is important to monitor the muscle condition of patients over time, especially following a diet change. Sarcopenia correlates with increased inflammation, decreased immune competence, and increased frailty. Declining LBM is a predictor of increased morbidity and mortality in aging pets; however, the rate and extent of sarcopenia may be modifiable through exercise and diet.

- Protein requirements in aging or senior pets are not established and can vary between individuals. Reducing protein intake is not recommended unless indicated for a specific disease; however, restricting intake below amounts adequate to maintain LBM is detrimental. The impact of altered digestive capacity in some senior pets is unclear. Increasing the digestibility of protein and fat, optimizing amino acid profiles, and specific amino acid supplementation may be beneficial as alternatives to increasing total protein intake.

- The omega-3 PUFAs EPA + DHA benefit aging pets through modulation of inflammation, supporting muscle mass and cognition, and disease management; however, increased total fat intake is contraindicated in fat-intolerant patients or those needing reduced energy intake. While EPA + DHA in both diet and supplements contribute to total daily intake, total omega-3 content is not an accurate reflection of EPA + DHA contents. Safe upper limits and recommendations for various disease management are available for dogs, but additional precautions are needed for cats.

- Diets marketed toward "senior" pets vary widely in nutrient profile and other attributes; therefore, patients should be asses to find a diet that is appropriate for their needs considering digestibility, energy density, protein and/or fat content, dietary fibers, omega-6 to 3 ratios, and concentration of EPA + DHA, phosphorus, calcium, sodium or other nutrients, as well as additions such as antioxidant blends or MCTs. Not every senior diet is appropriate for every senior pet.

- Evidence to support individual nutraceutical use in aging pets is limited. Many studies evaluated only proprietary blends of nutrients and diet formulations, complicating interpretation; however, supplementation of EPA + DHA, MCTs, SAMe, and support of gut microbial health with prebiotic fiber (± specific probiotics) have the most cumulative evidence to support their utility for aging pets.

DISCLOSURE

J. Stockman is a paid consultant for Petco Health and Wellness Company inc. and has received speaker honorarium by Hill's Pet Nutrition and research support from Royal Canin and Hill's Pet Nutrition. T.J. Owens has no disclosures.

REFERENCES

[1] National Research Council. Ad hoc committee on dog and cat nutrition. Nutrient requirements of dogs and cats. Washington DC: National Academies Press; 2006.

[2] Kerwin N. Packaged Facts details rise in senior pet ownership. In: Pet food processing. 2022. Available at: http://www.petfoodprocessing.net/articles/16313-packaged-facts-details-rise-in-senior-pet-ownership. [Accessed 9 May 2024] 2022.

[3] Hutchinson D, Freeman LM, Schreiner KE, et al. Survey of opinions about nutritional requirements of senior dogs and analysis of nutrient profiles of commercially available diets for senior dogs. Int J Appl Res Vet M 2011;9(1):68–79.

[4] Summers SC, Stockman J, Larsen JA, et al. Evaluation of nutrient content and caloric density in commercially available foods formulated for senior cats. J Vet Intern Med 2020;34(5):2029–35.

[5] Kamleh M, Khosa DK, Verbrugghe A, et al. A cross-sectional study of pet owners' attitudes and intentions

towards nutritional guidance received from veterinarians. Vet Rec 2020;187:e123.

[6] Di Micco R, Krizhanovsky V, Baker D, et al. Cellular senescence in ageing: from mechanisms to therapeutic opportunities. Nat Rev Mol Cell Biol 2021;22:75–95.

[7] Sándor S, Kubinyi E. Genetic pathways of aging and their relevance in the dog as a natural model of human aging. Front Genet 2019;10:268.

[8] Bernadotte A, Mikhelson VM, Spivak IM. Markers of cellular senescence. Telomere shortening as a marker of cellular senescence. Aging (Albany NY) 2016;8:3.

[9] McKevitt TP, Nasir L, Wallis CV, et al. A cohort study of telomere and telomerase biology in cats. Am J Vet Res 2003;64:1496–9.

[10] McKevitt TP, Nasir L, Argyle DJ, et al. Telomere lengths in dogs decrease with increasing donor age. J Nutr 2002; 132:1604S–6S.

[11] de Vos-Houben JM, Ottenheim NR, Kafatos A, et al. Telomere length, oxidative stress, and antioxidant status in elderly men in Zutphen and Crete. Mech Ageing Dev 2012;133:373–7.

[12] Tapp PD, Siwak CT. The canine model of human brain aging: cognition, behavior, and neuropathology. Handbook of Models for Human. Aging 2006;415–34.

[13] Horvath S, Lu AT, Haghani A, et al. DNA methylation clocks for dogs and humans. Proc Natl Acad Sci 2022; 119:e2120887119.

[14] Raj K, Szladovits B, Haghani A, et al. Epigenetic clock and methylation studies in cats. GeroScience 2021;43: 2363–78.

[15] Wang T, Ma J, Hogan AN, et al. Quantitative translation of dog-to-human aging by conserved remodeling of the DNA methylome. Cell Syst 2020;11:176–85. e176.

[16] Creevy KE, Austad SN, Hoffman JM, et al. The companion dog as a model for the longevity dividend. Cold Spring Harb Perspect Med 2016;6:a026633.

[17] Hawthorne AJ, Booles D, Nugent PA, et al. Body-weight changes during growth in puppies of different breeds. J Nutr 2004;134:2027S–30S.

[18] Creevy KE, Grady J, Little SE, et al. 2019 AAHA canine life stage guidelines. J Am Anim Hosp Assoc 2019;55: 267–90.

[19] Vogt AH, Rodan I, Brown M, et al. AAFP-AAHA: Feline life stage guidelines. J Fel Med Surg 2010;12:43–54.

[20] Hutchinson N. Evaluating the impact of environmental tobacco smoke on biological age markers: a canine model: PhD thesis. Glasgow, UK: University of Glasgow; 2017.

[21] Aydinonat D, Penn DJ, Smith S, et al. Social isolation shortens telomeres in African Grey parrots (Psittacus erithacus erithacus). PLoS One 2014;9:e93839.

[22] Tropf M, Nelson O, Lee P, et al. Cardiac and metabolic variables in obese dogs. J Vet Intern Med 2017;31: 1000–7.

[23] Teng K, McGreevy P, Toribio J, et al. Associations of body condition score with health conditions related to

overweight and obesity in cats. J Small Anim Pract 2018;59:603–15.

[24] Salt C, Morris PJ, Wilson D, et al. Association between life span and body condition in neutered client-owned dogs. J Vet Intern Med 2019;33:89–99.

[25] Johnson PR, Stern JS, Horwitz BA, et al. Longevity in obese and lean male and female rats of the Zucker strain: prevention of hyperphagia. Am J Clin Nutr 1997;66: 890–903.

[26] Kealy RD, Lawler DF, Ballam JM, et al. Effects of diet restriction on life span and age-related changes in dogs. J Am Vet Med Assoc 2002;220:1315–20.

[27] Gueugneau M, Coudy-Gandilhon C, Chambon C, et al. Muscle proteomic and transcriptomic profiling of healthy aging and metabolic syndrome in men. Int J Mol Sci 2021;22:4205.

[28] Lawler DF, Larson BT, Ballam JM, et al. Diet restriction and ageing in the dog: major observations over two decades. Br J Nutr 2008;99:793–805.

[29] Cupp CJ, Kerr WW, Jean-Philippe C, et al. The role of nutritional interventions in the longevity and maintenance of long-term health in aging cats. Int J Appl Res Vet 2008;6:69–81.

[30] Lawler DF, Evans RH, Larson BT, et al. Influence of lifetime food restriction on causes, time, and predictors of death in dogs. J Am Vet Med Assoc 2005; 226:225–31.

[31] Freeman L, Lachaud MP, Matthews S, et al. Evaluation of weight loss over time in cats with chronic kidney disease. J Vet Intern Med 2016;30:1661–6.

[32] Joskova V, Patkova A, Havel E, et al. Critical evaluation of muscle mass loss as a prognostic marker of morbidity in critically ill patients and methods for its determination. J Rehabil Med 2018;50:696–704.

[33] Freeman L. Cachexia and sarcopenia: emerging syndromes of importance in dogs and cats. J Vet Intern Med 2012;26:3–17.

[34] Murton AJ. Muscle protein turnover in the elderly and its potential contribution to the development of sarcopenia. Proc Nutr Soc 2015;74:387–96.

[35] Baum B, Meneses F, Kleinschmidt S, et al. Age-related histomorphologic changes in the canine gastrointestinal tract: a histologic and immunohistologic study. World J Gastroenterol: WJG 2007;13:152.

[36] Kienzle E, Rainbird A. Maintenance energy requirement of dogs: what is the correct value for the calculation of metabolic body weight in dogs? J Nutr 1991;121(11S): 39–40.

[37] Harper EJ. Changing perspectives on aging and energy requirements: aging and energy intakes in humans, dogs and cats. J Nutr 1998;128:S2623–6.

[38] Laflamme DP. Nutrition for aging cats and dogs and the importance of body condition. Vet Clin North Am Small Anim Pract 2005;35:713–42.

[39] Wall BT, Gorissen SH, Pennings B, et al. Aging is accompanied by a blunted muscle protein synthetic

[40] Kuzmuk KN, Swanson KS, Tappenden KA, et al. Diet and Age Affect Intestinal Morphology and Large Bowel Fermentative End-Product Concentrations in Senior and Young Adult Dogs. J Nutr 2005;135:1940–5.

[41] Gomes M, Beraldo M, Putarov T. Old Beagle dogs have lower faecal concentrations of some fermentation products and lower peripheral lymphocyte counts than young adult beagles. Br J Nutr 2011;106:S187–90.

[42] Benno Y, Nakao H, Uchida K, et al. Impact of the advances in age on the gastrointestinal microflora of beagle dogs. J Am Vet Med Assoc 1992;54:703–6.

[43] Bermingham E, Weidgraaf K, Hekman M, et al. Seasonal and age effects on energy requirements in domestic short-hair cats (Felis catus) in a temperate environment. J Anim Physiol an N 2013;97:522–30.

[44] Pérez-Camargo G. Cat nutrition: What is new in the old? Compend Contin Educ Vet 2003;26:5–10.

[45] Schauf S, Stockman J, Haydock R, et al. Healthy ageing is associated with preserved or enhanced nutrient and mineral apparent digestibility in dogs and cats fed commercially relevant extruded diets. Animals 2021;11:2127.

[46] Wakshlag J, Barr S, Ordway G, et al. Effect of dietary protein on lean body wasting in dogs: correlation between loss of lean mass and markers of proteasome-dependent proteolysis. J Anim Physiol an N 2003;87:408–20.

[47] Frantz NZ, Yamka RM, Friesen KG. The effect of diet and lysine: calorie ratio on body composition and kidney health in geriatric cats. Int J Appl Res Vet M 2007;5:25.

[48] Laflamme D, Gunn-Moore D. Nutrition of aging cats. Vet Clin North Am Small Anim Pract 2014;44:761–74.

[49] Freeman LM. Cachexia and sarcopenia in companion animals: An under-utilized natural animal model of human disease. JCSM Rapid Commun 2018;1:1–17.

[50] Li P, Wu G. Amino acid nutrition and metabolism in domestic cats and dogs. J Anim Sci Biotechnol 2023;14:19.

[51] Fahey Jr GC, Barry KA, Swanson KS. Age-related changes in nutrient utilization by companion animals. Annu Rev Nutr 2008;28:425–45.

[52] Jeromson S, Gallagher IJ, Galloway SD, et al. Omega-3 fatty acids and skeletal muscle health. Mar Drugs 2015;13:6977–7004.

[53] Freeman LM, Rush JE, Kehayias JJ, et al. Nutritional alterations and the effect of fish oil supplementation in dogs with heart failure. J Vet Intern Med 1998;12:440–8.

[54] Ghosh TS, Shanahan F, O'Toole PW. Toward an improved definition of a healthy microbiome for healthy aging. Nat Aging 2022;2:1054–69.

[55] Mizukami K, Uchiyama J, Igarashi H, et al. Age-related analysis of the gut microbiome in a purebred dog colony. FEMS Microbiol Lett 2019;366:fnz095.

[56] Hill C, Guarner F, Reid G, et al. Expert consensus document: The International Scientific Association for Probiotics and Prebiotics consensus statement on the scope and appropriate use of the term probiotic. Nat Rev Gastroenterol Hepatol 2014;11(8):506–14.

[57] Benyacoub J, Cavadini C, Sauthier T, et al. Supplementation of food with Enterococcus faecium (SF68) stimulates immune functions in young dogs. J Nutr 2003;133:1158–62.

[58] Yamazaki C, Rosenkrantz W, Griffin C. Pilot evaluation of Enterococcus faecium SF68 as adjunctive therapy for oclacitinib-responsive adult atopic dermatitis in dogs. J Small Anim Pract 2019;60:499–506.

[59] Lappin MR, Veir JK, Satyaraj E, et al. Pilot study to evaluate the effect of oral supplementation of Enterococcus faecium SF68 on cats with latent feline herpesvirus 1. J Fel Med Surg 2009;11:650–4.

[60] Boehme M, Rémond-Derbez N, Lerond C, et al. Bifidobacterium longum subsp. longum Reduces Perceived Psychological Stress in Healthy Adults: An Exploratory Clinical Trial. Nutrients 2023;15:3122.

[61] McGowan RT, Barnett HR, Czarnecki-Maulden G, et al. Tapping into those 'gut feelings': impact of BL999 (Bifidobacterium longum) on anxiety in dogs. Denver, CO: Veterinary Behavior Symposium Proceedings; 2018. p. 8–9.

[62] Yeh Y-M, Lye X-Y, Lin H-Y, et al. Effects of Lactiplantibacillus plantarum PS128 on alleviating canine aggression and separation anxiety. Appl Anim Behav Sci 2022;247:105569.

[63] Chapagain D, Virányi Z, Wallis LJ, et al. Aging of attentiveness in border collies and other pet dog breeds: the protective benefits of lifelong training. Front Age Neursci 2017;9:100.

[64] Landsberg GM, Denenberg S, Araujo JA. Cognitive dysfunction in cats: a syndrome we used to dismiss as 'old age'. J Fel Med Surg 2010;12:837–48.

[65] Levine M, Lloyd R, Fisher R, et al. Sensory, motor and cognitive alterations in aged cats. Neurobiol Aging 1987;8:253–63.

[66] Gunn-Moore D, Moffat K, Christie LA, et al. Cognitive dysfunction and the neurobiology of ageing in cats. J Small Anim Pract 2007;48:546–53.

[67] Hadley K, Bauer J, Milgram N. The oil-rich alga Schizochytrium sp. as a dietary source of docosahexaenoic acid improves shape discrimination learning associated with visual processing in a canine model of senescence. Prostaglandins Leukot Essent Fatty Acids 2017;118:10–8.

[68] Studzinski CM, MacKay WA, Beckett TL, et al. Induction of ketosis may improve mitochondrial function and decrease steady-state amyloid-β precursor protein (APP) levels in the aged dog. Brain Res 2008;1226:209–17.

[69] Pan Y, Landsberg G, Mougeot I, et al. Efficacy of a therapeutic diet on dogs with signs of cognitive dysfunction syndrome (CDS): a prospective double blinded placebo controlled clinical study. Front Nutr 2018;5:127.

[70] Chiang PK, Gordon RK, Tal J, et al. S-Adenosylmetliionine and methylation. Faseb J 1996;10:471–80.

[71] Shrubsole MJ, Wagner C, Zhu X, et al. Associations between S-adenosylmethionine, S-adenosylhomocysteine, and colorectal adenoma risk are modified by sex. Am J Cancer Res 2015;5:458.

[72] Wagner C, Koury MJ. S-Adenosylhomocysteine—a better indicator of vascular disease than homocysteine? Am J Clin Nutr 2007;86:1581–5.

[73] Kerins DM, Koury MJ, Capdevila A, et al. Plasma S-adenosylhomocysteine is a more sensitive indicator of cardiovascular disease than plasma homocysteine. Am J Clin Nutr 2001;74:723–9.

[74] Cachon T, Frykman O, Innes J, et al. Face validity of a proposed tool for staging canine osteoarthritis: Canine OsteoArthritis Staging Tool (COAST). Vet J 2018;235:1–8.

[75] Barbeau-Grégoire M, Otis C, Cournoyer A, et al. A 2022 systematic review and meta-analysis of enriched therapeutic diets and nutraceuticals in canine and feline osteoarthritis. Int J Mol Sci 2022;23:10384.

[76] Morley JE. Decreased food intake with aging. J Gerontol A Biol Sci Med Sci 2001;56:81–8.

[77] Giezenaar C, Chapman I, Luscombe-Marsh N, et al. Ageing is associated with decreases in appetite and energy intake—a meta-analysis in healthy adults. Nutrients 2016;8:28.

[78] Eyre R, Trehiou M, Marshall E, et al. Aging cats prefer warm food. J Vet Behav 2022;47:86–92.

[79] Alexander J, Stockman J, Atwal J, et al. Effects of the long-term feeding of diets enriched with inorganic phosphorus on the adult feline kidney and phosphorus metabolism. Br J Nutr 2019;121:249–69.

Advances in Small Animal Care 5 (2024) 165–178

ADVANCES IN SMALL ANIMAL CARE

Rational Approach and Dietary Considerations for Managing Dogs with Swallowing Impairment (Dysphagia)

Stanley L. Marks, BVSc, PhD, Diplomate ACVIM (Small Animal Internal Medicine, Oncology, Nutrition)*,
Tarini V. Ullal, DVM, MS, Diplomate ACVIM (Small Animal Internal Medicine)
Department of Medicine and Epidemiology, University of California, Davis, School of Veterinary Medicine, One Shields Avenue, Davis, CA 95616, USA

KEYWORDS
- Dysphagia • Swallowing impairment • Megaesophagus • Oropharyngeal • Aspiration • Regurgitation
- Malnutrition • Food texture

KEY POINTS
- The anatomic categorization of the dog's swallowing impairment into oropharyngeal and esophageal causes followed by determination of the pathophysiologic process (structural vs impaired motility) is pivotal for optimizing medical and dietary therapy.
- Utilization of swallowing fluoroscopy helps optimize the selection of different foods, food consistencies, and liquid intake for patients with swallowing impairment and helps to monitor their response to therapy.
- Increasing bolus viscosity has anecdotally been observed to improve clinical signs and reduce laryngeal penetration and aspiration in dogs with pharyngeal weakness and cricopharyngeus muscle dysfunction.
- There is no specific consistency of ingesta that has been shown to be most reliable for facilitating the transit of esophageal contents into the stomach of dogs with megaesophagus and diet consistency should be optimized for individual patients.
- Gravity-assisted feeding is indispensable for facilitating esophageal bolus transit in dogs with megaesophagus.

INTRODUCTION

Deglutition is the process of swallowing, which enables the transport of food and liquids from the oral cavity and pharynx to the esophagus and stomach. Deglutition (Fig. 1A–C) begins with the oral phase, which involves muscles of mastication and salivary glands that facilitate mastication, mixing, and lubrication of the bolus with saliva. After bolus preparation, the tongue, jaw, and hyoid muscles execute the movement of the bolus to the pharynx. Once the bolus has reached the pharynx, the pharyngeal phase begins with contraction of the pharyngeal muscles and relaxation of the cricopharyngeus muscle of the upper esophageal sphincter

(UES) to facilitate passage of the bolus into the proximal esophagus. Concurrently, the epiglottis closes the laryngeal opening and the soft palate elevates to prevent inappropriate entry of the bolus into the airways or nasal passages [1,2]. As the bolus reaches the esophagus, the esophageal phase is characterized by peristaltic contractions that drive the bolus in waves down the esophageal body, across the esophagogastric junction (EGJ) through the lower esophageal sphincter (LES), and into the stomach. Primary persistaltic contractions spearhead bolus transit, and secondary contractions clear any residual ingested material that is not cleared by the primary contractions [3]. The sequence of events

*Corresponding author, E-mail address: slmarks@ucdavis.edu

https://doi.org/10.1016/j.yasa.2024.06.010
2666-450X/24/

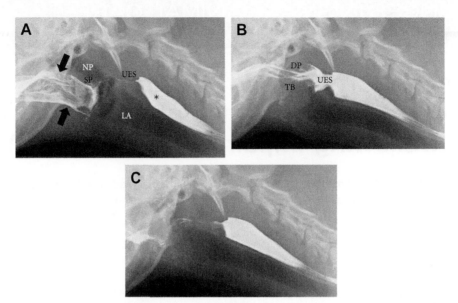

FIG. 1 Phases of deglutition. Digital images from a swallow fluoroscopy study in a healthy dog show the phases of deglutition. **(A)** Oral phase: Liquid barium contrast in the oral cavity (designated by *black arrows*). There is also remaining barium from a previous swallow in the cervical esophagus (*asterisk*). At the start of the pharyngeal phase, the soft palate will rise to close the nasopharynx while the epiglottis closes the larynx to prevent nasopharyngeal reflux and laryngeal penetration, respectively. LA, larynx; NP, nasopharynx; SP, soft palate; UES, upper esophageal sphincter. **(B)** As a continuation of the pharyngeal phase, the pharyngeal muscles contract and the dorsal pharyngeal wall (DP) meets the tongue base (TB) while the cricopharyngeus muscle relaxes to open the upper esophageal sphincter (UES). Liquid barium contrast can then pass through the open UES into the proximal esophagus. **(C)** After the contrast reaches the esophagus, esophageal peristalsis (primary and secondary) can occur to move the bolus through the lower esophageal sphincter (LES) to the stomach. (Pollard, Rachel E., Imaging Evaluation of Dogs and Cats with Dysphagia, International Scholarly Research Notices, 2012, 238505, 15 pages, 2012. https://doi.org/10.5402/2012/238505.)

that comprise deglutition from the oral cavity to the stomach is highly complex and coordinated by the actions and functions of 31 pairs of striated muscles, 5 cranial nerves, and the brainstem nuclei. Any disruption to this intricate process results in swallowing impairment, also known as "dysphagia" in humans. The term "dysphagia" has traditionally been used in veterinary medicine to describe swallowing impairment; however, "dysphagia" refers to the symptoms of swallowing impairment that can only be expressed by people. The authors have thus elected to use the term "swallowing impairment" in this article because animals cannot convey their symptoms [4].

Swallowing impairment is a common and potentially life-threatening disorder in dogs that can result in malnutrition, dehydration, regurgitation, aspiration pneumonia, and compromised quality of life [5–8]. The exact prevalence of swallowing impairment in dogs is unknown, but at the University of California, Davis, nearly

1% of 105,000 dogs presenting to the Small Animal Clinic over a 10-year period between 2003 and 2013 were evaluated for a swallowing abnormality. Swallowing impairment can be categorized anatomically into oropharyngeal or esophageal disorders. Common oropharyngeal disorders that affect dogs include pharyngeal weakness, characterized by poor pharyngeal contraction and ineffective clearance of pharyngeal contents, and cricopharyngeus muscle dysfunction (CPMD), characterized by a failure of the UES to relax (achalasia) or a lack of coordination between pharyngeal contraction and UES relaxation (asynchrony) [9,10]. Common esophageal disorders include esophagitis typically secondary to gastroesophageal reflux disease (GERD) [11,12] under general anesthesia or sliding hiatal herniation (SHH) [13], esophageal strictures [14], and megaesophagus (ME) [15]. ME is characterized by impaired to absent esophageal peristalsis with or without failure of the LES to relax in dogs (esophageal achalasia-like syndrome) [16–18].

Clinical signs of swallowing impairment differ based on the anatomic region involved, the severity of the disorder, and the underlying etiology. Dogs with oral disease have difficulty with prehension, which can manifest as dropping of food from the mouth [10,19]. Dogs with pharyngeal weakness exhibit signs of gagging, retching, coughing, multiple swallowing attempts, and nasal reflux of water or ingesta within seconds of swallowing [20]. Dogs with CPMD manifest with signs similar to those observed in dogs with pharyngeal weakness, but also have more difficulty swallowing liquids than solids [6,10,21]. Common clinical signs observed in dogs with esophageal diseases include hard swallowing, odynophagia, hypersalivation, lip-licking, or regurgitation [11,22]. Dogs with esophageal strictures or esophagitis are more likely to present with odynophagia (painful swallowing), hard swallowing, and regurgitation seconds to minutes after eating [12,14] compared to dogs with ME or SHH that can regurgitate anytime from the immediate postprandial period to hours after ingestion of a meal [23,24].

Recognizing the subtle differences in clinical presentation helps localize and ascertain the likely cause of swallowing impairment. It is thus important to obtain a comprehensive clinical and dietary history as highlighted in Table 1 [4]:

A thorough physical examination including an observation of the pet eating (ideally both canned and kibble consistencies) and drinking should also be performed. This can be accomplished by observing video recordings captured by the pet owner or performing a feeding trial in the hospital setting. Physical examination of the oral cavity can identify dental disease, oral tumors, cleft palate, macroglossia, glossal weakness, or oropharyngeal foreign bodies [10]. Cervical palpation can identify a distended esophagus in some dogs with megaesophagus. A neurologic examination and assessment of muscle condition can reveal neurologic abnormalities (cranial nerve deficits, weakness), a stiff gait, muscle atrophy, and muscle contracture indicative of a neuropathy, myopathy, or junctionopathy that might warrant subsequent testing for myasthenia gravis, masticatory muscle myositis, laryngeal examination, electrodiagnostics (electromyography, nerve conduction velocity), and nerve and muscle biopsies [4]. Assessment of hydration and body condition score is also important to recognize dehydration and malnutrition consequent to chronic regurgitation and swallowing impairment [10,22].

Upon completion of a comprehensive history and physical examination, further diagnostic testing including imaging and endoscopy can further localize and determine the underlying etiology of the swallowing disorder. Diagnostic imaging with survey thoracic and cervical radiographs can identify foreign bodies, a vascular ring anomaly, neoplasia, megaesophagus, SHH, and concurrent aspiration pneumonia. Swallowing fluoroscopy enables examination of pharyngeal contraction, UES and LES relaxation, esophageal peristalsis, gastroesophageal reflux (GER), and aspiration (passage of material past vocal cords) or penetration (passage of material past larynx) [4,5]. It can also evaluate which liquid and food consistencies optimize bolus transit and minimize aspiration or penetration. The standard swallowing fluoroscopy protocol consists of 5 swallows of 3 different consistencies typically starting with 60% weight (60 g of barium/100 mL volume of suspension) barium sulfate paste alone, followed by barium mixed with canned food, and concluding with barium mixed with kibble. In each bolus, approximately 5 mL of barium sulfate is administered orally via syringe or mixed into a canned food or kibble bolus [25]. Survey radiographs can be repeated 30 minutes and 1 h after the swallowing fluoroscopy to assess poor or delayed esophageal clearance in dogs with ME and suspected esophageal achalasia-like syndrome. Esophagoscopy requires anesthesia, but can facilitate the diagnosis of esophagitis, neoplasia, strictures, webs, or rings, and SHH. Endoscopy can also facilitate feeding tube placements (esophagostomy tube or percutaneous endoscopically placed gastrostomy tubes (PEG)) or interventional procedures such as foreign body removal, balloon dilation of esophageal strictures, and brush cytology or biopsy of the esophagus [22]. Additionally, with endoscopic guidance, targeted interventions of the UES or LES in dogs with cricopharyngeus muscle achalasia or esophageal achalasia-like syndrome such as botulinum toxin administration to relax the UES [22] or LES [26], double balloon dilation of the UES [27], and pneumatic balloon dilation of the LES can be performed [26]. If therapeutic response following endoscopic interventions is suboptimal, dogs with CPMD and esophageal achalasia-like syndrome can benefit from surgical interventions including cricopharyngeus myectomy [6] or Heller's myotomy with fundoplication [26], respectively.

Prior to interventional or surgical procedures of esophageal achalasia-like syndrome, medical treatment with the phosphodiesterase 5 inhibitor, sildenafil, can be trialed to promote nitric oxide mediated relaxation of the LES [28,29]. Other pharmacologic therapies commonly used in dogs with swallowing impairment include medications to treat esophagitis such as omeprazole for acid suppression, sucralfate to inactivate pepsin and adsorb bile salts,

TABLE 1
Important Aspects of the Clinical and Dietary History that Should Be Ascertained by the Clinician [4]

	Pertinent History Information	Clinical Relevance
Signalment	• Age of onset • Breed	• Congenital vs acquired swallowing disorder such as megaesophagus • Brachycephalic with brachycephalic obstructive airway syndrome, hiatal herniation, and GER • Breed predispositions such as Golden retriever breed with crico-pharyngeus muscle dysfunction or muscular dystrophy [4]
Onset, duration, timing, and severity of clinical signs	• Onset of swallowing problem (sudden vs gradual) • Duration of signs (acute vs subacute vs chronic) • Frequency of signs (intermittent vs persistent) • Progression of signs (static vs progressive) • Associations with meals, activity, or sleep	• Oropharyngeal swallowing impairment will occur within seconds of food or water consumption • Esophageal swallowing impairment will occur seconds to hours following food or water consumption • Activity exacerbates SHH • Association with sleep could be because of nocturnal GER
Clinical signs with varying bolus consistency	• Difficulty with solids, liquids, or both	• Canine patients with cricopharyng-eus muscle dysfunction and pharyngeal weakness typically experience exacerbation with liquids whereas patients with esophageal strictures experience exacerbation with solid foods
Signs of neuromuscular disease	• Weakness, painful, or stiff gait exercise intolerance • Dysphonia and dyspnea, history of laryngeal paralysis	• Suggestive of polymyopathy, poly-neuropathy, or junctionopathy
Sequelae of swallowing impairment	• Weight loss vs weight gain • Sarcopenia • Recurrent episodes of aspiration pneumonia	• Weight loss, sarcopenia suggests chronic, severe disorder causing malnutrition • Weight gain/obesity can exacerbate GER • Recurrent aspiration pneumonia suggestive of aerodigestive disorder
Exposure to medications, anesthesia, change in diet	• Recent administration of medications • Recent general anesthesia • Change in diet	• Pill-esophagitis or stricture forma-tion secondary to clindamycin, doxycycline, tetracycline, ampicillin or non-steroidal anti-inflammatory drug administration • Recent anesthesia causing GER and subsequent esophagitis or stricture formation • Change in diet triggering inflamma-tory bowel disease or eosinophilic esophagitis or increased dietary fat content that could precipitate de-layed gastric emptying

Abbreviations: GER, gastroesophageal reflux; SHH, sliding hiatal herniation.

induce mucous and bicarbonate secretion, and provide a protective barrier to the esophageal mucosa [30], and lidocaine-diphenhydramine-magnesium hydroxide solution, known as "magic mouthwash," to provide analgesia and esophageal mucosal barrier protection [31]. Cisapride, a serotonin 5-hydroxytryptamine 4 receptor (5HT4) agonist, increases lower esophageal sphincter tone and is the preferred prokinetic to increase gastric emptying and treat GER [32,33,34] although a recent study contradicted its enhancement of gastric emptying in healthy Beagle dogs administered the drug at 1mg/kg q 12h for 7 days [35]. In conjunction with interventional procedures and pharmacologic therapies, dietary therapy is vital to the management of dogs with swallowing impairment to optimize bolus transit, minimize aspiration and penetration, and provide adequate nutritional support. This article will highlight dietary modifications and nutritional strategies to implement in the treatment of common oropharyngeal and esophageal swallowing disorders in dogs.

DISCUSSION
Oropharyngeal Disorders
In dogs with oral diseases, administering softer food in the form of soaked kibble, canned food, slurries (milkshake consistency), or liquefied foods can optimize prehension and minimize pain in dogs with severe dental disease, ulcerative stomatitis, and oral neoplasia. Dogs with severe trismus [36] or masticatory weakness caused by myopathies (masticatory muscle myositis, muscular dystrophy) [19,36,37] or a trigeminal neuropathy [38] can benefit from an esophagostomy tube to bypass the oropharynx. Forced syringe feeding should be avoided to prevent food aversion and aspiration pneumonia. Foods that increase the risk of choking, such as hard, dry, and sharp kibble, rawhide, and tough, jerky treats should not be offered. Specific human food items such as carrots, fibrous and stringy foods such as green beans or psyllium husks, fruits with sharp or large seeds, and sticky treats such as peanut butter, marshmallows, and cheese are also not advised because of the choking hazard and because they require effective chewing and lingual movements that are often lacking in dogs with oropharyngeal disease [39].

Dogs with CPMD require definitive surgical treatment involving surgical myotomy or myectomy of the cricopharyngeus muscle [6]. Less invasive therapeutic modalities for temporary resolution involve injection of botulinum toxin into the cricopharyngeus muscle [10] or serial double-balloon dilations of the UES [27]. In addition to obtaining a comprehensive clinical history and observing the dog drinking and eating,

swallowing fluoroscopy can further optimize which liquid or food consistencies are best tolerated to minimize swallowing impairment and aspiration in dogs with pharyngeal or cricopharyngeal disease. Most dogs with pharyngeal weakness or CPMD have difficulty swallowing water in contrast to swallowing kibble or foods with a firm consistency and therefore, hydration should be carefully monitored in these patients. Increasing the viscosity of water by adding cornstarch-based formulas to create a mildly thick (nectar) or moderately thick (honey) consistency can improve swallowing function in affected dogs immensely. In addition, flavored ice cubes with beef or chicken broth can be used to facilitate water intake and optimize hydration status. Melons containing high moisture contents such as watermelon and cantaloupe (>90% moisture content) can also be used to augment water intake in affected dogs. For dogs with cricopharyngeus muscle asynchrony, paced and slower feeding of smaller liquid volumes or diminutive boluses of kibble (4–5 pieces of kibble or meatballs of canned food per mouthful every 30 seconds) can also help with coordination of the pharynx and UES and reduce clinical signs. Alternating between liquid and solid boluses can also facilitate improved bolus transfer.

Similarly, in human patients that are elderly [40], or afflicted by stroke [41], progressive neurologic diseases (Parkinson's, Alzheimer's) [42], or head and neck cancer [43], strategies to thicken liquid and modify food texture are typically recommended to slow bolus velocity and allow more time for glottic closure and airway protection [44]. However, the evidence supporting recommendations for thickened liquids in human patients with oropharyngeal dysphagia is conflicting. Higher viscosity liquids reduce airway aspiration or penetration but also require more oropharyngeal propulsive forces, which can ultimately increase oral or pharyngeal residue and result in greater post-swallow airway penetration [44–46]. There is also no evidence to document that thicker liquids reduce the rate of pneumonia or improve the quality of life in dysphagic human patients [47]. Rather, thickened nectar and honey-like liquids can affect palatability and increase dehydration and weight loss [48]. Texture-modified foods are suggested in the management of human patients with oropharyngeal dysphagia, but there are myriad textural properties and rheological factors to consider including whether food is whole, diced or chopped, minced, or pureed, hard, cohesive, and slippery [39,46]. Only recently was a standardized framework established for human patients that includes definitions and descriptive characteristics of 5 different levels of liquid thickness (thin, slightly thick, mildly thick, moderately thick, and extremely thick) and 5 levels of food texture (liquidized, pureed, minced and moist, soft, and regular) [39]. Bolus viscosity standardization and the effects of thickened liquids and texture modified diets on swallowing physiology have not yet been studied in dogs. Further study could demonstrate the utility of these methods to manage dogs with swallowing impairment.

An esophagostomy tube can bypass the oropharyngeal swallowing disorder and provide necessary hydration, nutrition, and medications temporarily or long-term. Enteral feeding via a gastrostomy tube, surgically or endoscopically placed, is also a viable alternative in dogs with pharyngeal weakness or CPMD. However, aspiration of saliva with subsequent pneumonia can occur despite the implementation of enteral feeding devices [49].

ESOPHAGEAL DISORDERS
Esophagitis and Gastroesophageal Reflux Disease

Esophagitis is an acute or chronic inflammatory disorder of the esophageal mucosa that occasionally involves the underlying submucosa and muscularis (Fig. 2). Esophagitis in dogs is most frequently associated with GERD [12], but can also result from pill-induced esophagitis (eg, doxycycline hyclate or clindamycin), esophageal foreign bodies, and ingestion of caustic substances. Dogs with GERD have compromised anti-reflux barrier integrity either due to an anatomic or functional abnormality of the EGJ. The integrity of the EGJ is maintained by the gastroesophageal flap valve (musculomucosal fold and acute angle of His created by the distal esophagus as it enters the stomach and the gastric fundus where it is attached by the phrenoesophageal ligament), tonic pressure of the LES, diaphragmatic crura, and gastric sling fibers [50]. An SHH is defined by disruption of the gastroesophageal flap valve and axial displacement of the stomach through the esophageal hiatus of the diaphragm into the thoracic cavity (Fig. 3). Sliding hiatal hernias have been well-documented in brachycephalic breeds and their nasofacial conformation and unique respiratory anatomy predisposes these breeds to Brachycephalic Obstructive Airway Syndrome (BOAS), which increases negative intrathoracic pressure and causes subsequent SHH and GER during inspiration [51,52]. Hiatal herniation reduces LES pressure and leads to GER, esophagitis, and segmental or diffuse esophageal hypomotility. Esophageal dysmotility with or without delayed gastric emptying can further contribute to GERD [13].

In conjunction with pharmacologic therapies to provide acid suppression, analgesia, and esophageal mucosal barrier protection, feeding softened food can alleviate discomfort associated with esophagitis. Lower esophageal sphincter contractions are weaker in response to liquid meals compared to solid foods and therefore might not be optimal for GERD [53]. However, liquid diets are often necessary if the esophagus is narrowed by a peptic esophageal stricture caused by GERD [14]. Upright, elevated feeding in a Bailey chair (Fig. 4) can assist with gravity-assisted esophageal acid clearance in dogs with esophageal dysmotility. Dietary recommendations for dogs with GER and delayed gastric emptying include feeding smaller, more frequent meals to prevent gastric overdistension and secondary transient lower esophageal sphincter relaxations [54,55]. Smaller volume, more frequent meals also enhance gastric emptying [56] as do lower viscosity, lower fiber [57], fat-restriction (<24% fat on ME basis) [58], and protein-restriction [34] in favor of more highly digestible starches [59]. While liquid diets [60] and warmer temperature liquids [61] improve gastric emptying, gastric emptying in dogs does not differ between canned and kibble diets [62]. In humans, increased osmolarity and acidic gastric contents also delay gastric emptying [63] and this phenomenon should be taken into consideration for dogs with GERD as well [64]. Gastritis, pyloroduodenal obstruction, and other gastric pathology can impair gastric emptying, which can be further exacerbated by pain, stress, and inactivity during hospitalization [65]. Because obesity is an important risk factor for GERD in humans, calorie restriction to facilitate weight loss should be considered in dogs with GERD to reduce intra-abdominal pressure and normalize the LES pressure gradient [66]. Weight management is especially important in dogs with BOAS because obesity is significantly associated with BOAS [67], which contributes to SHH and GERD [68]. In humans, improvements in lifestyle and diet such as incorporating proper exercise, separating meal times from sleep by at least 3 hours, antioxidant intake, reducing simple sugars, and restricting dietary fat are associated with reduced reflux and could be applicable strategies in dogs with GERD [69,70].

In dogs with chronic enteropathy and suspected GERD, hydrolyzed or novel protein source diets can improve clinical signs of GERD [11,12]. Additionally, in dogs with eosinophilic esophagitis, prescription hydrolyzed diets can help eliminate food allergens and address the suspected hypersensitivity in combination with corticosteroid therapy [71]. Eosinophilic esophagitis is infrequently

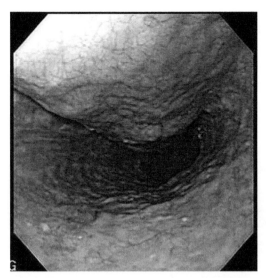

FIG. 2 Severe reflux esophagitis showing marked erythema, granularity, and erosive lesions of the mucosa in a 3-year male Labrador retriever following anesthesia for a dental procedure.

observed in dogs compared to humans, but in humans, dietary therapy with elemental or elimination diets (exclusion of milk, wheat, egg, soy-legumes) is an important first-line treatment and can be as effective as medical management [72].

When assisted nutrition is required, enteral nutrition is preferred over parenteral nutrition and can be administered via nasogastric, nasoesophageal, esophagostomy, gastrostomy, or jejunostomy tubes [49]. Although nasogastric tubes traverse the LES and constant stimulation of the pharynx by the tube can trigger LES relaxation, there is no evidence that either nasogastric or nasoesophageal tubes exacerbate GERD and esophagitis [73,74]. Additionally, nasogastric tubes permit intermittent evacuation, sampling, and pH testing of gastric contents [75]. Nasogastric or nasoesophageal tubes are typically short-term and require liquid enteral diets. There are a variety of fat-restricted elemental human liquid formulas and commercially-available fat-restricted veterinary diets to facilitate gastric emptying and minimize GER [49]. Both intermittent bolus and continuous feeding provide adequate nutritional support [76]. Gastrostomy tube feeding is preferred over esophagostomy tubes for the management of patients with severe, intractable esophagitis. Jejunostomy tube feeding of liquid fat-restricted enteral formulas can be implemented in patients with pancreatitis to avoid pancreatic stimulation [77] or to bypass

the stomach in patients with severe gastroparesis or gastric disease [78].

Megaesophagus

ME is one of the most common causes of regurgitation in dogs and is characterized by focal or diffuse esophageal dilation and concurrent esophageal dysmotility (Fig. 5A). The disorder can be congenital or acquired; however, the acquired form is more common and can be idiopathic or secondary to an underlying disease [15]. Myasthenia gravis is the most common secondary cause of acquired megaesophagus in dogs accounting for 25% of cases. Up to 67% of dogs with ME have esophageal achalasia-like syndrome resulting in marked retention of oral feedings, despite gravity-assisted feeding [16]. Rare cases of acquired megaesophagus associated with hypoadrenocorticism and hypothyroidism have also been reported in dogs [23].

The treatment of megaesophagus should be focused on addressing the underlying etiology such as treatment of the myasthenia gravis with pyridostigmine [79], modifying diet consistency, and implementing targeted therapies of the LES in dogs with esophageal achalasia-like syndrome, including sildenafil [28,29], pneumatic balloon dilation, botulinum toxin injection of the LES, or Heller's myotomy with fundoplication [26,80]. In addition, feeding practices designed to maximize food delivery to the stomach and minimize the risk of aspiration are pivotal in dogs with megaesophagus. The application of gravity-assisted feeding whereby the dog is fed in an elevated position with the head and neck of the animal elevated or in a specialized feeding chair such as a Bailey chair facilitates bolus transit from the hypopharynx to the LES. Fluoroscopic swallowing assessment in dogs with megaesophagus should be performed with the dogs seated upright in a Bailey chair to evaluate esophageal motility and LES function more safely. Gravity-assisted feeding also allows the clinician to determine which food consistency (liquid, canned meatballs, slurry, or kibble) most reliably facilitates bolus transit and LES relaxation in affected dogs. There is no specific consistency of ingesta that most reliably ensures transit of esophageal contents in dogs with megaesophagus, but 2 studies confirmed that swallowing fluoroscopic assessment led to alterations in food consistency in 50% and 29% of the dogs, respectively [17,18]. Additionally, in the latter study, swallowing fluoroscopy led to informed recommendations to alter water delivery in all dogs evaluated. Adjustments in the treatment plan and management of these dogs resulted in improved quality of life in 16/21 (76%) of dogs according to the pet owner. Thus, performing swallowing

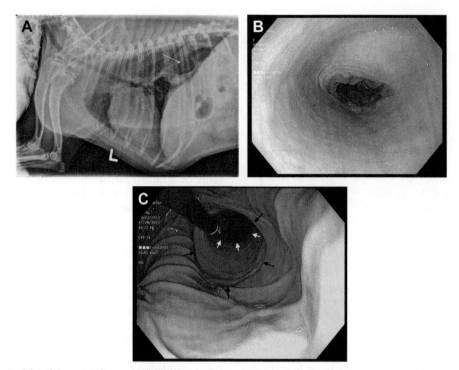

FIG. 3 **(A)** Left lateral radiograph obtained on a 5-year female spayed Boston terrier with a sliding hiatal hernia showing the stomach herniating into the craniodorsal thorax (*arrow*). **(B)** Endoscopic view of the herniated portion of the gastric fundus beyond the esophagogastric junction in a 9-month female German shepherd puppy. **(C)** Retroflexed view of the gastric cardia showing complete disruption of the esophagogastric junction in the 9-month female German shepherd puppy from Fig. 3B. The black arrows highlight the large diaphragmatic aperture observed after full insufflation and the white arrows highlight the lower esophageal sphincter.

fluoroscopy is critical not only for the diagnosis and assessment of ME, but also in the guidance of treatment. A contrast static esophagram with post-study radiographs can be performed by veterinarians who do not have access to a videofluoroscopy unit. The protocol is conducted by feeding a dog barium slurry in an upright position (in a Bailey chair) and obtaining a lateral thoracic radiograph after the dog has been maintained upright for 15 minutes. The barium slurry is followed by barium mixed with canned meatballs if the dog has successfully emptied the barium slurry into the stomach after which the dog is held upright for another 15 minutes and radiographs are repeated. The canned meatballs are followed by feeding barium mixed with kibble if the dog has successfully emptied the barium-coated meatballs into the stomach followed by the same 15-min protocol and radiographs. This feeding trial should help determine which food consistency is associated with the shortest esophageal transit time allowing the veterinarian to make recommendations to the pet owner. Repeating radiographs 30 to 60 minutes after the swallowing fluoroscopy (Fig. 5B) or after the described feeding trial with serial lateral thoracic radiographs can also help determine if delayed esophageal clearance occurs and can guide the clinician to make recommendations regarding the duration for maintaining the dog in an upright position after feeding and the addition of post-meal activity [17]. Feeding trials with different consistencies paired with fluoroscopic or contrast static esophagram imaging can also assess treatment response in dogs with esophageal achalasia-like syndrome. Human patients with esophageal achalasia are advised to consume smaller volume, lower fiber, and higher liquid content foods to improve bolus passage through the LES while awaiting targeted definitive therapeutic interventions of the LES [81]. The same recommendations can be translated and applied to dogs with ME [64], but should be guided by the swallowing

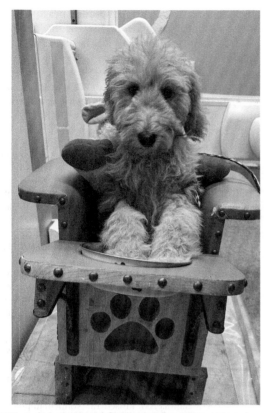

FIG. 4 A 4-month-old Goldendoodle puppy undergoing a swallowing fluoroscopy examination in a Bailey chair due to history of regurgitation. The Bailey chair acts as a restraining device and maintains the dog in an upright position, enabling gravity to assist with passage of boluses from the oropharynx into the stomach.

fluoroscopy assessment and tailored to the patient [17,18].

Severely malnourished animals or animals suffering repeated bouts of aspiration pneumonia should have a temporary or permanent gastrostomy tube placed for enteral nutritional support. Gastrostomy tube feeding reduces the risk of aspiration pneumonia and enables the administration of medications that would have otherwise been regurgitated; however, dogs with ME can still aspirate saliva or ingesta refluxed from the stomach into the esophagus. Intermittent at-home suctioning of esophageal content via placement of a fenestrated esophagostomy tube for prevention of recurrent aspiration pneumonia is a viable consideration for dogs with a giant sigmoid esophagus [82].

FUTURE CONSIDERATIONS

It is standard practice to only evaluate 3 phases (liquid, canned food, and kibble) during feeding trials or swallowing fluoroscopy of dogs, but a wider range of different viscosities and food textures are evaluated to screen and assess human patients. For example, in people with oropharyngeal dysphagia, a volume-viscosity swallowing test (V-VST) or modified V-VST is used, which administers swallow boluses of incrementally increasing volumes and viscosity, adjusted by starch, or xanthan-gum thickener [83]. Both the routine and modified V-VST are safe, quick, and accurate with high sensitivity and specificity for impaired swallowing safety (laryngeal penetration or aspiration) and efficacy [83,84]. Ongoing use of the V-VST also serves as a tool for monitoring patient progress over time, suggesting the need to adjust volume

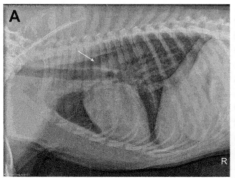
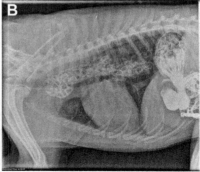

FIG. 5 (**A**) Right lateral survey thoracic radiograph of a 1-year male castrated Australian Kelpie mix-breed dog with congenital megaesophagus showing diffuse gas dilation of the thoracic esophagus (*arrow*) and interstitial pulmonary infiltrates in the dependent aspect of the caudal segment of the left cranial lung lobe. (**B**) Right lateral survey thoracic radiograph of the same dog in Fig. 5A with congenital megaesophagus (ME) 30 minutes after completion of a swallowing fluoroscopy study with the dog maintained in a Bailey chair during the study. The esophagus is filled with retained kibble, but canned food and barium liquid has cleared into the stomach.

and viscosity recommendations or to order further tests such as swallowing fluoroscopy [84].

The swallowing fluoroscopy procedure for humans is also more standardized in the bolus volumes administered, viscosities tested, and the contrast agent used [85]. For human patients with oropharyngeal disease, a standardized modified barium swallow test involving 6 different consistencies starting with thin liquid barium (2 trials of 5-mL cup sip, sequential swallows from cup), then nectar-thick barium (5-mL cup sip), honey-thick barium (5 mL), pudding-thick barium (5 mL), and ending with a 1-half shortbread cookie with 3 mL pudding thick barium. A standard barium sulfate product Varibar is used, which has a full line of products that meets the criteria for each consistency defined by the International Dysphagia Diet Standardization Initiative Framework (thin, mildly thick, moderately thick, extremely thick, and pureed). Barium products, such as Varibar, or thickening agents, could be incorporated into clinical swallowing tests and standardized swallowing fluoroscopy protocols that test different consistencies and enhance the assessment and management of dogs with swallowing impairment.

SUMMARY

Swallowing impairment in dogs is highly prevalent and potentially life-threatening. The diagnosis of swallowing impairment requires obtaining a thorough clinical history, performing a comprehensive physical examination including an observation of the pet drinking and eating, and completion of diagnostic testing such as cervical and thoracic radiographs, swallowing fluoroscopy, and esophagoscopy. The results of these diagnostic steps localize the swallowing impairment, determine the etiology, and help guide treatment decisions. While pharmacologic therapy and surgical interventions are important, dietary management is equally pivotal in the management of dogs with swallowing impairment. Liquefied foods or soaked kibble minimize pain in dogs with oropharyngeal disease (stomatitis, dental disease, and pharyngitis) or esophagitis. Liquid and dietary texture modifications can improve bolus transit and minimize aspiration and penetration in dogs with oropharyngeal disease and ME. In dogs with pharyngeal weakness or cricopharyngeus muscle dysfunction, increasing bolus, increasing bolus viscosity from liquid to pudding consistency can reduce laryngeal penetration and aspiration, but might increase post-swallow oropharyngeal residue similar to humans with oropharyngeal dysphagia. There is no reliable bolus viscosity or food consistency known to benefit dogs with ME, but

feeding trials and swallowing fluoroscopy can help tailor the feeding plan and selection of the optimal liquid or food bolus consistency that facilitates esophageal clearance. Follow-up fluoroscopic or radiographic images can also determine the ideal duration to maintain the dog in an upright position after feeding and to evaluate whether postprandial activity facilitates esophageal clearance. Smaller food volume, more frequent meals, dietary fat restriction, and treatment of obesity and BOAS should be implemented in the treatment of dogs with GERD and SHH. In any dog with severe malnourishment or repeated bouts of aspiration pneumonia, assisted enteral feeding with esophagostomy or gastrostomy tubes can be invaluable for nutrition, hydration, and effective administration of medications.

CLINICS CARE POINTS

- Performing a thorough diagnostic workup to anatomically categorize the dog's swallowing impairment and determine the underlying etiology is pivotal to developing the appropriate medical and dietary treatment plan.
- Utilization of swallowing fluoroscopy is invaluable for optimizing selection of liquid and food consistencies in affected patients and for monitoring response to therapy.
- Increasing bolus viscosity has anectodally been shown to improve clinical signs and reduce laryngeal penetration and aspiration in dogs with cricopharyngeus muscle dysfunction and pharyngeal weakness.
- Swallowing fluoroscopy guides recommendations that maximize esophageal clearance and improve the management of dogs with megaesophagus by altering oral fluid delivery, food consistency, duration of keeping the animal upright in the Bailey chair, and addition of postprandial activity.
- Smaller volume, more frequent meals, dietary fat restriction, and treatment of obesity and BOAS promote gastric emptying in dogs with GERD secondary to SHH and BOAS.

DISCLOSURE

The authors have nothing to disclose.

FUNDING

The authors are appreciative of Nestlé Purina's support of Dr Tarini Ullal's Gastroenterology and Hepatology

Fellowship at the University of California, Davis, School of Veterinary Medicine.

REFERENCES

[1] Venker-van-Haagen A, Washabau RJ, Day MJ, editors. Canine and feline gastroenterology. Saint Louis: W.B. Saunders; 2013. p. 570–605.

[2] Sasegbon A, Hamdy S. The anatomy and physiology of normal and abnormal swallowing in oropharyngeal dysphagia. Neuro Gastroenterol Motil 2017;29. https://doi.org/10.1111/nmo.13100.

[3] Goyal RK, Chaudhury A. Physiology of normal esophageal motility. J Clin Gastroenterol 2008;42:610–9. https://doi.org/10.1097/MCG.0b013e31816b444d.

[4] Ullal TV, Marks SL, Belafsky PC, et al. A Comparative Assessment of the Diagnosis of Swallowing Impairment and Gastroesophageal Reflux in Canines and Humans. Front Vet Sci 2022;9:889331. https://doi.org/10.3389/fvets.2022.889331.

[5] Pollard RE, Marks SL, Cheney DM, et al. Diagnostic outcome of contrast videofluoroscopic swallowing studies in 216 dysphagic dogs. Vet Radiol Ultrasound 2017;58:373–80. https://doi.org/10.1111/vru.12493.

[6] Warnock JJ, Marks SL, Pollard R, et al. Surgical management of cricopharyngeal dysphagia in dogs: 14 cases (1989-2001). J Am Vet Med Assoc 2003;223:1462–8. https://doi.org/10.2460/javma.2003.223.1462.

[7] Darcy HP, Humm K, Ter Haar G. Retrospective analysis of incidence, clinical features, potential risk factors, and prognostic indicators for aspiration pneumonia in three brachycephalic dog breeds. J Am Vet Med Assoc 2018; 253:869–76. https://doi.org/10.2460/javma.253.7.869.

[8] McBrearty AR, Ramsey IK, Courcier EA, et al. Clinical factors associated with death before discharge and overall survival time in dogs with generalized megaesophagus. J Am Vet Med Assoc 2011;238:1622–8. https://doi.org/10.2460/javma.238.12.1622.

[9] Pollard RE. Videofluoroscopic Evaluation of the Pharynx and Upper Esophageal Sphincter in the Dog: A Systematic Review of the Literature. Front Vet Sci 2019;6:117. https://doi.org/10.3389/fvets.2019.00117.

[10] Marks SL, Bonagura JD, Twedt DC, editors. Kirk's current veterinary therapy. 15th edition. St. Louis, Mo: Elsevier/Saunders; 2014. p. 3450–75.

[11] Kook PH, Kempf J, Ruetten M, et al. Wireless ambulatory esophageal pH monitoring in dogs with clinical signs interpreted as gastroesophageal reflux. J Vet Intern Med 2014;28:1716–23. https://doi.org/10.1111/jvim.12461.

[12] Kook PH. Esophagitis in Cats and Dogs. Vet Clin Small Anim Pract 2021;51:1–15. https://doi.org/10.1016/j.cvsm.2020.08.003.

[13] Eivers C, Chicon Rueda R, Liuti T, et al. Retrospective analysis of esophageal imaging features in brachycephalic versus non-brachycephalic dogs based on videofluoroscopic swallowing studies. J Vet Intern Med 2019;33:1740–6. https://doi.org/10.1111/jvim.15547.

[14] Leib MS, Dinnel H, Ward DL, et al. Endoscopic balloon dilation of benign esophageal strictures in dogs and cats. J Vet Intern Med 2001;15:547–52. https://doi.org/10.1892/0891-6640(2001)015<0547:ebdobe>2.3.co;2.

[15] Haines JM. Survey of owners on population characteristics, diagnosis, and environmental, health, and disease associations in dogs with megaesophagus. Res Vet Sci 2019;123:1–6. https://doi.org/10.1016/j.rvsc.2018.11.026.

[16] Grobman ME, Schachtel J, Gyawali CP, et al. Videofluoroscopic swallow study features of lower esophageal sphincter achalasia-like syndrome in dogs. J Vet Intern Med 2019;33:1954–63. https://doi.org/10.1111/jvim.15578.

[17] Lyngby JG, Haines JM, Guess SC. Use of a videofluoroscopic feeding evaluation to guide management of dogs with congenital idiopathic megaoesophagus. Veterinary Medicine and Science 2022;8:1434–42.

[18] Haines JM, Khoo A, Brinkman E, et al. Technique for Evaluation of Gravity-Assisted Esophageal Transit Characteristics in Dogs with Megaesophagus. J Am Anim Hosp Assoc 2019;55:167–77. https://doi.org/10.5326/JAAHA-MS-6711.

[19] Shelton GD, Cardinet IIIGH, Bandman E. Canine masticatory muscle disorders: A study of 29 cases. Muscle Nerve 1987;10:753–66. https://doi.org/10.1002/mus.880100812.

[20] Pollard RE, Marks SL, Davidson A, et al. Quantitative videofluoroscopic evaluation of pharyngeal function in the dog. Vet Radiol Ultrasound 2000;41:409–12. https://doi.org/10.1111/j.1740-8261.2000.tb01862.x.

[21] Davidson AP, Pollard RE, Bannasch DL, et al. Inheritance of cricopharyngeal dysfunction in Golden Retrievers. Am J Vet Res 2004;65:344–9. https://doi.org/10.2460/ajvr.2004.65.344.

[22] Marks SL, Feldman EC, Côté E, et al, editors. Textbook of veterinary internal medicine: diseases of the dog and the cat. 8th edition. St. Louis, Missouri: Elsevier, Inc; 2017. p. 8501–76.

[23] Mace S, Shelton GD, Eddlestone S. Megaesophagus. Compend Contin Educ Vet 2012;34:E1.

[24] Mayhew PD, Marks SL, Pollard R, et al. Prospective evaluation of surgical management of sliding hiatal hernia and gastroesophageal reflux in dogs. Vet Surg 2017;46:1098–109. https://doi.org/10.1111/vsu.12684.

[25] Pollard RE. Imaging evaluation of dogs and cats with Dysphagia. ISRN Vet Sci 2012;2012:238505. https://doi.org/10.5402/2012/238505.

[26] Grobman ME, Hutcheson KD, Lever TE, et al. Mechanical dilation, botulinum toxin A injection, and surgical myotomy with fundoplication for treatment of lower esophageal sphincter achalasia-like syndrome in dogs. J Vet Intern Med 2019;33:1423–33. https://doi.org/10.1111/jvim.15476.

[27] Jo YS, Cha JH, Kim YK, et al. Simultaneous double balloon dilatation using double channel therapeutic endoscope in patients with cricopharyngeal muscle

dysfunction: An observative study. Medicine (Baltimore) 2020;99:e21793. https://doi.org/10.1097/md.0000000 000021793.

[28] Quintavalla F, Menozzi A, Pozzoli C, et al. Sildenafil improves clinical signs and radiographic features in dogs with congenital idiopathic megaoesophagus: a randomised controlled trial. Vet Rec 2017;180:404. https://doi.org/10.1136/vr.103832.

[29] Mehain SO, Haines JM, Guess SC. A randomized crossover study of compounded liquid sildenafil for treatment of generalized megaesophagus in dogs. Am J Vet Res 2022;83:317–23. https://doi.org/10.2460/ajvr.21.02.0 030.

[30] Marks SL, Kook PH, Papich MG, et al. ACVIM consensus statement: Support for rational administration of gastrointestinal protectants to dogs and cats. J Vet Intern Med 2018;32:1823–40. https://doi.org/10.1111/jvim.15337.

[31] Dodd MJ, Dibble SL, Miaskowski C, et al. Randomized clinical trial of the effectiveness of 3 commonly used mouthwashes to treat chemotherapy-induced mucositis. Oral Surg Oral Med Oral Pathol Oral Radiol Endod 2000;90:39–47. https://doi.org/10.1067/moe.2000.105 713.

[32] Zacuto AC, Marks SL, Osborn J, et al. The influence of esomeprazole and cisapride on gastroesophageal reflux during anesthesia in dogs. J Vet Intern Med 2012;26: 518–25. https://doi.org/10.1111/j.1939-1676.2012.009 29.x.

[33] Ullal TV, Kass PH, Conklin JL, et al. High-resolution manometric evaluation of the effects of cisapride on the esophagus during administration of solid and liquid boluses in awake healthy dogs. Am J Vet Res 2016;77: 818–27. https://doi.org/10.2460/ajvr.77.8.818.

[34] Hall JA, Washabau RJ. Diagnosis and treatment of gastric motility disorders. Vet Clin North Am Small Anim Pract 1999;29:377–95.

[35] Schmitz S, Fink T, Failing K, et al. Effects of the neurokinin-1 antagonist maropitant on canine gastric emptying assessed by radioscintigraphy and breath test. Tierarztl Prax Ausg K Kleintiere Heimtiere 2016;44: 163–9. https://doi.org/10.15654/tpk-150039.

[36] Gatineau M, El-Warrak AO, Marretta SM, et al. Locked jaw syndrome in dogs and cats: 37 cases (1998-2005). J Vet Dent 2008;25:16–22. https://doi.org/10.1177/089 875640802500106.

[37] Costanzo G, Minei S, Zini E, et al. Radiographic, MRI, and CT findings in a young dog with Becker-like muscular dystrophy. Vet Radiol Ultrasound 2023;64: E19–22. https://doi.org/10.1111/vru.13200.

[38] Carmichael S, Griffiths IR. Case of isolated sensory trigeminal neuropathy in a dog. Vet Rec 1981;109:280–2. https://doi.org/10.1136/vr.109.13.280.

[39] Cichero JA, Lam P, Steele CM, et al. Development of International Terminology and Definitions for Texture-Modified Foods and Thickened Fluids Used in Dysphagia Management: The IDDSI Framework. Dysphagia 2017;32:293–314. https://doi.org/10.1007/s 00455-016-9758-y.

[40] Wirth R, Dziewas R, Beck AM, et al. Oropharyngeal dysphagia in older persons - from pathophysiology to adequate intervention: a review and summary of an international expert meeting. Clin Interv Aging 2016;11: 189–208. https://doi.org/10.2147/cia.S97481.

[41] Dziewas R, Michou E, Trapl-Grundschober M, et al. European Stroke Organisation and European Society for Swallowing Disorders guideline for the diagnosis and treatment of post-stroke dysphagia. Eur Stroke J 2021;6. https://doi.org/10.1177/23969873211039721:Lxxxix-cxv.

[42] Ueha R, Cotaoco C, Kondo K, et al. Management and Treatment for Dysphagia in Neurodegenerative Disorders. J Clin Med 2023;13. https://doi.org/10.3390/ jcm13010156.

[43] Kuhn MA, Gillespie MB, Ishman SL, et al. Expert Consensus Statement: Management of Dysphagia in Head and Neck Cancer Patients. Otolaryngol Head Neck Surg 2023;168:571–92. https://doi.org/10.1 002/ohn.302.

[44] Newman R, Vilardell N, Clave P, et al. Effect of Bolus Viscosity on the Safety and Efficacy of Swallowing and the Kinematics of the Swallow Response in Patients with Oropharyngeal Dysphagia: White Paper by the European Society for Swallowing Disorders (ESSD). Dysphagia 2016;31:232–49. https://doi.org/10.1007/s00455-016-9696-8.

[45] Clave P, de Kraa M, Arreola V, et al. The effect of bolus viscosity on swallowing function in neurogenic dysphagia. Aliment Pharmacol Ther 2006;24:1385–94. https://doi.org/10.1111/j.1365-2036.2006.03118.x.

[46] Steele CM, Alsanei WA, Ayanikalath S, et al. The influence of food texture and liquid consistency modification on swallowing physiology and function: a systematic review. Dysphagia 2015;30:2–26. https://doi.org/10.1007 /s00455-014-9578-x.

[47] Hansen T, Beck AM, Kjaersgaard A, et al. Second update of a systematic review and evidence-based recommendations on texture modified foods and thickened liquids for adults (above 17 years) with oropharyngeal dysphagia. Clin Nutr ESPEN 2022;49:551–5. https://doi.org/10.1016/j.clnesp.2022.03.039.

[48] Beck AM, Kjaersgaard A, Hansen T, et al. Systematic review and evidence based recommendations on texture modified foods and thickened liquids for adults (above 17 years) with oropharyngeal dysphagia - An updated clinical guideline. Clin Nutr 2018;37:1980–91. https://doi.org/10.1016/j.clnu.2017.09.002.

[49] Marks SL. The principles and practical application of enteral nutrition. Vet Clin North Am Small Anim Pract 1998;28:677–708. https://doi.org/10.1016/s0195-5616 (98)50062-9.

[50] Nguyen NT, Thosani NC, Canto MI, et al. The American Foregut Society White Paper on the Endoscopic Classification of Esophagogastric Junction Integrity. Foregut 2022;2:

339–48. https://doi.org/10.1177/2634516122 1126961.

[51] Reeve EJ, Sutton D, Friend EJ, et al. Documenting the prevalence of hiatal hernia and oesophageal abnormalities in brachycephalic dogs using fluoroscopy. J Small Anim Pract 2017;58:703–8. https://doi.org/10.1111 /jsap.12734.

[52] Poncet CM, Dupre GP, Freiche VG, et al. Long-term results of upper respiratory syndrome surgery and gastrointestinal tract medical treatment in 51 brachycephalic dogs. J Small Anim Pract 2006;47:137–42.

[53] Sanmiguel CP, Ito Y, Hagiike M, et al. The effect of eating on lower esophageal sphincter electrical activity. Am J Physiol Gastrointest Liver Physiol 2009;296:G793–7. https://doi.org/10.1152/ajpgi.90369.2008.

[54] Franzi SJ, Martin CJ, Cox MR, et al. Response of canine lower esophageal sphincter to gastric distension. Am J Physiol 1990;259:G380–5. https://doi.org/10.1152/aj pgi.1990.259.3.G380.

[55] Pettersson GB, Bombeck CT, Nyhus LM. The lower esophageal sphincter: mechanisms of opening and closure. Surgery 1980;88:307–14.

[56] Miyabayashi T, Morgan JP. Gastric emptying in the normal dog a Contrast Radiographic Technique. Vet Radiol 1984;25:187–91.

[57] Russell J, Bass P. Canine gastric emptying of fiber meals: influence of meal viscosity and antroduodenal motility. Am J Physiol 1985;249:G662–7. https://doi.org/10.11 52/ajpgi.1985.249.6.G662.

[58] Palerme JS, Silverstone A, Riedesel EA, et al. A pilot study on the effect of fat loading on the gastrointestinal tract of healthy dogs. J Small Anim Pract 2020;61:732–7. https: //doi.org/10.1111/jsap.13216.

[59] Richards TL, Rankovic A, Cant JP, et al. Effect of total starch and resistant starch in commercial extruded dog foods on gastric emptying in Siberian huskies. Animals 2021;11:2928.

[60] Gruber P, Rubinstein A, Li VHK, et al. Gastric Emptying of Nondigestible Solids in the Fasted Dog. J Pharmac eut Sci 1987;76:117–22.

[61] Teeter BC, Bass P. Gastric Emptying of Liquid Test Meals of Various Temperatures in the Dog. PSEBM (Proc Soc Exp Biol Med) 1982;169:527–31. https://doi.org/10. 3181/00379727-169-41384.

[62] Burrows CF, Bright RM, Spencer CP. Influence of dietary composition on gastric emptying and motility in dogs: potential involvement in acute gastric dilatation. Am J Vet Res 1985;46:2609–12.

[63] Thomas JE. Mechanics and regulation of gastric emptying. Physiol Rev 1957;37:453–74.

[64] Washabau RJ. Gastrointestinal motility disorders and gastrointestinal prokinetic therapy. Veterinary Clinics: Small Animal Practice 2003;33:1007–28.

[65] Warrit K, Boscan P, Ferguson LE, et al. Effect of hospitalization on gastrointestinal motility and pH in dogs. J Am Vet Med Assoc 2017;251:65–70.

[66] Chang P, Friedenberg F. Obesity and GERD. Gastroenterol Clin North Am 2014;43:161–73. https://doi.org/10 .1016/j.gtc.2013.11.009.

[67] Liu NC, Adams VJ, Kalmar L, et al. Whole-Body Barometric Plethysmography Characterizes Upper Airway Obstruction in 3 Brachycephalic Breeds of Dogs. J Vet Intern Med 2016;30:853–65. https://doi.org/10.111 1/jvim.13933.

[68] Luciani E, Reinero C, Grobman M. Evaluation of aerodigestive disease and diagnosis of sliding hiatal hernia in brachycephalic and nonbrachycephalic dogs. J Vet Intern Med 2022;36:1229–36. https://doi.org/10.1111/jvi m.16485.

[69] Surdea-Blaga T, Negrutiu DE, Palage M, et al. Food and Gastroesophageal Reflux Disease. Curr Med Chem 2019;26:3497–511. https://doi.org/10.2174/09298673 24666170515123807.

[70] Zhang M, Hou ZK, Huang ZB, et al. Dietary and Lifestyle Factors Related to Gastroesophageal Reflux Disease: A Systematic Review. Ther Clin Risk Manag 2021;17: 305–23. https://doi.org/10.2147/tcrm.S296680.

[71] Mazzei MJ, Bissett SA, Murphy KM, et al. Eosinophilic esophagitis in a dog. J Am Vet Med Assoc 2009;235: 61–5. https://doi.org/10.2460/javma.235.1.61.

[72] Votto M, De Filippo M, Lenti MV, et al. Diet Therapy in Eosinophilic Esophagitis. Focus on a Personalized Approach. Front Pediatr 2021;9:820192. https: //doi.org/10.3389/fped.2021.820192.

[73] Yu MK, Freeman LM, Heinze CR, et al. Comparison of complication rates in dogs with nasoesophageal versus nasogastric feeding tubes. J Vet Emerg Crit Care (San Antonio) 2013;23:300–4. https://doi.org/10.1111/vec. 12048.

[74] Dumont R, Lemetayer J, Desquilbet L, et al. Tolerability of naso-esophageal feeding tubes in dogs and cats at home: Retrospective review of 119 cases. J Vet Intern Med 2023;37:2315–21. https://doi.org/10.1111/j vim.16732.

[75] Crowe DT Jr. Use of a nasogastric tube for gastric and esophageal decompression in the dog and cat. J Am Vet Med Assoc 1986;188:1178–82.

[76] Holahan M, Abood S, Hauptman J, et al. Intermittent and continuous enteral nutrition in critically ill dogs: a prospective randomized trial. J Vet Intern Med 2010; 24:520–6. https://doi.org/10.1111/j.1939-1676.2010.0 487.x.

[77] Ragins H, Levenson SM, Signer R, et al. Intrajejunal administration of an elemental diet at neutral pH avoids pancreatic stimulation: Studies in dog and man. Am J Surg 1973;126:606–14.

[78] Wang Z, Song Q-Z, Jiang J-X, et al. Nutritional therapy for gastroparesis. Journal of Nutritional Oncology 2023;8.

[79] Shelton GD, Willard MD, Cardinet GH, Lindstrom J. Acquired myasthenia gravis. Selective involvement of esophageal, pharyngeal, and facial muscles. J Vet Intern

Med 1990;4:281–4. https://doi.org/10.1111/j.1939-16 76.1990.tb03124.x.

[80] Winston JM 3rd, Mann FAT, Dean L. Management and outcomes of 13 dogs treated with a modified Heller myotomy and Dor fundoplication for lower esophageal sphincter achalasia-like syndrome. Vet Surg 2023;52: 315–29. https://doi.org/10.1111/vsu.13912.

[81] Montoro-Huguet MA. Dietary and Nutritional Support in Gastrointestinal Diseases of the Upper Gastrointestinal Tract (I): Esophagus. Nutrients 2022;14. https://doi.org/10.3390/nu14224819.

[82] Manning K, Birkenheuer AJ, Briley J, et al. Intermittent At-Home Suctioning of Esophageal Content for Prevention of Recurrent Aspiration Pneumonia in 4 Dogs with Megaesophagus. J Vet Intern Med 2016;30: 1715–9. https://doi.org/10.1111/jvim.14527.

[83] Lin Y, Wan G, Wu H, et al. The sensitivity and specificity of the modified volume-viscosity swallow test for dysphagia screening among neurological patients. Front Neurol 2022;13:961893. https://doi.org/10.3389/fneur.2022.961893.

[84] Clavé P, Arreola V, Romea M, et al. Accuracy of the volume-viscosity swallow test for clinical screening of oropharyngeal dysphagia and aspiration. Clin Nutr 2008;27: 806–15. https://doi.org/10.1016/j.clnu.2008.06.011.

[85] Harris RA, Grobman ME, Allen MJ, et al. Standardization of a Videofluoroscopic Swallow Study Protocol to Investigate Dysphagia in Dogs. J Vet Intern Med 2017;31: 383–93. https://doi.org/10.1111/jvim.14676.

SECTION V - UROLOGY

Advances in Small Animal Care 5 (2024) 179–188

ADVANCES IN SMALL ANIMAL CARE

New Therapeutic Approaches to Management of Anemia and Iron Metabolism in Chronic Kidney Disease

Shelly L. Vaden, DVM, PhD, DACVIM (SAIM)[a],*, Jessica Quimby, DVM, PhD, DACVIM (SAIM)[b], Cathy E. Langston, DVM, DACVIM (SAIM)[b]

[a]Department of Clinical Sciences, College of Veterinary Medicine, North Carolina State University, 1052 William Moore Drive, Raleigh, NC 27607, USA; [b]Department of Veterinary Clinical Sciences, College of Veterinary Medicine, The Ohio State University, 601 Vernon Tharp Street, Columbus, OH 43210, USA

KEYWORDS

- Anemia of chronic kidney disease • HIF-PH inhibitor (hypoxia-inducible factor-prolyl hydroxylase inhibitor) • Iron
- Hepcidin • Erythropoietin • Molidustat • Hypoxia

KEY POINTS

- Anemia, a common sequela of chronic kidney disease (CKD), is a negative predictor of survival and has the potential to exacerbate progression of CKD, even with decreases in hematocrit.
- Available treatments include blood transfusion, human recombinant erythropoietin products (not labeled for use in animals), and hypoxia-inducible factor-prolyl hydroxylase inhibitors.
- Hypoxia-inducible factor-prolyl hydroxylase inhibitors block the enzyme that degrades hypoxia-inducible factor, thus stabilizing it and stimulating the body to produce more erythropoietin.
- Patients with CKD may have an absolute (eg, from gastrointestinal blood loss or blood sampling) or functional iron deficiency, likely mediated by excess hepcidin.
- Hepcidin is increased by inflammation and CKD, leading to decreased intestinal iron absorption and decreased release of iron from storage cells.

INTRODUCTION

Anemia is common in cats and dogs with chronic kidney disease (CKD) and is typically characterized as normocytic, normochromic nonregenerative in nature. Approximately 30% to 65% of cats and 60% of dogs with CKD will develop anemia associated with CKD, and the incidence and severity increases with International Renal Interest Society (IRIS) stage (Table 1) [1–5]. Clinical signs attributed to anemia may include mucous membrane pallor, heart murmur, fatigue, listlessness, lethargy, weakness, and inappetence.

Anemia of CKD is usually multifactorial in origin. The primary cause is inadequate production of erythropoietin (EPO), which regulates red blood cell (RBC) production. EPO stimulates RBC production in the bone marrow by binding to a receptor on erythroid progenitors that stimulate those cells to differentiate into normoblasts and then mature erythrocytes [1]. Other factors that contribute to the anemia of CKD include absolute and functional iron deficiency (FID), poor nutrition, chronic inflammation or infection, effects of medications, reduced RBC lifespan, excessive blood taken for testing,

*Corresponding author, *E-mail address:* slvaden@ncsu.edu

https://doi.org/10.1016/j.yasa.2024.06.013
2666-450X/24/

TABLE 1
Incidence of Anemia by International Renal Interest Society Chronic Kidney Disease Stage [3,4]

IRIS Stage	2	3	4
Cats[a]	4.8%	17.7%	53.3%
Dogs[b]	47%	71%	82%

[a] Anemia defined as hematocrit <25%.
[b] Anemia defined as hematocrit <37%.

and spontaneous bleeding [1,6]. Cats with CKD have a relative iron deficiency and excess hepcidin [7]. Hepcidin, a key regulator in iron homeostasis, is upregulated in inflammatory environments and leads to sequestration of iron in cells. In addition to the activities of hepcidin, proinflammatory cytokines also inhibit erythropoiesis in inflammatory states. Although gastric ulceration is less common in dogs and cats than humans [8], chronic low-grade gastrointestinal (GI) hemorrhage from mucosal friability and uremic thrombocytopathy may also contribute to anemia [6,9]. Lastly, RBC lifespan may be shortened due to the deleterious effects of uremic toxins [10].

CONSEQUENCES OF ANEMIA

Several studies have identified anemia as a negative predictor of survival in CKD [3,5,11,12], and even relatively small reductions in PCV have been associated with progression (median PCV 31% vs 35%) [13]. Anemia triggers physiologic adaptations that can be detrimental, including an increased release of norepinephrine, renin, angiotensin II, and aldosterone that can lead to increased heart workload and hypertension [14]. Anemia may also cause left heart enlargement that could predispose patients to heart failure and fluid overload [1,14,15]. In patients where high-output heart failure has occurred secondary to anemia, prompt correction of the anemia is key to clinical resolution [14].

Anemia has the potential to exacerbate progression of CKD as it compromises oxygen delivery to the kidney. Hypoxia is a driver in the formation of fibrosis and is thus thought to be a critical mediator in the progression of CKD [13,16,17]. The inflammation and fibrosis associated with tubulointerstitial disease results in the expansion of interstitium, and the subsequent increased diffusion distance compromises tubular cell access to peritubular capillary blood supply. Glomerular damage and vasoconstriction of afferent arterioles

decrease postglomerular peritubular capillary blood flow [16]. Vascular endothelial growth factor (VEGF) is integral to vascular health, and VEGF concentrations are decreased in CKD [18–20]. These processes result in capillary rarefaction, which is loss of peritubular capillaries and thus reduction in the density of blood supply surrounding the tubule [21]. If the already compromised blood supply reaching tubular cells is anemic, with poor oxygen carrying capacity, the consequence is hypoxia. Hypoxia results in fibrosis, tubular cell transdifferentiation and activation of fibroblasts, further exacerbating the diseased state [16,17]. Thus, the resolution of anemia, particularly in late stage disease where fibrosis and capillary rarefaction are pronounced, is a key therapeutic goal [13,21–23].

Importantly, when assessing the patient as a whole, moderate-to-severe anemia likely has the potential to affect quality of life in feline patients due to weakness, lethargy, and inappetence. Anemia (packed cell volume [PCV] <27%) was associated with poorer health-related quality of life scores in cats with CKD [24].

PHYSIOLOGY OF RED BLOOD CELL PRODUCTION

RBC production in the bone marrow is regulated by the hormone EPO, which is mainly produced by peritubular interstitial cells called renal erythropoietin-producing (REP) cells in the corticomedullary region of the kidney. As kidney disease progresses, it is thought that the number of active REP cells decrease and anemia can result due to lack of stimulation of RBC progenitors in the bone marrow by erythropoietin. EPO is controlled by hypoxia-inducible factor (HIF), a master gene regulator that is responsible for the physiologic response to reduced tissue oxygenation. It activates key genes to restore oxygen balance and protect against cellular damage [17,25]. Under normoxic conditions, HIFα is hydroxylated, and this allows it to be recognized by von Hippil-Lindau E3 ubiquitin ligase, resulting in ubiquitination [25]. This is a signal to the cell that permits degradation by lysosomes. Under hypoxic conditions, HIFα cannot be hydroxylated and instead translocates to the nucleus where it combines with HIFβ and induces the transcription of erythropoietin [25]. The regulation of EPO has only recently been described in detail, and many aspects of this pathophysiology still remain to be explained. It is not clear why REP cells fail to produce EPO in CKD despite tissue hypoxia, as recent studies have demonstrated it is not simply due to a loss of functional tissue [26,27]. One theory is microenvironmental relative hyperoxia, whereupon the immediate environment surrounding the REP cells is saturated with oxygen due to the loss of neighboring cells, with a resultant decrease in local oxygen utilization [26,27]. In people it is well established that CKD is associated with inflammation. The degree of inflammation worsens with the severity of CKD, but even patients who are not dialysis dependent have evidence of inflammation [28]. CKD in dogs and cats has also been associated with inflammation [29,30], and inflammation can suppress the effects of EPO, causing or worsening anemia. Additional factors that result in the suppression of EPO include mediators of fibrosis (transforming growth factor [TGF]-β, nuclear factor kappa light chain enhancer of activated B cells [NFkβ], and interleukin [IL]-6), fibroblast growth factor 23 (FGF-23) and uremic toxins [10,31,32]. Although complex, the regulation of HIF and EPO is important to understand due to the availability of a class of drugs referred to as HIF-PHIs (HIF-prolyl hydroxylase inhibitors). These drugs have been utilized in human medicine for some time and recently have become available in veterinary medicine [33]. Mechanistically, HIF-PHIs work to inhibit hydroxylation of HIFα even in the normoxic state, resulting in the increased production of endogenous EPO [34].

TREATMENT OPTIONS

Blood Transfusion

Blood transfusion has long been available to treat severe, symptomatic anemia (Table 2). This may arise in patients with recent diagnosis of advanced CKD, in patients with untreated (or ineffectively treated) anemia of CKD, and in patients with an acute hemorrhagic condition such as GI bleeding. Blood transfusion has the benefit of rapid correction of anemia. Downsides of blood transfusion include the risk of hypersensitivity reactions or acute lung injury, volume overload with rapid administration, and shortened survival of red blood cells in a uremic environment. If a transfusion is needed, the goal is to restore the packed cell volume to the low end of the normal range, and then follow with a longer term therapy (see later discussion) to sustain the red cell mass.

Erythropoiesis Stimulating Agents

Erythropoiesis stimulating agents (ESAs) including erythropoietin analogs, such as epoetin and darbepoetin, have been used by veterinarians for decades. Epoetin alpha (Epogen, Amgen, Thousand Oaks, CA; Procrit, Janssen, Beerse, Belguim) is a human recombinant erythropoietin that has been associated with an immunogenic reaction leading to pure red cell aplasia in 20% to 25% of dogs and cats and is no longer recommended. Darbepoetin is a human recombinant erythropoietin that is hyperglycosylated, which prolongs the half-life and appears to reduce the immunogenicity. Darbepoetin is commonly used in the management of anemia associated with CKD (Fig. 1) [35,36]. In a retrospective study of 25 cats with CKD receiving darbepoetin, 56% were considered to have responded to the drug, with response defined as reaching and maintaining a PCV of 25% or greater at day 56 [35]. The median increase in PCV was 8%. The majority of cats (21 of 25) were treated with a maximum dose of 1 μg/kg subcutaneously weekly at some point during treatment. In responder cats, the median time to response was 21 days (range, 7–47 days). In a retrospective study of 33 dogs with CKD receiving darbepoetin, 85% responded, defined as reaching a PCV of 30% or higher [36]. The median maximum dose administered was 0.8 μg/kg subcutaneously weekly. The median time to response was 29 days (range, 6–106 days). Complications were common. In the cats, the blood pressure increased by a median of 30 mm Hg, and 2 cats were started on antihypertensive medications. Four cats had

TABLE 2 Anemia Treatments		
Agent	**Mechanism of Action**	**Dose**
Blood transfusion		Packed RBCs: 6–10 mL/kg IV Whole Blood: 12–20 mL/kg IV
Darbepoetin	Hyperglycosylated human recombinant erythropoietin	Starting dose: 0.45–1 mcg/kg subcutaneous (SQ) weekly Maintenance dose: 0.45–1 mcg/kg SQ q 2–3 wk
Feline erythropoietin	Feline recombinant erythropoietin	Not available
Feline erythropoietin gene therapy	AAV gene therapy	Not available (studies involved 1–2 IM injections)
Molidustat	HIF-PHI	5 mg/kg PO daily for 28 d, stop for 7 d, repeat cycle

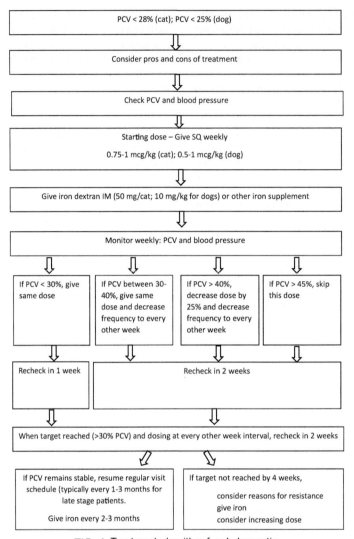

FIG. 1 Treatment algorithm for darbepoetin.

seizures or acute neurologic events. Two cats had nonresponsive anemia without an identifiable cause, but these were not consistent with pure red cell aplasia. In the dogs, hypertension was noted during treatment in 24 of 25 dogs with blood pressure monitoring and required treatment in 13 dogs. Mild hyperkalemia developed in 42% but did not need treatment. Seizures occurred in 5 dogs. Pure red cell aplasia was considered likely in one dog. Darbepoetin is not Food and Drug Administration (FDA)-approved for use in dogs or cats. Feline and canine recombinant erythropoietin products have been tested in pilot studies, but these products are not commercially available [37,38].

Hypoxia Inducible Factor-Prolyl Hydroxylase Inhibitors

A novel drug to treat anemia of CKD in cats (molidustat, Varenzin-CA1, Elanco, Indianapolis, IN) was conditionally approved by the FDA in 2023. This drug is an HIF-PHI. As mentioned earlier, HIF is composed of an HIF-1 β subunit and an HIFα subunit, which could be HIF-1α, HIF-2α, or HIF-3α. Among the α subunits, HIF-2α is believed to be of greatest importance for the regulation of hypoxia-inducible EPO expression in the mammalian kidney [39–42]. Regulation of the HIF-2α subunit is controlled by HIF-prolyl hydroxylase (PH) expressed in multiple tissues including renal epithelial cells. HIF-PH enzymes use oxygen and 2-oxoglutarate as substrates, and thus their activity is controlled by changes in oxygen levels. In normoxic conditions, HIF-PH enzymes deactivate HIF by the hydroxylation of proline residues, followed by ubiquitination and proteasomal degradation [42]. Under hypoxic conditions, HIF-PH enzymes become inactive, and HIF is no longer degraded, thereby activating transcription of the EPO gene in REP cells located in the peritubular interstitium of kidneys, increasing EPO production and its release into the circulation [39–43]. HIF-PHIs inhibit prolyl hydroxylase activity, even in normoxic conditions, leading to persistence of HIFα and continued production of EPO.

A study of molidustat in healthy cats showed a robust increase in hematocrit [44]. At a daily oral dose of 5 mg/kg, the hematocrit was significantly higher than placebo treated cats at day 14 (54.4% vs 40.3%), and treatment was stopped at day 23 because the hematocrit exceeded 60%. The hematocrit slowly decreased to baseline over the next 5 weeks. Mean erythropoietin concentrations were significantly increased at 6 hours after molidustat administration but returned to baseline by 24 hours. Vomiting was more frequent in the treated group compared to the placebo group.

In a pilot study of client-owned cats with CKD and a hematocrit under 28%, 15 cats were treated with 5 mg/kg molidustat daily and 6 cats were treated with placebo [33]. The hematocrit was higher in treated cats compared to placebo cats at 21 days. However, in this 28 day study, only 50% of molidustat-treated cats reached the criteria of treatment success, defined as an increase in hematocrit of 4% or a 25% increase from baseline. In the treated group, hematocrit increased from 23.6% ± 3.23 at day 0 to 27.8% ± 5.25 at day 28. Eight cats continued receiving molidustat after the 28 day study, at doses of 2.5 to 5 mg/kg daily. Six of 8 cats (75%) were considered treatment successes at day 56. Vomiting was the most frequently reported adverse event and occurred in 6 of 15 cats. Three cats vomited once, 1 cat vomited twice, 1 cat vomited three times, and 1 cat vomited 9 times. None of the cats in the study developed hypertension or seizures.

As of the time of this report, molidustat is conditionally approved by the FDA, which prohibits off-label use. The label instructions include daily treatment for 28 days, then a 7 day discontinuation, followed by repeated cycles if needed (Fig. 2). Although healthy cats were at risk for polycythemia without a break in administration, polycythemia has not been noted in cats with CKD.

In addition to their effect on increasing erythropoietin, HIF-PHIs have been shown to suppress hepatic hepcidin and upregulate iron metabolism and transport genes in rats [45]. In contrast to darbepoetin, which has been associated with increases in blood pressure, molidustat decreased blood pressure in rats and had no effect in cats in a pilot study [33,36,39]. Treatment has also ameliorated kidney damage, inflammation, and fibrosis in rats [39,41,42].

Gene Therapy

Recently, the use of an adeno-associated virus vectored (AAV)-based gene therapeutic agent that allows for the expression of feline erythropoietin was evaluated in 23 cats [46]. A single intramuscular injection led to the desired increase in PCV within 28 to 70 days in 86% of cats. Polycythemia developed in 3 cats. Although the therapy was generally well tolerated, hypertension and encephalopathy were noted in some cats, as has been reported in association with administration of other ESAs. Further study of this agent will be needed to determine its full efficacy and safety, including an assessment of whether repeat doses are required or not to maintain an adequate response.

IRON HOMEOSTASIS, ASSESSMENT AND TREATMENT

Iron is essential for oxygen transport, cellular respiration, and DNA synthesis and repair, largely because of its ability to donate and accept electrons. Iron is abundant and the body must tightly regulate its absorption and storage because iron excess leads to the generation of toxic reactive oxygen species. The concentration of iron in the blood is controlled by 3 key areas: dietary iron absorption in the duodenum and upper jejunum; iron recycling by the reticuloendothelial system; and iron release from hepatocytes [47]. Ingested iron is absorbed by the enterocyte in the ferrous form (Fe^{2+}) [48]. Iron that is ingested as ferric iron (Fe^{3+}) is reduced to ferrous iron by the ascorbate-dependent hemoprotein duodenal cytochrome b before uptake [47]. Some compounds found in the diet can bind iron and prevent its absorption. Most of the absorbed iron is not needed and is stored in the enterocyte as ferritin until the cell is shed and the iron is excreted in the feces. When iron is needed, it is transported through the enterocyte basolateral membrane by ferroportin where it becomes bound to plasma transferrin and is transported to one of many sites. Iron is stored in the form of ferritin (the major intracellular iron storage protein) or hemosiderin in the liver, spleen, bone marrow, duodenum, and skeletal muscles. However, the largest source of iron in the body is found within

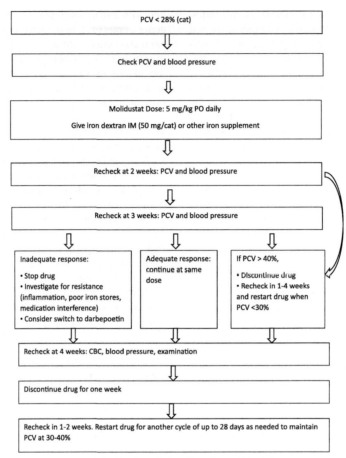

FIG. 2 Treatment algorithm for molidustat.

heme (hemoglobin, myoglobin, and hemoproteins). Iron loss from the body is not regulated but occurs mainly from shedding of enterocytes, uroepithelial cells, and epidermal cells.

Iron regulatory proteins help to maximize iron supply when there is a deficit and restrict iron absorption and promote storage when the cells are replete. Importantly, when the body is replete, the system is downregulated by hepcidin, an acute phase reactant protein produced in the liver. Hepcidin inhibits intestinal iron absorption and intracellular iron transport including iron release from macrophages and hepatocytes, leading to sequestration of iron. Hepcidin concentrations are reduced when there is anemia, hypoxia, or iron deficiency. Hepcidin concentrations are increased when the body iron stores are replete (ie, ferritin is high), during systemic inflammatory states or when the glomerular filtration rate is reduced (because hepcidin undergoes renal elimination and metabolism) [49,50].

Absolute iron deficiency (AID) is defined by reduced iron stores whereas FID (aka iron-restricted erythropoiesis) is defined by adequate iron stores but insufficient iron availability. Hepcidin excess is a main contributor to disordered iron homeostasis that occurs in CKD, most likely causing impaired dietary iron absorption and reticuloendothelial cell iron blockade (ie, anemia of chronic inflammation) leading to FID [50]. In addition, patients with CKD may have AID from increased iron losses due to platelet dysfunction-induced chronic hemorrhage and blood sample collections. Dialysis patients may lose additional iron via blood trapping in the dialysis apparatus. ESA administration further depletes the iron pools by increasing erythropoiesis but also causes FID by causing a supply/demand mismatch. FID related to ESAs can be difficult to differentiate from anemia of chronic disease.

The classic means of assessing iron stores is problematic in patients with CKD (Table 3) [51–53]. Serum iron

TABLE 3
Assessment of Iron Stores

Parameter	AID	Functional Iron Deficiency	Caveats in Patients with CKD
Serum iron	Reduced	Reduced	Does not reflect total body iron
Transferrin	Normal to increased	Normal to decreased	Indirectly measured by TIBC Inflammation obscures AID
Percent saturation	Decreased	Normal to decreased	Represents serum iron:TIBC ratio When decreased, does not differentiate AID from FID Increased consistent with iron overload
Ferritin	Decreased	Normal to increased	Assay not readily available for dogs and cats
Bone marrow iron	Decreased	Increased	Semiquantitative Gold standard
Hepcidin	Decreased	Increased	Assay not readily available for dogs and cats

Abbreviations: AID, absolute iron deficiency; FID, functional iron deficiency; TIBC, total iron binding capacity.

concentrations do not accurately reflect total body iron. Ferritin, an acute phase reactant, is a better indicator of total body iron in health; low ferritin concentrations indicate AID, but normal or increased ferritin concentrations do not exclude AID because inflammation increases ferritin. Transferrin concentrations, indirectly measured as total iron binding capacity (TIBC), can be normal to increased with AID. However, transferrin is a negative acute phase reactant and decreases with inflammation, potentially masking iron deficiency. Percent saturation (ie, transferrin saturation, TSAT) is the ratio of serum iron to TIBC, or the percentage of transferrin that is occupied by iron. Low TSAT is suggestive of iron deficiency and does not discriminate between absolute versus functional, whereas increased TSAT is suggestive of iron overload. ESAs can strip iron from transferrin faster than it can be mobilized leading to decreased TSAT. While patients with FID would be expected to have low serum transferrin and high-to-normal ferritin, none of these parameters consistently differentiate between absolute and FID. Semiquantitative assessment of iron stores in bone marrow or liver with Prussian blue staining is the gold standard for assessing iron stores. An animal with AID should have an absence of iron fragments in bone marrow whereas absence of erythroid precursors with the presence of iron stores suggests FID.

Novel biomarkers have been proposed to assess iron stores in patients with CKD, including soluble transferrin receptor, percentage of hypochromic RBCs, reticulocyte hemoglobin content, hepcidin, and plasma neutrophil gelatinase-associated lipocalin [51]. The percentage of hypochromic RBC and the content of hemoglobin in reticulocytes may be indicators of iron deficiency and

anticipated response to iron administration. In a study of reticulocyte indices and iron status in cats with CKD, reticulocyte hemoglobin concentration was found to add some value to the diagnosis of iron deficiency diagnosed by TSAT, whereas the mean corpuscular volume (MCV) of reticulocyte and standard erythrocyte indices did not contribute to the diagnosis [54].

Iron supplementation is an important part of the treatment of anemia of CKD and has been shown to improve physical, cognitive, and immune functions in people with CKD [55]. However, optimal management is problematic and unclear. Iron therapy is recommended in people who have low serum ferritin and TSAT [53]. Several oral iron preparations are available, but iron citrate may offer an advantage of also acting as a phosphate binder. Oral iron supplementation can cause GI upset and anorexia as well as alter the microbiome, promoting the growth of potentially pathogenic bacteria while reducing the population of protective lactobacilli and bifidobacteria [48]. Parenteral iron (typically intravenous [IV] for people, intramuscular [IM] for dogs and cats) circumvents poor iron absorption and GI adverse effects of oral iron but poses a small, yet real, risk of iron overload. In people, an iron-administered IV may be more effective than oral therapy, but the comparable safety remains debatable [56].

Therapeutically blocking hepcidin might improve dietary iron absorption from the gut and iron mobilization within the body [57]. This could potentially occur if one were to inhibit the molecules leading to production of hepcidin with agents such as IL-6 antibodies, tumor necrosis factor alpha and transforming growth factor gamma (TGFγ inhibitors, or pentoxifylline. Direct hepcidin antagonists and hepcidin-ferroportin stabilizers are being evaluated for use in people.

FUTURE DIRECTIONS

Due to the risks and expense of previously available treatments for anemia, treatment has frequently been delayed until anemia is severe or symptomatic. Given the evidence that even mild anemia is associated with progression, future research should be directed to determine if earlier treatment of anemia will preserve renal function. With the advent of new drugs to treat anemia, therapy can be individualized. Darbepoetin has been successful for the majority of patients treated. HIF-PH inhibitors may prove to be a valuable tool to prevent mild anemia from progressing. The importance of FID is gaining more attention. New biomarkers may help to determine iron status more precisely in patients with anemia, and better understanding of hepcidin may lead to the development of more effective iron-replacement strategies.

CLINICS CARE POINTS

- Anemia of CKD, even if mild, likely warrants treatment.
- Darbepoetin is effective in about 50% to 85% of cats and dogs, whereas molidustat is effective in about 75% of cats.
- Differentiation of FID from AID in patients with CKD is difficult with the diagnostic tests that are standardly available.
- Reticulocyte hemoglobin content may add value to diagnosing iron deficiency, but more study is needed.
- Oral iron citrate also acts as a phosphate binder.

DISCLOSURE

S.L. Vaden: consultant for Elanco US Inc (VarenzinTM-CA-1); received research funding from Scout Bio, Inc (SB-101). C.E. Langston: consultant for Elanco US Inc (VarenzinTM-CA-1) J.M. Quimby: consultant for Elanco US Inc (VarenzinTM-CA-1).

REFERENCES

[1] Chalhoub S, Langston C, Eatroff A. Anemia of renal disease: what it is, what to do and what's new. J Feline Med Surg 2011;13:629–40.

[2] Elliott J, Barber PJ. Feline chronic renal failure: clinical findings in 80 cases diagnosed between 1992 and 1995. J Small Anim Pract 1998;39:78–85.

[3] King JN, Tasker S, Gunn-Moore DA, et al. Prognostic factors in cats with chronic kidney disease. J Vet Intern Med 2007;21:906–16.

[4] Lippi I, Perondi F, Lubas G, et al. Erythrogram patterns in dogs with chronic kidney disease. Vet Sci 2021;8:123.

[5] King LG, Giger U, Diserens D, et al. Anemia of chronic renal failure in dogs. J Vet Intern Med 1992;6:264–70.

[6] Borin-Crivellenti S, Crivellenti LZ, Gilor C, et al. Anemia in canine chronic kidney disease is multifactorial and associated with decreased erythroid precursor cells, gastrointestinal bleeding. Systemic Inflammation 2023; 84:1–6.

[7] Gest J, Langston C, Eatroff A. Iron Status of Cats with Chronic Kidney Disease. J Vet Intern Med 2015;29: 1488–93.

[8] McLeland SM, Lunn KF, Duncan CG, et al. Relationship among serum creatinine, serum gastrin, calcium-phosphorus product, and uremic gastropathy in cats with chronic kidney disease. J Vet Intern Med 2014;28: 827–37.

[9] Benson KK, Quimby JM, Shropshire SB, et al. Evaluation of platelet function in cats with and without kidney disease: a pilot study. J Feline Med Surg 2020;23(8):1098612X20972069.

[10] Lau WL, Savoj J, Nakata MB, et al. Altered microbiome in chronic kidney disease: systemic effects of gut-derived uremic toxins. Clin Sci (Lond) 2018;132:509–22.

[11] Chakrabarti S, Syme HM, Elliott J. Clinicopathological variables predicting progression of azotemia in cats with chronic kidney disease. J Vet Intern Med 2012;26: 275–81.

[12] Geddes RF, Elliott J, Syme HM. Relationship between Plasma Fibroblast Growth Factor-23 Concentration and Survival Time in Cats with Chronic Kidney Disease. J Vet Intern Med 2015;29:1494–501.

[13] Elliott J. Therapeutics of managing reduced red cell mass associated with chronic kidney disease - Is there a case for earlier intervention? J Vet Pharmacol Ther 2023;46: 145–57.

[14] Hammond H, Pierce KV. Treatment of high-output cardiac failure secondary to anemia in three cats. J Fel Med Surg 2023;9(1).

[15] Wilson HE, Jasani S, Wagner TB, et al. Signs of left heart volume overload in severely anaemic cats. J Feline Med Surg 2010;12:904–9.

[16] Nangaku M. Chronic hypoxia and tubulointerstitial injury: a final common pathway to end-stage renal failure. J Am Soc Nephrol 2006;17:17–25.

[17] Spencer S, Wheeler-Jones C, Elliott J. Hypoxia and chronic kidney disease: Possible mechanisms, therapeutic targets, and relevance to cats. Vet J 2021;274:105714.

[18] Mayer G. Capillary rarefaction, hypoxia, VEGF and angiogenesis in chronic renal disease. Nephrol Dial Transplant 2011;26:1132–7.

[19] Habenicht LM, Webb TL, Clauss LA, et al. Urinary cytokine levels in apparently healthy cats and cats with chronic kidney disease. J Feline Med Surg 2013;15:99–104.

[20] Lourenco BN, Coleman AE, Tarigo JL, et al. Evaluation of profibrotic gene transcription in renal tissues from cats with naturally occurring chronic kidney disease. J Vet Intern Med 2020;34:1476–87.

[21] Paschall RE, Quimby JM, Cianciolo RE, et al. Assessment of peritubular capillary rarefaction in kidneys of cats with chronic kidney disease. J Vet Intern Med 2023;37:556–66.

[22] Chakrabarti S, Syme HM, Brown CA, et al. Histomorphometry of feline chronic kidney disease and correlation with markers of renal dysfunction. Vet Pathol 2013;50:147–55.

[23] McLeland SM, Cianciolo RE, Duncan CG, et al. A comparison of biochemical and histopathologic staging in cats with chronic kidney disease. Vet Pathol 2015;52:524–34.

[24] Lorbach S, Quimby J, Nijveldt E, et al. Evaluation of Health-Related Quality of Life in Cats with Chronic Kidney Disease. 2022;88.

[25] Sugahara M, Tanaka T, Nangaku M. Prolyl hydroxylase domain inhibitors as a novel therapeutic approach against anemia in chronic kidney disease. Kidney Int 2017;92:306–12.

[26] Dahl SL, Bapst AM, Khodo SN, et al. Fount, fate, features, and function of renal erythropoietin-producing cells. Pflugers Arch 2022;474:783–97.

[27] Dahl SL, Pfundstein S, Hunkeler R, et al. Fate-mapping of erythropoietin-producing cells in mouse models of hypoxaemia and renal tissue remodelling reveals repeated recruitment and persistent functionality. Acta Physiol 2022;234:e13768.

[28] Gupta J, Mitra N, Kanetsky PA, et al. Association between albuminuria, kidney function, and inflammatory biomarker profile in CKD in CRIC. Clin J Am Soc Nephrol 2012;7:1938–46.

[29] Nentwig A, Schweighauser A, Maissen-Villiger C, et al. Assessment of the expression of biomarkers of uremic inflammation in dogs with renal disease. Am J Vet Res 2016;77.218–24.

[30] Javard R, Grimes C, Bau-Gaudreault L, et al. Acute-Phase Proteins and Iron Status in Cats with Chronic Kidney Disease. J Vet Intern Med 2017;31:457–64.

[31] Shih HM, Pan SY, Wu CJ, et al. Transforming growth factor-beta1 decreases erythropoietin production through repressing hypoxia-inducible factor 2alpha in erythropoietin-producing cells. J Biomed Sci 2021;28:73.

[32] Afsar B, Kanbay M, Afsar RE. Interconnections of fibroblast growth factor 23 and klotho with erythropoietin and hypoxia-inducible factor. Mol Cell Biochem 2022;477:1973–85.

[33] Charles S, Sussenberger R, Settje T, et al. Use of molidustat, a hypoxia-inducible factor prolyl hydroxylase inhibitor, in chronic kidney disease-associated anemia in cats. J Vet Intern Med 2024;38(1):197–204.

[34] Locatelli F, Minutolo R, De Nicola L, et al. Evolving Strategies in the Treatment of Anaemia in Chronic Kidney Disease: The HIF-Prolyl Hydroxylase Inhibitors. Drugs 2022;82:1565–89.

[35] Chalhoub S, Langston CE, Farrelly J. The use of darbepoetin to stimulate erythropoiesis in anemia of chronic kidney disease in cats: 25 cases. J Vet Intern Med 2012;26:363–9.

[36] Fiocchi EH, Cowgill LD, Brown DC, et al. The Use of Darbepoetin to Stimulate Erythropoiesis in the Treatment of Anemia of Chronic Kidney Disease in Dogs. J Vet Intern Med 2017;31:476–85.

[37] Randolph JE, Scarlett J, Stokol T, et al. Clinical efficacy and safety of recombinant canine erythropoietin in dogs with anemia of chronic renal failure and dogs with recombinant human erythropoietin-induced red cell aplasia. J Vet Intern Med 2004;18:81–91.

[38] Randolph JE, Scarlett JM, Stokol T, et al. Expression, bioactivity, and clinical assessment of recombinant feline erythropoietin. Am J Vet Res 2004;65:1355–66.

[39] Flamme I, Oehme F, Ellinghaus P, et al. Mimicking hypoxia to treat anemia: HIF-stabilizer BAY 85-3934 (Molidustat) stimulates erythropoietin production without hypertensive effects. PLoS One 2014;9:e111838.

[40] Beck H, Jeske M, Thede K, et al. Discovery of Molidustat (BAY 85-3934): A Small-Molecule Oral HIF-Prolyl Hydroxylase (HIF-PH) Inhibitor for the Treatment of Renal Anemia. ChemMedChem 2018;13:988–1003.

[41] Haase VH. Hypoxia-inducible factor-prolyl hydroxylase inhibitors in the treatment of anemia of chronic kidney disease. Kidney Int Suppl 2021;11:8–25.

[42] Hirota K. HIF-α Prolyl Hydroxylase Inhibitors and Their Implications for Biomedicine: A Comprehensive Review. Biomedicines 2021;9:468.

[43] Gupta N, Wish JB. Hypoxia-Inducible Factor Prolyl Hydroxylase Inhibitors: A Potential New Treatment for Anemia in Patients With CKD. Am J Kidney Dis 2017;69:815–26.

[44] Boegel A, Flamme I, Krebber R, et al. Pharmacodynamic effects of molidustat on erythropoiesis in healthy cats. J Vet Intern Med 2024;38:381–7.

[45] Barrett TD, Palomino HL, Brondstetter TI, et al. Prolyl hydroxylase inhibition corrects functional iron deficiency and inflammation-induced anaemia in rats. Br J Pharmacol 2015;172:4078–88.

[46] Vaden SL, Kendall AR, Foster JD, et al. Adeno-associated virus-vectored erythropoietin gene therapy for anemia in cats with chronic kidney disease. J Vet Intern Med 2023;37:2200–10.

[47] Lane DJ, Bae DH, Merlot AM, et al. Duodenal cytochrome b (DCYTB) in iron metabolism: an update on function and regulation. Nutrients 2015;7:2274–96.

[48] Anderson GJ, Frazer DM. Current understanding of iron homeostasis. Am J Clin Nutr 2017;106:1559s–66s.

[49] Zaritsky J, Young B, Wang HJ, et al. Hepcidin–a potential novel biomarker for iron status in chronic kidney disease. Clin J Am Soc Nephrol 2009;4:1051–6.

[50] Babitt JL, Lin HY. Mechanisms of anemia in CKD. J Am Soc Nephrol 2012;23:1631–4.

[51] Batchelor EK, Kapitsinou P, Pergola PE, et al. Iron deficiency in chronic kidney disease: updates on pathophysiology, diagnosis, and treatment. J Am Soc Nephrol 2020;31:456–68.

[52] Gaweda AE. Markers of iron status in chronic kidney disease. Hemodial Int 2017;21(Suppl 1):S21–7.

[53] Gafter-Gvili A, Schechter A, Rozen-Zvi B. Iron Deficiency Anemia in Chronic Kidney Disease. Acta Haematol 2019; 142:44–50.

[54] Betting A, Schweighauser A, Francey T. Diagnostic value of reticulocyte indices for the assessment of the iron status of cats with chronic kidney disease. J Vet Intern Med 2022;36:619–28.

[55] Hanna RM, Streja E, Kalantar-Zadeh K. Burden of Anemia in Chronic Kidney Disease: Beyond Erythropoietin. Adv Ther 2021;38:52–75.

[56] Shepshelovich D, Rozen-Zvi B, Avni T, et al. Intravenous Versus Oral Iron Supplementation for the Treatment of Anemia in CKD: An Updated Systematic Review and Meta-analysis. Am J Kidney Dis 2016;68:677–90.

[57] Begum S, Latunde-Dada GO. Anemia of Inflammation with An Emphasis on Chronic Kidney Disease. Nutrients 2019;11:2424.

Advances in Small Animal Care 5 (2024) 189–197

ADVANCES IN SMALL ANIMAL CARE

The Future of Veterinary Nephrology and Urology

Historical and Editorial Perspective

Larry D. Cowgill, DVM, PhD, Dipl ACVIM (SAIM), ACVNU (President)*

Department of Medicine and Epidemiology, University of California, Davis School of Veterinary Medicine, Davis, CA 95616, USA

KEYWORDS

- Nephrology • Urology • ACVNU • Specialty veterinary medicine

KEY POINTS

- Overview of how urinary disease has advanced and become more specialized over the past 40 years.
- Review of the veterinarians and organizations that have focused their professional interests to the advancement of urinary disease.
- Contributions of nephrology and urology to the advancement of general and specialized veterinary health care.
- Recognition of the evolution and establishment of the American College of Veterinary Nephrology and Urology (ACVNU).
- The promise and the future of urinary disease specialization and the roll of the ACVNU

INTRODUCTION

Nephrology may be defined as the medical discipline concerned with the structure, function, clinical diseases, and pathology of the kidneys. Urology is defined similarly as the medical discipline concerned with the structure, function, clinical diseases, and pathology of the urinary or urogenital organs inclusive or exclusive of the kidneys. In human medicine nephrology is concerned with the diseases of kidneys exclusively, and urology is a distinct surgical discipline focused on diseases of the urogenital system generally exclusive of the kidneys. In contrast, veterinarians who focus on their professional activities as nephrologist or as urologist, typically are broader base and concerned with the structure, function, clinical diseases, and pathology of the collective urinary system. Although some may emphasize upper versus lower urinary tract disorders, at this time, it is reasonable to define veterinary nephrology or veterinary urology with singular emphasis to urinary disease—veterinary nephrology and urology.

The question could be asked, "Has veterinary medicine changed sufficiently to rank veterinary nephrology and urology as a unique specialty discipline in veterinary medicine?", and "How would specialty designation help veterinarians provide better patient-care?" For the past 50 to 70 years, we have witnessed the transition of veterinary medicine from "the romance of James Herriot", with physical diagnosis as the nearly singular diagnostic tool, to x-ray, sophisticated clinical chemistries, ultrasound, computed tomography (CT), MRI, and linear accelerators as standard features of general and multispecialty practice. Similarly, nephrology and urology has changed from urinalysis and blood urea nitrogen to sophisticated diagnostics including immunofluorescence and electron microscopy for the evaluation of glomerular disease, kidney-specific biomarkers for early

---

*P.O. Box 221658, Sacramento, CA 95822. *E-mail address:* ldcowgill@ucdavis.edu

https://doi.org/10.1016/j.yasa.2024.07.001
2666-450X/24/

detection of clinically occult disease, and state-of-the-art interventional technologies and extracorporeal therapies. Yes, veterinary medicine has changed and will change exponentially in the future to advance clinical disciplines and ignite experts with the insights and interest to harness these exponential changes. All past advances promoting development of clinical specialties were doubted and criticized at first by conventional standards but have become expectations of today's veterinarians and pet owners.

Routine and even some complex urinary diseases will continue to be managed effectively by the existing general and specialty expertise within the profession. Specialists in nephrology and urology will serve as an advanced tier of expertise for the diagnosis of urinary diseases and management of patients with urinary disease beyond the experience, interest, or technical capabilities of non-specialists. More importantly, as with all specialties, these more urinary focused individuals will continuously and more rapidly transfer their newly discovered knowledge back to the profession at large to update old theories, conventional diagnostics and therapies, and dispel old dogmas, so future patients will be managed more expertly by everyone than patients of today. As with all the medical disciplines, individuals with dedicated interest and passion will advance their discipline—more quickly and more precisely—than those with lesser opportunities to focus (non-specialists). The fruits of such directed effort and passion are the discovery and advancement of new knowledge, application of new technologies, and more effective therapies that raise the standards of the profession as a whole.

In human medicine, evidence has demonstrated the management of urologic diseases by individuals with advanced expertise provides better outcomes than those managed by more generalized practitioners. Many of the routine needs of dogs and cats with urinary diseases will continue to be met adequately in the future, by veterinarians without specialty expertise in urinary disease. In all medical disciplines, clinical specialties based on scientific advancement and disease discovery have expanded the foundations of veterinary medicine, established management strategies for previously unmanageable diseases, and kept pace with increasingly higher pet owner expectations. Veterinary science advances in an atmosphere of curiosity, query, necessity, commitment, and most importantly, a dedicated critical mass. The most effective way to generate and capture these advances is through the focused energy and vision embedded in discipline-oriented clinical specialties. A specialty directed to nephrology and urology would establish an advanced level of expertise in veterinary medicine to fulfill current unmet needs, to recognize unidentified disease, and to provide health care to patients whose needs cannot be met by conventional standards-of-care or non-specialists.

Historic Progress of Veterinary Nephrology and Urology

Has veterinary nephrology and urology matured sufficiently and earmarked a niche in the profession to warrant consideration as a clinical specialty? The concept of a urinary specialty has not been based on whim, professional trends, or possession of unique clinical toys. It is a concept of considered deliberation for over 40 years. Why should and how could specialty designation be established in nephrology and urology? The answer is this discipline now has the culmination of dedicated leadership, proven training visions, critical mass, an established infrastructure, and a collaborative vision. It also faces unmet clinical needs and emerging therapeutic and diagnostic agendas, which are not being addressed adequately in conventional training programs as its future.

Veterinary nephrology and urology have been evolving and gaining clinical distinction over the past 70 years. Among a small handful of veterinarians who began to focus their clinical interests on urinary disease in the 1950s, Dr. Donald G. Low (University of Minnesota) is arguably regarded as the intellectual spark and "Grandfather" of veterinary urinary disease and established the initial pedigree for the foundations of today's discipline. The "Big Bang" for veterinary nephrology likely can be traced to the publication of *Canine and Feline Urology* by Carl Osborne, Donald Low, and Delmar Finco as the definitive textbook devoted to urinary disease in companion animals in 1972 [1]. Subsequently, Drs. Kenneth Bovee (University of Pennsylvania), Carl Osborne (University of Minnesota), and Delmar Finco (University of Georgia) established the second generation of training programs directed specifically to urinary disease and became the recognized experts in the field. Contemporary veterinary nephrology has been forged by these early giants who stewarded development of the discipline and ignited the torches their trainees have faithfully carried to bring the discipline to its current state of maturity.

Over subsequent years, urinary disease began to establish a clinical identity: early nephrologists and urologists characterized new urinary diseases, expanded urinary-directed literature, and envisioned new therapeutic strategies and procedures to address the most perplexing and formidable urinary diseases. In the late

1970s and 1980s, veterinary nephrology and urology introduced evidence-based medicine to the profession to discard forever the acceptance of anecdotal opinion and market claims as acceptable foundations for therapeutic directions. It was an era of dynamic research, specialized clinical training, well-financed clinical trials, exponential scientific discovery, and therapeutic strategies directed to understanding the dietary and therapeutic requirements for the management of progressive chronic kidney disease and urolithiasis [2–7]. The clinical and basic science literature related to veterinary nephrology and urology has been robust, evidence-based, and relevant to both animal care and One Health. A PubMed search conducted in 2020 to document the scientific foundations for a veterinary specialty yielded 45,033 relevant citations using companion animal-specific search terms. Importantly, this evaluation was performed using a single database, and the scope of significant literature in 2024 unquestionably is even more extensive. There also has been a progressive and extensive compilation of authoritative textbooks and topical reviews devoted to urinary disease since the benchmark work of Osborne, Low, and Finco [8–24].

From its early history to the current day, nephrology and urology, in concert with the pet food industry, generated the therapeutic hypotheses, conducted validating clinical trials, and promoted the evidence-based recommendations to establish the dietary management of progressive kidney disease and a variety of lower-tract urinary maladies including urolithiasis. These early efforts brought nutritional therapy to the forefront of disease management, and subsequently established dietary strategies and nutritional products as the therapeutic tenets for urinary and other organ system diseases and now are applied uniformly by all segments of the profession. From the 1970s, veterinary nephrology dragged and ultimately convinced the profession that blood pressure assessment was a vital component of patient evaluation, which has become routine in veterinary practice. With the advent of blood pressure assessment, systemic hypertension became an identifiable pathologic component (or cause) of nearly every progressive kidney disease, as well as many endocrine and other organ system diseases. These discoveries necessitated introduction and routine use of antihypertensive agents as standard-of-care for kidney-associated systemic hypertension and hypertension of other etiologies[d] [25]. Similarly, veterinary nephrology transformed the relatively banal assessment of proteinuria on routine urinalysis to its current status as both a predictor and promoter of kidney disease and its progression. Today, throughout the profession, proteinuria commands more deserved diagnostic respect and directed therapeutic management[d] [26].

The application of hemodialysis as an extracorporeal (outside of the body) therapy for the management of kidney failure in veterinary patients started in the early 1970s by 2 independent veterinary nephrologists [27]. Veterinary developments paralleled those of human medicine and were proven to be effective and safe for the management of uremia in dogs and cats [28]. However, despite these developments, it took 35 years before hemodialysis became mainstream as an advanced standard-of-care for acute uremia and toxin removal. Interest and application of extracorporeal therapies has risen substantially with expanding interest in critical care and was supported by fellowship training programs beginning in the 1993 [27] and establishment of the Hemodialysis Academy in 2014[a]. The Hemodialysis Academy provides in-depth instruction on the theoretic foundations, indications, and veterinary applications of all extracorporeal therapies and is taught by the most notable international authorities in the field. To date, over 500 veterinarians from 32 countries have attended the Hemodialysis Academy and expanded the availability of hemodialysis worldwide.

More recently, hemadsorption (hemoperfusion), an extracorporeal blood-based therapy first used by veterinary nephrologists since the 1980s, was revitalized for the management of life-threatening endogenous and exogenous intoxications where there exist no effective antidotes, despite its virtual abandonment in human medicine about this same time. Hemadsorption uses selective or nonselective adsorbents (eg, charcoal, carbon, macroporous cross-linked, or functionalized polymers) to capture pathologic solutes or circulating pathogens from the flowing blood. Because of the continued interest and application of legacy of hemadsorptive devices in veterinary medicine, this technology recently has reemerged with newer adsorbents as an effective, safe, and important blood purification strategy in which veterinary medicine is leading its reintroduction into human medicine. Current hemadsorptive devices have a broad range of blood purifying potential including drug overdosage or intoxication (eg, non-steriodal anti-inflammatory drug, chemotherapeutics), central nervous system depressants (baclofen, phenobarbital, etc.), inflammatory mediators, inflammatory cytokines, metabolic solutes (bilirubin, ammonia), and even circulating viruses

---

[a]Hemodialysis Academy. https://www.hemodialysisacademy.com/.

and bacteria [29,30,31]. New generations of carbon-based sorbents have potential for adsorption of solutes with the molecular dimensions of immunoglobulins. Veterinary hemoperfusion delivery systems have been introduced recently, providing greater simplicity of operation than other extracorporeal platforms, which will expand the application and availability for this life-saving therapy [30].

In 2008, apheresis medicine (therapeutic plasma exchange [TPE], plasma adsorption, and cytapheresis) became the newest entry in the veterinary extracorporeal portfolio. TPE became a gateway to unmet therapies for the acute management of a variety of immune-mediated diseases (eg, myasthenia gravis, immune-mediated hemolytic anemia and thrombocytopenia, immune-mediated polyarthritis) otherwise difficult or impossible to control. It became a first-line strategy for blood purification of endogenous and exogenous toxins too large for clearance by hemodialysis. Therapeutic cytapheresis involves collection or removal of specific cellular components of a patient's blood. It is an emerging extracorporeal procedure in veterinary therapeutics for leukoreduction in patients with pathologic increased white blood cell or platelet counts or autologous collection of immune cells or stem cells required for innovative immunologic approaches to cancer therapy or bone marrow transplantation, respectively [32]. Nephrology-based extracorporeal programs have been instrumental in the collection of immune cells for these innovative technologies.

Another field that is rapidly evolving in veterinary urology is the application of minimally invasive urologic procedures and endourology. These include, but are not limited to, placement of subcutaneous bypass devices and ureteral stents for ureteral obstruction, laser ablation of ectopic ureters, urethral stenting, laser lithotripsy, and profilometry, urethral bulking and placement of hydraulic urethral occluders to control urinary incontinence. All these procedures require special skills and training embodied in veterinary urology.

For these many decades, nephrology and urology has decidedly influenced the advancement of both general and specialized health care throughout the profession. From these limited examples of today's advanced standards-of-practice and public expectations, it is clear the clinical insight and sophistication of today's therapies for many patients with urinary (and non-urinary) disease is beyond the training, clinical acumen, interest, and skills of even veterinary specialists outside this focused discipline. In the future, the well-being of animals with advanced or complicated urinary disease, those requiring sophisticated extracorporeal or endourologic procedures, and the increasing expectations of the public for advanced pet health only will be met by a level of specialization and advanced expertise in nephrology and urology that is greater than currently provided in the profession.

THE ORGANIZATION AND EDUCATIONAL FUTURE OF VETERINARY NEPHROLOGY

The American Society of Veterinary Nephrology and Urology[b] and the European Society of Veterinary Nephrology and Urology[c] are long-established specialty interest groups actively supporting a community of veterinarians directed to advancing the standards-of-care for kidney and urinary disease of companion animals. These interest groups are closely affiliated and broadly include veterinarians from many fields, specialties, and disciplines including internal medicine, critical care, nutrition, anesthesia, interventional radiology/endoscopy, nephropathology and cardiology, as well as industry partners with an interest in the comparative pathogenesis and management of urinary disease. Their educational missions are supported by annual business meetings and specialty symposia, which have become standards in the profession.

The International Renal Interest Society (IRIS)[d] was founded in 1998 to advance the scientific understanding of kidney disease in small animals. The IRIS Board is composed of 16 of the world's leading authorities of kidney disease form 8 countries throughout the world. The directed goals of IRIS are to promote a uniform international understanding of existing and emerging kidney diseases and to better standardize the diagnosis and treatment of kidney disease in cats and dogs. To this goal, IRIS has become the internationally recognized standard for the classification and diagnosis of acute and chronic kidney disease, as well as best practice guidelines for the treatment of these diseases. Notable contributions from the IRIS Board include the annually updated IRIS Staging and Treatment Recommendations for Chronic Kidney Disease[d] [33] the IRIS Grading of Acute Kidney Injury[d] [33], The IRIS Canine Proteinuria Classification and Consensus Project [34], consensus guidelines for the diagnosis and

---

[b]American Society of Veterinary Nephrology and Urology. https://www.asvnu.org/.

[c]European Society of Veterinary Nephrology. https://www.facebook.com/ESVNU/.

[d]International Renal Interest Society. http://www.iris-kidney.com/.

management of acute kidney injury [35], and best-practice guidelines for the management of animals with intermittent hemodialysis [36].

IRIS agendas are ongoing with guidelines for the delivery of continuous renal replacement therapy and extracorporeal hemadsorption (hemoperfusion) nearing publication. In 2016, IRIS established its first Biennial IRIS Renal Week and Extracorporeal Boot Camp, which over the past 8 years has become recognized internationally as the premier educational offering in veterinary nephrology and extracorporeal therapies. The 3 1/2-day Renal Week program provides state-of-the-art presentations on topical issues in veterinary and human nephrology and a diverse array of interactive laboratory sessions devoted to extracorporeal therapies. The formal Renal Week meeting is joined by a two-and-a-half-day lecture/laboratory Extracorporeal Boot Camp experience for those seeking an introduction to extracorporeal therapies.

Nephropathology is another example of an expanding field initiated with the collaborative vision and direction of veterinary nephrologists and pathologists. With competition of the World Small Animal Veterinary Association (WSAVA) Standardization Project, the characterization, understanding, diagnosis, and management of proteinuric kidney diseases in dogs have been better defined for the benefit of the entirety of the profession who confront these diseases [34]. Veterinary nephrologists through IRIS and the WSAVA established the International Veterinary Renal Pathology Service (IVRPS)[e] and the European Veterinary Renal Pathology Service[f], which have become the genesis for specialized expertise in nephropathology available to all levels of veterinary health care. These centers incorporated state-of-the-art light, immunofluorescent, and electron microscopic imaging and trained nephropathologists to exploit the diagnostic utility of routine kidney biopsy and establish the advanced standard for kidney and urinary pathology. The IVRPS is integrated with specialized clinical pathology and nephrology consultative resources to provide an inclusive clinicopathologic diagnosis and therapeutic recommendations for glomerular and uncharacterized kidney diseases. The IVRPS is actively engaged with established anatomic pathology training programs to promote future generations of nephropathologists.

THE FUTURE OF VETERINARY NEPHROLOGY AND UROLOGY AS A CLINICAL SPECIALTY

Some might argue specialization has driven the profession to become too narrowly focused, too costly, and has compromised delivery of basic or even specialized veterinary care. However, denying specialty development, with its attendant advances in diagnostic and therapeutic innovations, just as effectively stifles therapeutic opportunities for animals whose diseases are unresponsive to conventional "basic medicine" but responsive to specialized care. It denies pet owners, who desire more effective outcome-directed therapeutics, the opportunities for renewed quality-of-life or solution for their pet's urinary disease. Regrettably, despite the best efforts of our profession, veterinary care will not be equally and universally available to all pet owners. Some specialized veterinary care will be available to a population who has the financial means, pet insurance, or allocation of discretionary income to access more advanced care. This also is the reality for veterinary care as it exists today. The establishment of additional clinical expertise and advanced health care delivery will not corrupt veterinary health care further but expand opportunity for better care across the entire spectrum of the profession by the translation of improved diagnostics and therapeutics to both basic and specialty medicine. Greater sophistication of veterinary medicine often comes with an increased price for some services but just as often brings innovations applicable to all levels of veterinary care. Should the advancement of veterinary nephrology and urology be curtailed due to the costs or unavailability of care to all? Should some pet owners and animal patients be denied these advancements because they are not universally available or desired by all? Historically, advancements in veterinary science and novel diagnostics and treatments have not escaped criticism over their cost or accessibility (CT and MRI imaging, radiation therapy, or joint replacement as examples), yet their medical benefits have become routine, effective, embraced by the profession, financially feasible, and well-accepted by the public.

Perhaps the most significant development for the future of veterinary nephrology and urology occurred on Tuesday, 08 March, 2022, when the American Board of Veterinary Specialties (ABVS) granted provisional recognition to the American College of Veterinary Nephrology and Urology (ACVNU)[g] as a Registered Veterinary Specialty Organization (RVSO). As such, the

---

[e]International Veterinary Renal Pathology Service. https://vetmed.tamu.edu/ivrps/.

[f]European Veterinary Renal Pathology Service. https://www.evrps.net/.

[g]American College of Veterinary Nephrology and Urology. https://acvnu.org/.

ACVNU became the newest specialty college of the ABVS and veterinary nephrology and urology was officially established as a distinct veterinary discipline. The ACVNU became the American Veterinary Medical Association's recognized certifying organization for Veterinary Nephrologist and Urologist. Provisional recognition authorized immediate establishment of the college, the ability to train residents, and the authority to certify Diplomates and Affiliate Members in Nephrology and Urology.

The journey to this important milestone for urinary disease began over 40 years ago and came to fruition only after a long and bumpy journey. The earliest concept and momentum to create specialty recognition for nephrology and urology originated from members of the Small Animal Internal Medicine specialty of the American College of Veterinary Internal Medicine (ACVIM-SAIM) in the late 1970s and early 1980s; however, the timing for a new specialty was premature, critical mass was too small, and the structure and economics for new specialty training programs in academia were insufficient. As a result, the concept smoldered but was not extinguished. Many models have been proposed subsequently to facilitate its development.

Renewed efforts to this initial vision began again in 2003. From 2003 to 2008, a small steering committee established the foundational structure for subspecialty recognition as Small Animal Nephrology and Urology under the auspices of ACVIM-SAIM. Between 2011 and 2015, the steering committee worked diligently with the ACVIM Board of Regents to establish the subspecialty, but unpredicted changes in existing ABVS Policies and Procedures suddenly eliminated subspecialties as a recognition option in 2015. At the invitation of the ACVIM Board of Regents, the steering committee changed direction to establish Small Animal Nephrology and Urology as the 6th Registered Veterinary Specialty (RVS) under the ACVIM umbrella. However, in 2019, the now matured proposal was rejected by ACVIM membership, and the opportunities for specialty designation once again appeared lost.

With sustained commitment for the growing and unmet needs for urinary health care, the advancement of specialty training in urinary disease, and an opportunity to better serve the public, an Organizing Committee (Founders) from a broad-base of leadership in nephrology, urology, critical care, clinical pathology, nephropathology, and pharmacology was established in 2020 to petition the ABVS to recognize the proposed ACVNU as an independent RVSO. Many of these founders had been committed to the vision of specialty designation in nephrology and urology since its inception more than

30 years earlier. Others came to this initiative to embrace the intersection of urinary disease with existing specialty colleges, for example, the European College of Veterinary Internal Medicine-Companion Animal, American College of Veterinary Emergency and Critical Care, American College of Veterinary Pathology, and the American College of Veterinary Nutrition. As an RVSO, the college would have greater freedom and flexibility to achieve its firmly held visions of inclusivity with established specialties and a novel training structure not possible if affiliated under another specialty organization. As a provisional RVSO, the long-held objectives and missions of the college were on a recognized path to.

1. Advance the scientific knowledge and clinical practice of veterinary nephrology and urology through the promotion of basic and clinical investigation and communication and dissemination of this knowledge.
2. Establish standards of excellence and advance innovative clinical practices to evaluate and alleviate diseases of the urinary system.
3. Promote continued professional development of its membership and promote the Specialty among the scientific, professional, and lay communities.
4. Approve and oversee training programs and guidelines for specialty education and clinical competency prerequisites for certification of clinical specialists in nephrology and urology.
5. Examine candidate Diplomates and Affiliate Members for competencies and clinical proficiencies required by ABVS standards for certification as a specialist in veterinary nephrology and urology.
6. Certify the qualifications of Resident candidates as Diplomates or Affiliate Members of the College to elevate the quality, competency, and scope of practice of the Specialty.

Certification of ACVNU Diplomates would not preclude other veterinarians or specialists from the management of urinary diseases, just as certification does not preclude Diplomates of other specialties from management of cardiovascular disease, skin disease, neurologic disease, or cancer when it overlaps their certified discipline. It would, however, provide an advanced level of expertise for consultation or referral of patients with advanced urinary needs. One of the foundational goals of the ACVNU was to embrace and incorporate a broad array of clinical specialties that meaningfully intersect with nephrology and urology into the ACVNU. This diversification provides unification with other specialty colleges and enriches the expertise in the ACVNU. To facilitate this goal, the ACVNU uniquely proposed 2 certification pathways for specialty designation, Diplomate status and Affiliate Member status. Diplomate Certification is established for individuals who satisfy all credentialing criteria and are concurrently certified in an approved *patient care* veterinary specialty, for example, internal medicine, emergency and critical care, surgery, and cardiology. Diplomate Certification confers "Specialist" status in nephrology and urology. Affiliate Member status is conferred to candidates who satisfy all credentialing criteria and have prerequisite board certification in an approved *non-patient care* veterinary specialty, for example, pathology, clinical pathology, nutrition, and so forth. Affiliate Members are not designated as "Specialist" but provide specialized recognition and expertise in related disciplines essential to nephrology and urology and hold equal membership status in the ACVNU. Through this approach, the ACVNU will extend the breadth of its knowledge base, clinical expertise, interdisciplinary collaborations, and the strength and advancement of the discipline and the college.

In 2023, the ACVNU established a robust, 2-year residency training program in advanced nephrology and urology. The training opportunities have been fortified by inclusion of a didactic, 2-year, web-based Core Curriculum available to every resident. Establishment of the Core Curriculum is unique among all specialty colleges. It provides 150 hours of advanced didactic instruction, divided into 9 modular domains of competency, and is delivered by 60 international authorities in veterinary and human nephrology and urology. The Core Curriculum spans the professional competencies expected of a Diplomate or Affiliate Member and assesses mastery of these competencies through a series of topical examinations delivered at the end of each module in addition to a terminal certifying examination required by the ABVS. The training requirements also include more than 50 clinical proficiencies specific to the urinary disease requiring mastery for certification. Instruction on unique interventional or extracorporeal procedures that may not be available at some residency training sites will be provided at centralized training centers or external rotations to facilities where instruction for these clinical proficiencies can be acquired and documented. The level of didactic instruction and scope of the clinical proficiencies required during residency training establish a degree of rigor and expertise that exceeds any currently available training in urinary disease.

Resident candidates for the ACVNU typically are newly certified or substantially established Diplomates of other specialties and actively engaged in their professional careers and personal lives. Consequently, reengagement of their careers into a traditional residency training structure might be financially and logistically problematic. The ACVNU envisioned the opportunity for an alternative virtual training program exploiting the candidate's advanced clinical experience and facilities without substantial disruption to their professional, financial, geographic, or personal lives. For resident candidates who do not have an onsite ACVNU Diplomate or Founder to supervise training face-to-face (traditional residency), the college assigns an off-site mentor who provides virtual mentorship and program oversight (virtual residency). The concept and effectiveness of virtual clinical training had been envisioned and tested for many years in extracorporeal fellowship training programs to document proof of concept and training validity, but virtual clinical training became immediately endorsed and routine at many academic centers during the coronavirus disease 2019 pandemic. The unique concept and expanded opportunities afforded with virtual clinical training reinforces and further justifies the requirement for ACVNU residents to have pre-existing board certification, as it provides the requisite clinical maturity, experience, and established facilities to function semi-independently. It seemed likely to the ACVNU a newly internship-trained resident candidate might struggle in a virtual training experience with the complexities of urinary disease. This approach for precedent clinical certification provides a unique foundation to materialize a breadth of expertise in ACVNU diplomates that is not materialized in other certified specialties.

SUMMARY

What is the future forecast for veterinary nephrology and urology? I believe the future looks promising, diversified, challenging, meaningful, contributory, visionary, trailblazing, and above all, collaborative. We are facing new opportunities in the understanding of urinary diseases. Nephrology and urology-orientated specialists will validate and bring new standards of practice to the profession for all to benefit. The diagnostic expertise and specialized therapies currently limited to a handful of focal centers will become increasingly available throughout the world by highly skilled urinary specialists, eliminating disease risk and providing diversified therapeutic benefits. The current advancement of novel directions in urinary diagnostics, extracorporeal procedures, interventional techniques, and innovative therapies has been achieved by the motivated urinary clinician-scientist, providing life-saving therapies to animals and pet owners worldwide through their directed efforts and focused expertise. One can only speculate on the future advancements to be realized for veterinary nephrology and urology as the regiment of urinary specialists expands from this small cadre of its early and current pioneers.

CLINICS CARE POINTS

- Veterinary nephrologists and urologists have provided improved definition to common urinary disease managed by all segments of the profession.
- Veterinary nephrologists and urologists have sought and established therapeutic solutions to the most formidable urinary diseases and innovative approaches to diseases beyond the urinary system.
- Specialized veterinary medicine should not be feared but embraced as it advances the quality and delivery of health care for animals for the entire veterinary profession.
- Establishment of the ACVNU portends a future of advanced discovery, innovative solutions, and compassionate resolution of urinary diseases in companion animals.

DISCLOSURE

The author has received materials and research funding from Aimalojic Animal Health.

REFERENCES

[1] Osborne CA, Low DG, Finco DR. Canine and feline urology. Philadelphia: W. B. Saunders Company; 1972.

[2] Morris ML Jr, Patton RS. Diet in renal disease. Vet Med Small Anim Clin 1976;71:773–9.

[3] Bovee KC, Joyce T. Clinical evaluation of glomerular function: 24-hour creatinine clearance in dogs. Am J Vet Med Assoc 1979;174:488–91.

[4] Bovee KC, Kronfeld DS, Ramberg C. Goldschmidt. Long-term measurement of renal function in partially nephrectomized dogs fed 56, 27, or 19% protein. Invest Urol 1979;16:378–84.

[5] Polzin DJ, Osborne CA. Influence of reduced protein diets on morbidity, mortality, and renal function in dogs with induced chronic renal failure. Am J Vet Res 1984; 45:506–17.

[6] Polzin DJ, Osborne CA, Hayden DW, et al. Effects of modified protein diets in dogs with chronic renal failure. J Am Vet Med Assoc 1983 Nov 1;183(9):980–6.

[7] Polzin DJ, Osborne CA, Stevens JB, et al. Influence of modified protein diets on electrolyte, acid base, and divalent ion balance in dogs with experimentally induced chronic renal failure. Am J Vet Res 1982;43:1978–86.

[8] Bovee DC. Canine nephrolgy. Media, PA: Harwall Publishing Company; 1984.

[9] Ackerman N. Radiology and ultrasound of urogenital diseases in dogs and cats. Ames, IA: Iowa State University Press; 1991.

[10] Chew DJ, DiBartola SP. Interpretation of canine and feline urinalysis (Nestle Purina clinical handbook series). Wilmingtion, DE: The Gloyd Group, Inc.; 1998.

[11] Stone EA, Barsanti JA. Urologic surgery of the dog and cat. Philadelphia, PA: Lea & Febiger; 1992.

[12] Holt PE. Color atlas of small animal urology. St. Louis, MO: Mosby Inc; 1994.

[13] Ling GV. Lower urinary tract diseases of dogs and cats: diagnosis, medical management, prevention. St. Louis, MO: Mosby Inc; 1995.

[14] Small animal practice - renal dysfunction. DJ Polzin, editor. Vet Clin North Am 1996;26 (6).

[15] Bainbridge J, Elliott J, editors. Manual of canine and feline nephrology and urology. 1st edition. Gloucester, UK: BSAVA; 1996.

[16] Lane IF, Forrester SD, Vaden SL. Clinical nephrology and Urology. Vet Clin North Am 2004;36. https://doi.org/10.1016/j.

[17] Elliott J, Grauer G, editors. BSAVA manual of canine and feline nephrology and urology. 2nd Edition. Gloucester, UK: BSAVA; 2007.

[18] Chew DJ, DiBartola SP. Canine and feline nephrology and urology. St. Louis, MO: Elsevier; 2010.

[19] Kidney diseases and renal replacement therapies. Acierno MF, Labato M, editors. Vet Clin North Am 2011;41(1).

[20] Bartges J, Polzin DJ, editors. Nephrology and urology of small animals. Oxford: Wiley; 2011.

[21] Bartges J, editor. Urology. Vet Clin North Am 2015;45(4).

[22] Chronic kidney disease. In: Polzin DJ, Cowgill LD, editors. Vet Clin North Am: Small An Practice 2016;46(6).

[23] Westropp J, Grauer GF, Elliott J, editors. BSAVA manual of canine and feline nephrology and urology. 3rd edition. Gloucester, UK: BSAVA; 2017.

[24] Cianciolo R, Brown C, Mohr C, et al. Atlas of renal lesions in proteinuric dogs. Athens, OH: Ohio State University; 2018. Available at: https://ohiostate.pressbooks.pub/vetrenalpathatlas/.

[25] Acierno MJ, Brown S, Coleman AE, et al. ACVIM consensus statement: Guidelines for the identification, evaluation, and management of systemic hypertension in dogs and cats. J Vet Intern Med 2018;32(6):1803–22.

[26] Lees GE, Brown SA, Elliott J, et al. Assessment and management of proteinuria in dogs and cats: 2004 ACVIM Forum Consensus Statement (small animal). J Vet Intern Med 2005;19(3):377–85.

[27] Cowgill LD, Langston CE. History of hemodialysis in dog and other companion animals. In: Ing TS, Rahman MA, Kjellstrand CM, editors. Dialysis: history, development and promise. Singapore: World Scientific Publishing Co. Pte. Ltd; 2012. p. 901–13.

[28] Cowgill LD, Francey T. Hemodial and extracorporeal blood purification. In: DiBartola SP, editor. Fluid, electrolyte, and acid-base disorders in small animal practice. 4th edition. St Louis: Elsevier (Saunders); 2012. p. 680–712. Available at: http://www.iris-kidney.com/ysis.

[29] Eden G, Schmidt JJ, Büttner S, et al. Safety and efficacy of the Seraph® 100 Microbind® Affinity Blood Filter to remove bacteria from the blood stream: results of the first in human study. Crit Care 2022;26(1):181.

[30] Barnes J, Cowgill LD, Aunon JD. Activated carbon hemoperfusion and plasma adsorption. Rediscovery and veterinary applications of these abandoned therapies. Advances in Small Animal Care 2021;2:131–42.

[31] McCrea K, Ward R, LaRosa SP. Removal of Carbapenem-Resistant Enterobacteriaceae (CRE) from Blood by Heparin Functional Hemoperfusion Media. PLoS One 2014; 9(12):e114242.

[32] Flesner BK, Wood GW, Gayheart-Walstern P, et al. Autologous cancer cell vaccination, adoptive T-cell transfer, and interleukin-2 administration results in long-term survival for companion dogs with osteosarcoma. J Vet Intern Med 2020;34(5):2056–67.

[33] Elliott J, Cowgill LD. Diagnostic algorithms for grading acute kidney injury and staging the chronic kidney disease patient. In: Westropp J, Grauer GF, Elliott J, editors. BSAVA manual of canine and feline nephrology and urology. 3rd Edition. BSAVA; 2017. p. 151–60.

[34] Polzin DJ, Cowgill LD. Development of clinical guidelines for management of glomerular disease in dogs. J Vet Intern Med 2013;27:S2–75.

[35] Segev G, Cortellini S, Foster JD, et al. International renal interest society best practice consensus guidelines for the diagnosis and management of acute kidney injury in cats and dogs. Vet J 2024;305:106068.

[36] Segev G, Foster JD, Francey T, et al. International renal interest society best practice consensus guidelines for intermittent hemodialysis in dogs and cats. Vet J 2024;305: 106092.

Advances in Small Animal Care 5 (2024) 199–206

ADVANCES IN SMALL ANIMAL CARE

Extracorporeal Removal of Viral and Bacterial Pathogens

Lakhmir S. Chawla, MD[a,b,c], Keith R. McCrea, PhD[c,*]

[a]Veterans Affairs Medical Center, San Diego, CA, USA; [b]Department of Anesthesiology and Critical Care Medicine, George Washington University Medical Center, Washington, DC, USA; [c]Department of Research and Development, ExThera Medical Corporation, Martinez, CA, USA

KEYWORDS
- Pathogenemia • Bacteremia • Viremia • Sepsis • Fungemia

KEY POINTS
- Sepsis is a disseminated infection that leads to a dysregulated immune response, which may be both hyper- and hypo-inflammatory.
- Adequate and rapid source control must be achieved to prevent multiple organ failure and death.
- Antimicrobial drugs are often insufficient for the treatment of sepsis or disseminated infections, and alternate strategies for source control should be evaluated.
- Rapid filtration of pathogens, damage-associated molecular patterns, and pathogen-associated molecular patterns may allow for a quicker clearance of disseminated pathogens allowing for recovery of the dysregulated immune system.

INTRODUCTION

Every day, healthy animals are exposed to microbial organisms that can lead to infectious disease. In the majority of cases, the innate and adaptive immune systems are sufficient to ward off serious disease [1]. However, if the immune response fails, the infectious organisms may be disseminated throughout the body, which often leads to sepsis or persistent infections. Antibiotics, antivirals, and antifungal drugs have given the medical community an essential arsenal to help the body fight infections when the immune response is either insufficient or dysregulated. These interventions are considered 'additive', in that drugs are added to the host to help inactivate or kill the infectious organisms. While overall outcomes improve with additive medicine, there are still a number of patients that do not sufficiently respond.

Antimicrobial drugs must be provided in a timely matter; however, there are multiple factors for why administration is challenging, and use of antimicrobials may lead to unwanted side effects.

1. Physicians rely primarily on empirical antimicrobial dosing strategies. If an adequate antimicrobial therapy is correctly chosen, then the patient may respond favorably. However, if the wrong antimicrobial drug is administered, then essentially, the patient was not provided a therapeutic to address the causative infection. Selecting the incorrect antimicrobial agent is associated with worse outcomes. Ideally, after empirical antimicrobial therapy, culture and susceptibility testing would be completed to help provide a more precise therapeutic strategy. However, a recent publication indicated that less than 4% of animals prescribed antibiotics have culture and susceptibility tests performed [2]. From the human clinical data, empirical antimicrobial therapy is incorrect up to 37% of cases [3] leading to an increase mortality from 28.4% to 61.9% [4].

---

*Corresponding author, E-mail address: keith@extheramedical.com

https://doi.org/10.1016/j.yasa.2024.06.011
2666-450X/24/

2. Increasing incidence of drug resistance is limiting available options. The World Health Organization has already declared that the world has entered the post antibiotic era. A 10-year study evaluating methicillin-resistant (MR) and multi-drug resistant (MDR) organisms in canine and feline patients revealed that between 56% and 63% of *Staphylococcus* spp. isolates were MR, while between 44.6% and 52.8% were MDR [5].

3. Some antimicrobial drugs may lead to serious adverse drug reactions, which may limit their use. While the benefits may outweigh the risk, a review article lists various side effects for canines for many different antibiotics, leading to adverse events such as diarrhea, vomiting, pemphigus vulgaris, hypersensitive reactions, Gray baby syndrome, ototoxicity, nephrotoxicity, and onset of arthropathy [6].

4. The use of antibiotics also may release pathogen-associated molecular patterns (PAMPs), which stimulate pattern recognition receptors that can exacerbate the dysregulated immune response of sepsis [7,8].

Prudent use of antimicrobial drug therapy will always be the standard-of-care; however, alternate adjunctive therapeutic approaches must be explored for the treatment of sepsis and infectious diseases [9]. A 'subtractive' approach through blood filtration is being explored for rapid blood source control. Instead of adding drugs to a patient, hemoperfusion physically removes pathogens, PAMPs, and damage-associated molecular patterns (DAMPs) from the bloodstream. In this review, we discuss the rationale for removing pathogens and toxins from the blood, provide relevant clinical experience, and offer examples of various companion animal diseases that may benefit from adjunctive 'subtractive' therapy.

Background

Infections can lead to sepsis and immunosuppression. Sepsis is defined as life-threatening organ dysfunction caused by a dysregulated host response to an infection. [10] The 'newer' 2016 definition was refined to include 'dysregulated host response' instead of the prior sepsis definition, which required two or more systemic inflammatory response criteria. The reason for the new definition pointed to the fact that in addition to a hyper-inflammatory stage, sepsis is often categorized as a hypo-inflammatory phase. Thus, the 2016 definition allows for the understanding that anti-inflammatory therapies may not always be appropriate, depending on the phenotype of sepsis. In some cases,

extreme inflammation may occur, while in others immunosuppression prevents homeostasis [11]. An uncontrolled infection triggers a cascade of events, including release of PAMPs and DAMPs, activation of the complement and coagulation systems, activation of vascular cells, tissue cells, and immune cells. This activation can lead to increase of cytokines, chemokines, and other signaling molecules [12]. If left untreated, organ dysfunction and failure will occur. If the infection can be controlled through effective source control, markers of disease will decrease, and the patient may recover. Without adequate source control, the patient will succumb to multiple organ failure. Within the spectrum of therapeutics that may impact various phases of the sepsis cascade, strategies focused on source control are essential.

Uncontrolled infections can lead to other non-sepsis diseases. It has been understood that infections can lead to immunodeficiency or disruption of normal immune function such as feline immunodeficiency virus and feline leukemia virus [13]. Patients are then at risk of secondary opportunistic infections. Outcomes for canine distemper virus (CDV) depend on how quickly the patient's immune system is able to clear the virus. Parvovirus diseases also lead to severe secondary superinfections [13]. As with sepsis, the earlier a patient receives antimicrobial therapies, the better the outcome.

ADDING AND ADJUNCTIVE OPTION TO DRUGS FOR THE MANAGEMENT OF INFECTIOUS DISEASES

While antimicrobial drugs remain the gold standard for treating infections, adjunctive therapies that can rapidly reduce the circulating concentration of pathogens, DAMPs, and PAMPs from the bloodstream through hemoperfusion could improve outcomes. While a few approaches have been proposed [14] and evaluated in animal and human clinical studies, this review focuses ExThera Medical's VM100, which is under development, (also known as Seraph 100 for human use) due to the availability of the human and animal data.

VM100 is a broad-spectrum hemoperfusion device that contains solid beads of ultrahigh molecular weight polyethylene copolymerized with endpoint-attached heparin. By copolymerizing heparin in a brush-like structure, the surface of the adsorbent of VM100 mimics the heparan sulfate (HS) structure (Fig. 1) that is found within the endothelial glycocalyx layer [15]. The glycocalyx surface is primarily made up of HS (>50%), and other molecules such as hyaluronan, sialic acid, chondroitin sulfate, and dermatan sulfate [16]. Many

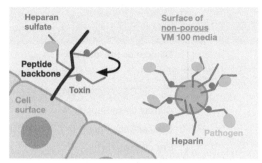

FIG. 1 Schematic of glycocalyx mimetic structure of VM100 adsorbent designed to bind pathogens.

pathogens, including bacteria, viruses, fungi, and parasites have evolved to target HS for attachment to the endothelium. VM100 utilizes this natural affinity of pathogens to target heparin or heparan sulfate by providing a high-surface area of covalently bonded, 'endpoint-attached' heparin, which exposes the entire heparin molecular chain to potential adsorbates. Pathogens are physically removed from the bloodstream by VM100, rapidly debulking the blood of pathogens *and* disease-causing molecules and cell fragments.

Over 60 pathogens and toxins have been identified in the literature that utilize HS during pathogenesis [17], and are therefore, able to bind to VM100 adsorption media. Based on multiple independent laboratory tests, over 20 drug-susceptible and drug-resistant bacteria, viruses, and fungi have been shown to bind to Seraph *in vitro* with high affinity [18–21]. Examples include both drug susceptible bacteria (*Staphylococcus aureus, E. coli, Streptococcus pneumoniae, K. pneumoniae*) and drug resistant (CRE *E coli*, CRE *K. pneumoniae*, CRE *A. baumannii*, MRSA, and ESBL *E. faecium*) [15]. Confirmed viral removal has been demonstrated for CMV, adenovirus, SARS-CoV-2, and Zika [15,22]. In a recirculation study evaluating several strains of *S. aureus* in human plasma at a flow rate of 60 mL per min, it was demonstrated that over 90% of the *S. aureus* was removed after 4 hours [23]. The specific surface protein expression of the various *S. aureus* strains had no impact on binding efficiency. Based on the challenge concentration, it was extrapolated that a Seraph 100 (VM100) filter is capable of binding 5×10^8 CFU of *S. aureus* cells. Table 1 shows a partial list of pathogens tested.

In addition to pathogens, DAMPs have also been shown to bind to the VM100's adsorbent material [32]. Septic plasma was exposed to the heparinized adsorbent material and the concentration of HMGB1, histones, and platelet factor 4 were reduced by 58.9%,

50%, and 89%, respectively. The reduction of these DAMPs may help in the reduction of immunothrombosis in sepsis and disseminated infections.

The Defense Advanced Projects Agency funded a good laboratory practice (GLP) non-human primate performed at Duke University to evaluate the effectiveness and safety of the VM100 technology in an established sepsis model [8]. The study was a randomized controlled baboon model of severe pneumococcal pneumonia and sepsis with organ dysfunction. Four non-septic animals were evaluated for safety. Twelve additional subjects were inhalationally exposed to 5×10^9 CFU of *S. pneumoniae*. Twenty four hours after the inoculation, animals had positive blood cultures and the subjects were dosed with ceftriaxone. Hemoperfusion with VM100 was initiated at 30 hours with an extracorporeal blood flow rate of 150 mL per min for a duration of 4 hours. Because the strain of *S. pneumoniae* was highly susceptible to ceftriaxone, all blood cultures were negative by initiation of hemoperfusion. Therefore, even though the subjects were septic, they were not bacteremic. Blood and urine samples were collected, along with additional patient monitoring, occurred at 0, 6, 24, 30, 36, and 48 hours, repectively. Results of the study concluded that the treatment with VM100 was safe in both healthy and septic animals. Additionally, while the acute lung injury was similar in both treatment and control animals, animals that underwent hemoperfusion had several significant measures of clinical improvement. Septic animals treated with VM100 displayed Less: kidney injury, metabolic acidosis, and hypoglycemia shock ($P<.5$). Additionally, the treated animals exhibited a reduced rise in peripheral blood *S. pneumoniae* DNA (PAMPs), had attenuated bronchoalveolar lavage CCL4, CCL2, and IL-18, exhibited reduced renal oxidative injury and classical NLRP3-inflammasome activation. The authors concluded that the observed improvement was likely due to reducing the PAMPs, reduced bronchoalveolar lavage fluid cytokines and renal inflammasome activation. Reducing PAMPs is an important consideration as studies have shown that PAMPs induce cytokine production, contribute to lactic acidosis, and shock.

Clinical Studies and Case Reports

VM100 is under development for the veterinary community and there are no published case reports on it use in small animals. However, there are many case reports and studies reporting clinical use and evaluation for Seraph 100. Considering septic mechanisms are similar, regardless of species, several relevant clinical publications will be summarized.

TABLE 1
List of Pathogens Evaluated Either in *in vitro* or Case Presentations/Studies

Target	Clinical or Pre-clinical
Viruses	
Epstein Barr Virus (EBV)	Clinical Case Report [24]
Hepatitis B	Clinical Case Report [24]
SARS-CoV-2	Clinical Case Report [25] Series [26]
CMV	Pre-clinical [15] Clinical Case Series [27]
Ebola	Pre-clinical
Zika	Pre-clinical [15]
Adenovirus	Pre-clinical [15] Clinical Case Report [28]
Bacteria	
S. aureus, MRSA, S. pneumoniae, E. faecalis, VRE, E. Faecium, S. epidermidis, S. pyrogenes, K. pneumoniae, E. coli, CRE, S. marcescens, A. baumannii	Pre-clinical [15]
S. aureus	Clinical Case Report [29]
K. pneumoniae, E. faecalis, P. aeruginosa	Clinical Case Series [30]
Enterobacter cloacae	Clinical Case Report [31]
Fungi	
C. albicans, C. auris, Saccharomyces	Clinical Case Series [30]
DAMPs or PAMPs	
PAMPs	Pre-clinical NHP study [8]
DAMPS (Histones, nucleosomes, PF4, HMGB1)	Pre-clinical [32]

Seraph 100 was evaluated in a first in human study that took place in Germany. Fifteen hemodialysis patients with confirmed positive blood cultures were enrolled in the study [33]. The study concluded that the treatment was well-tolerated, and blood cultures, as measured by thrombotic thrombocytopenic purpura were observed to decrease. There were no significant changes in hematology or blood chemistry, and blood pressure and heart rate remained stable. Interestingly, it was observed that there was a significant increase in oxygen saturation for all patients.

Shortly after Seraph 100 received CE mark in Europe, the COVID-19 pandemic began. Due to the lack of effective therapeutics, the technology began being used to treat severe and critically-ill COVID-19 patients in Europe, and shortly received Emergency Use Authorization in the United States after compassionate use at Walter Reed Army Memorial Hospital demonstrated encouraging results [22].

To evaluate the efficacy of Seraph 100 for the treatment of COVID-19 patients, the Department of Defense funded an observational clinical trial of Seraph 100. The 'PURIFY OBS' trial includes both retrospective and prospective arms with matched controls. Using multivariable regression analysis of the data from the first 106 patients (53 treated patients and 53 controls) a nearly 4X improvement in survivability odds was found for patients treated with Seraph versus control [34]. The Survival for Seraph-treated patients was 68% versus 36% for control patients ($P=.001$). Similar results were observed in a large patient registry in Europe [35].

Several case reports and case series have been published for other viral, bacterial, and fungal infections. A patient's, aged 17 years, immunosuppressed kidney transplant was treated with Seraph 100 with a disseminated adenovirus infection [28]. Prior to treatment, the patient was febrile to 40.2° C for 2 weeks with over 10 million viral copies per mL in the blood while her immunosuppression drugs were paused. The patient received 2 Seraph 100 treatments. After the first treatment, the patient became afebrile, and the viral load dropped from greater than 10 million copies per mL to 1.5 million copies per mL. The viral load continued to drop during and after the second treatment and was down to 20,000 copies per mL 3 days after the first treatment. The immunosuppression drugs were restarted, and the viral load was undetectable 1 week after discharge from the hospital. Several other viral diseases treated with Seraph 100 have been reported including cytomegalovirus [27], herpes simplex virus, and Epstein-Barr virus [24], and hepatitis B [24].

A significant number of COVID-19 patients treated with Seraph 100 had bacterial or fungal superinfections. A case series reported patient response for 9 septic shock patients with an average Sequential Organ Failure Assessment score of 13 +/- 2.3 [30]. Across all patients, the various causative pathogens included *S. aureus*, MRSA, *P. aeruginosa, Candida* spp., and *Saccharomyces*. Most patients received a single Seraph 100 treatment, while 2 patients received 2 treatments using either continuous renal replacement therapy or in parallel with extracorporeal membrane oxygenation. Clinical monitoring showed significant improvement for several variables after 24 hours. Mean arterial pressure increased from 64.2 to 76.2 mm Hg ($P<.0001$), heart rate decreased from 128 to 100 bpm ($P<.0001$), fraction of inspired oxygen delivery decreased from 74.4% to 60.3% ($P<.001$), and lactate dropped from 6.14 to 2.8 ($P = .001$). Significant reduction of vasopressor requirements were also observed for Norepinephrine ($P<.001$), Vasopressin ($P<.001$), and Angiotensin II ($P<.001$). In this extremely sick group of patients, 44.4% of the patients survived to discharge. Importantly, there were no documented adverse events.

While reduction of pathogens and toxins can provide benefit to patients, it is important that a 'subtractive' therapy does not remove 'good' things from the blood. One concern with extracorporeal treatments is the potential to remove drugs. For example, if a pathogen reduction technology is adjunctive to antibiotics, it is important to know whether drug concentrations are altered. Ideally, drug levels would not be impacted. However, if drug levels are impacted, physicians should be informed so dosing can be adjusted. Several studies have looked at the potential of Seraph 100 to remove antibiotics. Clinical case reports have shown no impact on vancomycin [36], remdesivir [37], or hydroxychloroquine [38]. An *in vitro* study evaluated the potential reduction of 18 antimicrobial drugs and found negligible impact for 16 and a potential adsorption for

tobramycin and gentamycin [39]. The clinical trial data reported 7 antibiotics, which included azithromycin, cefazolin, cefepime, ceftriaxone, linezolid, piperacillin, and vancomycin, were not significantly cleared by Seraph 100 [40].

Additional concern on whether Seraph 100 would impact antibody levels. Immunoglobulin (Ig) G, IgM, IgA, and IgE levels were measured in the first in-human study and showed no reduction after Seraph treatment [33]. Another interesting case study in which a critically ill COVID-19 patient was treated with Seraph 100 appeared to show seroconversion during the treatment regimen [25]. Prior to treatment, the SARS-CoV-2 N-protein was high in the blood while the spike IgG was low. During the course of treatment, the n-protein quickly dropped, while the anti-spike IgG increased. The data suggest that Seraph 100 did not remove the anti-spike IgG, and may have aided in accelerating seroconversion.

The aforementioned discussion provides examples of clinical experience of Seraph 100 for the treatment of several different types of infections, including bacterial, viral, and fungal. As VM100 is still under development, there are no published cases in which the therapy has been used to treat companion animals. The following are a few examples of infectious disease in which VM100 could improve outcomes based on the pathogenesis of the pathogen and whether the pathogen would bind to VM100.

CDV leads to high mortality in puppies and adult dogs. CDV is a Paramyxoviridae and can lead to a systemic disease. While vaccines are available for CDV, cases are increasing, even in vaccinated animals [41]. A Reverse Transcriptase-Polymerase Chain Reaction study showed viral RNA copies can be found in blood within a day after infection and persist well past 20 days [42]. The authors note that the virus is spread in the blood through cell-free virus or leukocyte-associated virus. Even though the animals seroconverted at 14 days post infection, persistent viremia indicates the immune response is inadequate. An investigation found that soluble heparin was able to inhibit CDV infection of several cell lines and that the F and H proteins of CDV will bind to immobilized heparin [43]. Based on this finding, it is highly likely that bloodborne CDV will bind to VM100. Considering the persistent viremia of CDV, hemoperfusion with VM100 could potentially reduce the duration of viremia, and potentially accelerate seroconversion by rapidly decreasing the viral load.

The fungal infection blastomycosis is caused by *B. dermatiditis or B. helicus*, which is endemic in various parts of the world [44]. A study showed 50% of human cases of *B. helices* were systemic with fungemia, while fungemia with *B. dermatitidis* may be rare [45]. Like other fungi, *Blastomyces* has been shown bind to heparan sulfate [44].

Canine parvovirus type-2 is a highly contagious pathogen that leads to significant morbidity and mortality in dogs. Common symptoms include severe intestinal hemorrhage, diarrhea, vomiting, and myocarditis [46]. Symptomatic dogs exhibit higher serum viral titers. Viremia has been identified as an important component of pathogenesis and precedes development of intestinal epithelial infection and fecal virus shedding [47]. Symptomatic dogs are viremic for greater than 5 days after infection [48,49]. *Parvoviridae* express glycan receptors that have been shown to bind to heparan sulfate and other components of the glycocalyx surface [50]. As with other viral diseases with a viremic phase, it is possible that a rapid clearance of circulating viral load could accelerate seroconversion.

SUMMARY

Sepsis remains a significant cause of morbidity and mortality. In addition, the increasing prevalence of antimicrobial resistance compels new innovations to treat sepsis. Extracorporeal pathogen reduction is a potential therapeutic option that offers a new approach to sepsis that leverages the safe removal of pathogens, DAMPs, and PAMPs in order to treat infectious disease. The data in both human and animal studies demonstrate a role for this approach. Larger studies with a broader variety of microorganisms are needed to further demonstrate the potential impact that pathogen reduction through blood filtration may have toward improving outcomes.

CLINICS CARE POINTS

- VM100 is being developed to be a pathogen-agnostic blood filtration technology and could be used to provide rapid blood source control prior to pathogen identification.
- Rapid source control can greatly reduce severe disease.
- Extracorporeal therapies require additional training and specialized equipment.
- More patient monitoring is required during treatment.
- Blood volume of the patient may limit treatment options.

DISCLOSURE

K.R. McCrea is Chief Science Officer of ExThera Medical. Dr.L.S. Chawla is a Board Member of ExThera Medical and is the Chair of the Scientific Advisory Board at ExThera Medical.

REFERENCES

[1] Dempsey PW, Vaidya SA, Cheng G. The Art of War: Innate and adaptive immune responses. Cell Mol Life Sci 2003;60(12):2604–21.

[2] Bollig ER, Granick JL, Webb TL, et al. A quarterly survey of antibiotic prescribing in small animal and equine practices—Minnesota and North Dakota, 2020. Zoonoses and Public Health 2022;69(7):864–74.

[3] Byl B, Clevenbergh P, Jacobs F, et al. Impact of Infectious Diseases Specialists and Microbiological Data on the Appropriateness of Antimicrobial Therapy for Bacteremia. Clin Infect Dis 1999;29(1):60–6.

[4] Ibrahim EH, Sherman G, Ward S, et al. The Influence of Inadequate Antimicrobial Treatment of Bloodstream Infections on Patient Outcomes in the ICU Setting. Chest 2000;118(1):146–55.

[5] Burke M, Santoro D. Prevalence of multidrug-resistant coagulase-positive staphylococci in canine and feline dermatological patients over a 10-year period: a retrospective study. Microbiology 2023;169(2). https://doi.org/10.1099/mic.0.001300.

[6] Arunvikram K, Mohanty I, Sardar KK, et al. Adverse drug reaction and toxicity caused by commonly used antimicrobials in canine practice. Vet World 2014;7(5): 299–305.

[7] Kagan JC. Infection infidelities drive innate immunity. Science 2023;379(6630):333–5.

[8] Chen L, Kraft BD, Roggli VL, et al. Heparin-based blood purification attenuates organ injury in baboons with *Streptococcus pneumoniae* pneumonia. Am J Physiol Lung Cell Mol Physiol 2021;321(2):L321–35.

[9] Opal SM. Non-antibiotic treatments for bacterial diseases in an era of progressive antibiotic resistance. Crit Care 2016;20(1). https://doi.org/10.1186/s13054-016-1549-1.

[10] Singer M, Deutschman CS, Seymour CW. The third international consensus definitions for sepsis and septic shock (sepsis-3). JAMA 2016;315(8):801–10.

[11] Cao M, Wang G, Xie J. Immune dysregulation in sepsis: experiences, lessons and perspectives. Cell Death Discovery 2023;9(1):1–11.

[12] Reinhart K, Bauer M, Riedemann NC, et al. New Approaches to Sepsis: Molecular Diagnostics and Biomarkers. Clin Microbiol Rev 2012;25(4):609–34.

[13] Sykes JE. Immunodeficiencies Caused by Infectious Diseases. Vet Clin Small Anim Pract 2010;40(3):409–23.

[14] Stewart IJ, McCrea K, Chawla L, et al. Adsorption of Pathogens and Blockade of Sepsis Cascade. Contrib Nephrol 2023;200:123–32, Epub 2023 Jun 22. PMID: 37348482.

[15] Seffer MT, Cottam D, Forni LG, et al. Heparin 2.0: A New Approach to the Infection Crisis. Blood Purif 2021;50(1): 28–34, Epub 2020 Jul 2. PMID: 32615569; PMCID: PMC7445380.

[16] Uchimido R, Schmidt EP, Shapiro NI. The glycocalyx: a novel diagnostic and therapeutic target in sepsis. Crit Care 2019;23(1). https://doi.org/10.1186/s13054-018-2292-6.

[17] Bartlett AH, Park PW. Heparan Sulfate Proteoglycans in Infection. Glycans in Diseases and Therapeutics 2011 Mar;19:31–62.

[18] LaRosa S, McCrea K, Ward R. 984: removal of cytomegalovirus from blood by heparin-functional hemoperfusion media. Crit Care Med 2014;42(12):A1597.

[19] Mattsby-Baltzer I, Bergstrom T, McCrea K, et al. Affinity apheresis for treatment of bacteremia caused by Staphylococcus aureus and/or methicillin-resistant S. aureus (MRSA). J Microbiol Biotechnol 2011 Jun;21(6): 659–64, PMID: 21715974.

[20] McCrea K, Ward R, LaRosa SP. Removal of Carbapenem-Resistant Enterobacteriaceae (CRE) from Blood by Heparin-Functional Hemoperfusion Media. In: Nguyen MH, editor. PLoS One 2014;9(12):e114242.

[21] McCrea KR, Ward RS. An affinity adsorption media that mimics heparan sulfate proteoglycans for the treatment of drug-resistant bacteremia. Surf Sci 2016;648:42–6.

[22] Olson SW, Oliver JD, Collen J, et al. Treatment for Severe Coronavirus Disease 2019 With the Seraph-100 Microbind Affinity Blood Filter. Critical Care Explorations 2020;2(8):e0180.

[23] Malin-Theres S, Weinert M, Molinari G, et al. Staphylococcus aureus binding to Seraph® 100 Microbind® Affinity Filter: Effects of surface protein expression and treatment duration. PLoS One 2023;18(3):e0283304.

[24] Andermatt R, Bloemberg GV, Ganter CC, et al. Elimination of Herpes Simplex Virus-2 and Epstein-Barr Virus With Seraph 100 Microbind Affinity Blood Filter and Therapeutic Plasma Exchange: An Explorative Study in a Patient With Acute Liver Failure. Critical Care Explorations 2022;4(8):e0745.

[25] Merrill KA, Krallman KA, Loeb D, et al. First-Time Use of the Seraph® 100 Microbind® Affinity Blood Filter in an Adolescent Patient with Severe COVID-19 Disease: A Case Report. Case Rep Nephrol Dial 2023;1–6. https://doi.org/10.1159/000527290.

[26] Kielstein JT, Borchina DN, Fühner T, et al. Hemofiltration with the Seraph® 100 Microbind® Affinity filter decreases SARS-CoV-2 nucleocapsid protein in critically ill COVID-19 patients. Crit Care 2021;25(1). https://doi.org/10.1186/s13054-021-03597-3.

[27] Votrico V, Grilli M, Ugo G, et al. Hemoperfusion with high-affinity polyethylene microbeads (Seraph-100®) for the removal of pathogens in chronic critically ill patients: Clinical experience. Int J Artif Organs 2024. https://doi.org/10.1177/03913988231221405.

[28] Li DS, Burke TM, Smith JM, et al. Use of the Seraph® 100 Microbind® Affinity Blood Filter in an adolescent patient with disseminated adenoviral disease. Pediatr Nephrol 2023;39(1):331–5.

[29] Malin-Theres S, Eden G, Engelmann S, et al. Elimination of *Staphylococcus aureus* from the bloodstream using a novel biomimetic sorbent haemoperfusion device. Case Reports 2020;13(8):e235262.

[30] Stoffel S, Boster J, Jarrett Z, et al. Single-Center Experience With the Seraph-100® Microbind® Affinity Blood Filter in Patients With SARS-CoV-2 Infection and Septic Shock at a Military Treatment Facility. Mil Med 2023. https://doi.org/10.1093/milmed/usad063.

[31] Pavlov M, Poljak D, Pavlović N, et al. Enterobacter cloacae septicemia in a triple-cannula extracorporeal membrane oxygenation circulatory support treated with Seraph-100 Microbind affinity blood filter. Croat Med J 2023;64(4):284–8.

[32] Ebeyer-Masotta M, Eichhorn T, Weiss R, et al. Heparin-Functionalized Adsorbents Eliminate Central Effectors of Immunothrombosis, including Platelet Factor 4, High-Mobility Group Box 1 Protein and Histones. Int J Mol Sci 2022;23(3):1823.

[33] Eden G, Schmidt JJ, Büttner S, et al. Safety and efficacy of the Seraph® 100 Microbind® Affinity Blood Filter to remove bacteria from the blood stream: results of the first in human study. Crit Care 2022;26(1). https://doi.org/10.1186/s13054-022-04044-7.

[34] Chitty SA, Mobbs S, Rifkin BS, et al. A Multicenter Evaluation of the Seraph 100 Microbind Affinity Blood Filter for the Treatment of Severe COVID-19. Critical Care Explorations 2022;4(4):e0662.

[35] Schmidt JJ, Borchina DN, van't Klooster M, et al. Interim analysis of the COSA (COVID-19 patients treated with the Seraph® 100 Microbind® Affinity filter) registry. Nephrol Dial Transplant 2021;37(4):673–80.

[36] Hilde ST, Hoek RAS, Henrik E, et al. The Seraph®-100 Microbind Affinity Blood Filter Does Not Affect Vancomycin, Tacrolimus, and Mycophenolic Acid Plasma Concentrations. Blood Purif 2021;50(6):971–5.

[37] Schmidt JJ, Bode-Böger SM, Martens-Lobenhoffer J, et al. Pharmacokinetics of Remdesivir and GS-441524 during PIRRT and Seraph 100 Therapy. Clin J Am Soc Nephrol 2021;16(8):1256–7.

[38] Seffer M, Martens-Lobenhoffer J, Schmidt JJ, et al. Clearance of chloroquine and hydroxychloroquine by the Seraph® 100 Microbinda Affinity Blood Filter - a device approved for the treatment of COVID -19 patients. Ther Apher Dial 2020. https://doi.org/10.1111/1744-9987.13549.

[39] Schmidt JJ, Eden G, Malin-Theres S, et al. In vitro elimination of anti-infective drugs by the Seraph® 100 Microbind® affinity blood filter. Ndt Plus 2020. https://doi.org/10.1093/ckj/sfaa063.

[40] DeLuca JP, Selig DJ, Vir P, et al. Seraph 100 Microbind Affinity Blood Filter Does Not Clear Antibiotics: An Analysis of Antibiotic Concentration Data from PURIFY-OBS. Blood Purif 2024;1–7. https://doi.org/10.1159/000531951.

[41] Martella V, Elia G, Buonavoglia C. Canine Distemper Virus. Vet Clin Small Anim Pract 2008;38(4):787–97.

[42] Sehata G, Sato H, Ito T, et al. Use of quantitative real-time RT-PCR to investigate the correlation between viremia and viral shedding of canine distemper virus, and infection outcomes in experimentally infected dogs. J Vet Med Sci 2015;77(7):851–5.

[43] Fujita K, Miura R, Yoneda M, et al. Host range and receptor utilization of canine distemper virus analyzed by recombinant viruses: Involvement of heparin-like molecule in CDV infection. Virology 2007;359(2): 324–35.

[44] Beaussart A, Brandhorst T, Dufrêne YF, et al. Blastomyces Virulence Adhesin-1 Protein Binding to Glycosaminoglycans Is Enhanced by Protein Disulfide Isomerase. mBio 2015;6(5). https://doi.org/10.1128/mBio.01403-15.

[45] Schwartz IS, Wiederhold NP, Hanson KE, et al. *Blastomyces helicus*, a New Dimorphic Fungus Causing Fatal Pulmonary and Systemic Disease in Humans and Animals in Western Canada and the United States. Clin Infect Dis 2018;68(2):188–95.

[46] Rabbani AH, Ullah Q, Naseer O, et al. Canine Parvo Virus: A Review on Current Perspectives in Seroprevalence, Diagnostics and Therapeutics. Global Vet 2021;23: 113–26.

[47] Meunier PC. The pathogenesis of canine parvovirus infection. Diss Abstr Int B 1983;44:1742.

[48] Meunier PC, Cooper BJ, Appel MJG, et al. Pathogenesis of Canine Parvovirus Enteritis: Sequential Virus Distribution and Passive Immunization Studies. Veterinary Pathology 1985;22(6):617–24.

[49] Meunier PC, Cooper BJ, Appel MJG, et al. Pathogenesis of Canine Parvovirus Enteritis: The Importance of Viremia. Veterinary Pathology 1985;22(1):60–71.

[50] Huang LY, Halder S, Agbandje-McKenna M. Parvovirus glycan interactions. Current Opinion in Virology 2014; 7:108–18.

Moving?

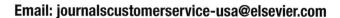

Make sure your subscription moves with you!

To notify us of your new address, find your **Clinics Account Number** (located on your mailing label above your name), and contact customer service at:

Email: journalscustomerservice-usa@elsevier.com

800-654-2452 (subscribers in the U.S. & Canada)
314-447-8871 (subscribers outside of the U.S. & Canada)

Fax number: 314-447-8029

Elsevier Health Sciences Division
Subscription Customer Service
3251 Riverport Lane
Maryland Heights, MO 63043

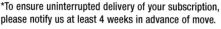

*To ensure uninterrupted delivery of your subscription, please notify us at least 4 weeks in advance of move.

ELSEVIER

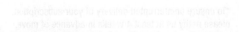

Printed and bound by CPI Group (UK) Ltd, Croydon, CR0 4YY

08/05/2025

01864751-0012